THE COMPLEMENTARY AND ALTERNATIVE MEDICINE INFORMATION SOURCE BOOK

FIRST EDITION

Edited by
Alan M. Rees

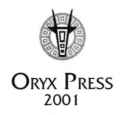

ORYX PRESS
2001

The rare Arabian Oryx is believed to have inspired the myth of the unicorn. This desert antelope became virtually extinct in the early 1960s. At that time several groups of international conservationists arranged to have 9 animals sent to the Phoenix Zoo to be the nucleus of a captive breeding herd. Today the Oryx population is over 800 and nearly 400 have been returned to reserves in the Middle East.

© 2001 by **The Oryx Press**
An imprint of Greenwood Publishing Group, Inc.
88 Post Road West
Westport, CT 06881-5007
(203) 226-3571
(800) 225-5800
http://www.oryxpress.com

Published simultaneously in Canada
Printed and Bound in the United States of America

♾ The paper used in this publication meets the minimum requirements of American National Standard for Information Science—Permanence of Paper for Printed Library Materials, ANSI Z39.48, 1984.

Library of Congress Cataloging-in-Publication Data

Rees, Alan M.
The complementary and alternative medicine information source book /
Alan M. Rees.— 1st ed.
        p. ; cm.
Includes bibliographical references and index.
    ISBN 1-57356-388-9 (alk. paper)
1. Alternative medicine—Popular works.
    [DNLM: 1. Alternative Medicine—Popular Works. 2. Alternative
Medicine—Resource Guides. WB 39 R328c 2001] I. Title.
R733 .R427 2001
615.5—dc21   00-012830

CONTENTS

Contents
iv

PREFACE

The increasing use of alternative medicine in the United States during the past decade has been well documented. Various studies have indicated that more than 40 percent of the U.S. population have used alternative therapies. This enthusiastic embrace of alternative medicine has been largely consumer- and market-driven, running counter to the doubts, disparagement, and negative judgment of the conventional medical community. The movement towards widespread acceptance of alternative medicine has evoked antagonism and hostility on the part of mainstream medicine. Derisory terminology used to characterize alternative medicine includes fringe medicine, folk medicine, medical cultism, and quackery. Many proponents of conventional medicine go so far as to deny the existence of alternative medicine, claiming that there is only scientifically proven, evidence-based medicine supported by solid data, or unproven medicine for which there is no scientific evidence. Advocates of alternative medicine rejoin that the scientific method of controlled studies is not well-suited for a holistic approach to healing and question whether conventional medicine is "scientific," in that it is a dogma of authority and not of science. How can one reasonably reject the richness of Chinese medicine, a coherent and independent system of thought and practice developed over two millennia? Much of the dialog between orthodoxy and non-orthodoxy is typically conducted in the form of a religious war, with "bunglers" and "charlatans" locked in battle with proponents of cold war, high-tech medicine. A fundamental divide separates two vastly different historical, philosophical, and theoretical traditions of medical practice.

To patients, complementary and alternative medicine (CAM) represents a new frontier in medical consumerism offering the ultimate in self-help and empowerment with a largely increased freedom of choice of treatment. Yet the free exercise of such extended choice may be hazardous. As the enthusiasm for CAM escalates, there is an impelling need for consumers and patients to be fully cognizant of the potential for harm posed by the use of alternative therapies and consumers should be aware of both benefits and risks. Considering what is at stake, regardless of one's viewpoint, there can be no doubt that Americans should be fully informed of the available evidence attesting to the safety and efficacy of CAM therapies.

The importance of access to reliable and authoritative CAM information is underscored by the need felt by many consumers to bridge the gap between their conventional and alternative providers. In so many cases, physicians lack the knowledge to provide guidance and counsel and patients are filling the void. If patients wish to receive truly integrative treatment it is necessary that they reconnoiter what is essentially the *terra incognita* of alternative medicine. Patients are forced to navigate through a morass of conflicting, contradictory, inconclusive, fragmented and undocumented information in order to assess whether an alternative treatment will be beneficial or detrimental to their health. The failure of patients to inform their conventional providers of alternative therapies stems in large part from the difficulties involved in performing a necessary bridging role.

It must be stated that the editor takes no position on the value and use of complementary and alternative (CAM) therapies. No attempt has been made either to "trash" alternative medicine or to extoll its merits. Nor has any effort been made to evaluate the reliability and credibility of the information content of the sources described. Instead, attention is focused on presenting the widest possible assortment of viewpoints and on evaluating the trustworthiness of the information sources. The focus of the book lies in its description and evaluation of the increasing amount of published evidence currently available. Informed individuals are better prepared to assess the value and appropriateness of CAM usage in their individual circumstances.

This volume is intended to supplement *The Consumer Health Information Source Book*, 6th edition (Oryx, 2000) by providing in-depth access to the growing literature relating to complementary and alternative medicine. It is more than a simple spinoff of *The Consumer Health Information Source Book* in that it represents an attempt to map the new landscape of complementary and alternative medicine as portrayed by the diverse information sources currently available. The book should be of use to consumers, patients, and others who wish to be more informed as to what the burgeoning field of alternative medicine has to offer. It should also contribute to improve communication between patients and their doctors.

In this connection, consumers contemplating, or actually using, alternative therapies are likely to encounter three types of mainstream physicians—those who are implacably opposed in light of their formal training and clinical experience to alternative medicine in any shape or form; those who dabble in alternative and complementary medicine while seeking further evidence of efficacy and safety; and those, trained in conventional medicine, who are now actively involved in integrative clinical practice. While the number of physicians who practice integrative medicine is still quite small, there exists a growing body of physicians committed to drawing upon the best of conventional and alternative therapies. These physicians believe that integrative medicine will bring the best knowledge of traditional and non-traditional medicine into a common space where the patient's welfare becomes paramount. Consumers are also engaged in dialog with many alternative practitioners who have a variety of professional qualifications in naturopathy, herbal medicine, acupuncture, chiropractic, traditional Chinese medicine, homeopathy, and massage.

The present popularity of CAM therapies and the burgeoning public interest and expenditure, largely out-of-pocket, has convinced the federal establishment—the National Institutes of Health, National Library of Medicine and other bulwarks of mainstream medicine—that investment in research is desirable. Professional associations, such as the American Medical Association, and previous foes of alternative medicine such as the Arthritis Foundation, have jumped on the bandwagon, whether out of conviction or expediency. The final endorsement of the policy of subjecting CAM therapies to scientific scrutiny came in the form of the appointment by President Clinton in April 2000 of a White House Commission on Complementary and Alternative Medicine charged with the mandate of preparing a report to the president on "legislative and administrative recommendations for assuring that public policy maximizes the benefits to Americans of complementary and alternative medicine." Both the National Center for Complementary and Alternative Medicine (NCCAM) and the White House Commission articulate the need to determine whether the pervasive use of untested alternative health practices poses any threat to public health and to determine "What works, and what does not?" In these initiatives, public opinion and widespread usage of CAM therapies has prevailed over the hesitancy, reluctance, foot-dragging, and opposition of mainstream medicine.

The volume brings together a large collection of information sources in the form of popular books, magazines and newsletters, supportive professional books and journals, CD-ROM databases, Internet resources, pamphlet materials, together with several hundred resource organizations with addresses, phone numbers, e-mail addresses, and Web sites. As more research and clinical experience are reported, the amount of reliable information will increase.

The book is divided into twelve sections. Section 1 provides a number of definitions of complementary and alternative medicine (CAM) that describe the general context. This section discusses problems of terminology; reasons for, and extent of, popular usage of CAM; safety concerns; the shifting relationship between mainstream medicine and CAM; the role of the National Center for Complementary and Alternative Medicine of the National Institutes of Health in funding CAM research and education; the vocal critics of CAM; the extent and availability of information resources; the movement towards integrative medicine in terms of a number of innovative clinical programs; consumer empowerment; and what the future holds.

Section 2 lists The Best of Complementary and Alternative Medicine Information Resources and includes 22 popular books, 2 book series, 8 consumer magazines and newsletters, 9 professional books, 7 professional journals and newsletters, 3 CD-ROM products, and 10 Web sites.

Section 3 lists several hundred CAM associations, professional groups, educational institutions, trade associations, accrediting agencies, clearinghouses, research institutions, clinical centers, and research organizations. Each entry supplies the name, address, phone and fax numbers, e-mail address, and Web site. A vigorous effort has been made to contact organizations to verify addresses and phone numbers.

Section 4 lists and describes consumer magazines and newsletters covering a wide assortment of subject content. A number of general magazines have established a beachhead in the consumer marketplace alongside more specialized publications focusing on specific areas such as herbal medicine, massage, and the like.

Section 5 lists pamphlets, booklets, leaflets, and brochures. The number of these currently available is still quite small due to the modest federal sponsorship of research. Doubtless, as the tempo of federal funding picks up more of these publications will become available both from federal agencies and the NCCAM-sponsored research centers.

Section 6 contains reviews of some 35 professional texts and reference publications on CAM and integrative medicine which can be used to supplement a popular collection. An increasing number of professional books published both in the United States and the United Kingdom are now devoted to integrative medicine Section 6 also lists 50 related professional journals and newsletters. The—as yet—small number of CD-ROM CAM-related products are described in Section 7.

The importance of the Internet as a source of CAM-related information is discussed by Tom Flemming in Section 8 from the point of view of usage, quality, evidence of efficacy, use of MEDLINE for searching, availability of other bibliographic databases, use of search engines and catalogs, the need to adopt a critical approach to CAM information, and the future of CAM on the Internet. Flemming also provides detailed descriptions and evaluations of more than 60 sites, utilizing a four-star ranking system. A list of "Tom's Ten Best Internet Picks" is included in Section 2. Tom Flemming is head of public services at McMaster University Health Sciences Library, Hamilton, Ontario, Canada.

Section 9 contains reviews of 355 popular books on CAM, mainly published in 1999 and 2000. A few earlier, classic titles are also included. The criteria used in selecting books for review involve credibility, clarity, comprehensiveness, and substantive content. No attempt was made to superimpose prior judgment. Instead, books were selected to represent the widest diversity of approach and opinion. Particular attention was paid to reviewing those books that reflect an integrative approach. A large number of current books deal with herbal medicine and phytomedicine with multiple publications on, for example, St. John's wort, kava, and echinacea. Other topics such as traditional Chinese medicine, Ayurvedic medicine, and mind-body medicine are well represented. Surprisingly, there are comparatively few books devoted to chiropractic and homeopathy.

To facilitate access, books are arranged according to broad topics (Acupuncture and Reflexology), by area of application (Alternative Medicine … and Breast Cancer, Heart Disease), and in the case of herbal medicine by name of specific herb (Kava, Saw Palmetto, Echinacea.)

The last section of the book contains appendices that reprint a number of valuable publications produced by the National Center for Complementary and Alternative Medicine and relate to the major domains of CAM, fields of practice, frequently asked questions, judicious choice of alternative therapies, and suggestions for searching the medical literature.

My thanks are due to a number of individuals and organizations. To Cynthia Strong for successfully transcribing and keyboarding textual material that went far beyond traditional medical terminology; to Tom Flemming for his expertise and knowledge of Internet resources; to the numerous publishers who contributed review copies; to Sherry Thompson and colleagues at Major's Scientific Books for providing access to many new professional and consumer books; to the Cleveland Heights-University Heights Public Library and to the Cuyahoga County Library for use of their resources; and to the editorial staff at Oryx Press—Jennifer Ashley, Susan Slesinger, and Anne Thompson.

Alan M. Rees
Cleveland Heights, OH
December 2000

SECTION 1

Complementary and Alternative Medicine: A New Dimension in Medical Consumerism

A Short History of Medicine

I have an earache ....

2000 B.C.	Here, eat this root.
1000 A.D.	That root is heathen. Here, say this prayer.
1850 A.D.	That prayer is superstition. Here, drink this potion.
1940 A.D.	That potion is snake oil. Here, swallow this pill.
1985 A.D.	That pill is ineffective. Here, take this antibiotic.
2000 A.D.	That antibiotic is artificial. Here, eat this root.

(Author unknown)

- "The complementary and alternative medicine of today will be the conventional medicine of tomorrow." Stephen E. Straus M.D. Director of the National Center for Complementary and Alternative Medicine, NIH. January 2000.
- "Alternative medicine is here to stay. It is no longer an option to ignore it or treat it as something outside of the normal processes of science and medicine. The challenge is to move forward carefully, using both reason and wisdom, as we attempt to separate the pearls from the mud." Wayne B. Jonas M.D. JAMA 1998. 280. 1618
- "We need to commit ourselves to a rigorous but open minded evaluation of practice in all aspects of health care, and to finding ways of trans-

lating ideas into action in the most effective manner." HRH Charles, Prince of Wales. May 1998. *Journal of Alternative and Complementary Medicine: Research on Paradigm, Practice, and Policy.* 1998. 4 (2) 209.

- "The quackbusters say they're protecting public health, but in fact, they're abandoning the public to their own suffering to protect the financial interests of conventional medicine, which has no interest or ability to produce benefits for their condition. The quackbusters say they're serving the public, but the truth is they're grossly disserving patients." Burton Goldberg. Publisher's Statement #24. *Alternative Medicine Magazine* (alternativemedicine. com).

1. PROBLEMS OF TERMINOLOGY

A number of terms are often used loosely and interchangeably to describe what is popularly known as alternative medicine. Contemporary usage recognizes the following: *Alternative Medicine*—treatment modalities used to substitute for mainstream or conventional medicine; *Complementary Medicine*—use of therapies in addition to treatment offerings of conventional medicine; *Complementary and Alternative Medicine (CAM)*—combined use of mainstream and alternative treatment modalities; *Integrative Medicine*—a synergistic combination of therapies without preference given to any one system—clinical care that is a synthesis or blend of alternative, complementary, and mainstream medicine; *Holistic Medicine*—the art and science that treats and prevents disease, while focusing on empowering patients to create a condition of optimal health. Clinical care that focuses on the integration of body, mind, and spirit.

Variations in definition reflect differing points of view among clinicians and researchers. Zollman and Vickers[1] consider that "Complementary medicine refers to a group of therapeutic and diagnostic disciplines that exist largely outside the institutions where conventional health care is taught and provided." Eisenberg[2] offers a similar definition: "Alternative therapies can be defined as medical interventions that are neither taught widely in U.S. medical schools nor generally available in U.S. hospitals." These two definitions, with their focus on physical locale, do not adequately describe essential concepts and content.

A more detailed, though somewhat academic, definition is provided by the Cochrane Collaboration:

> Complementary and alternative medicine (CAM) is a broad domain of healing resources that encompasses all health systems, modalities, and practices and their accompanying theories and beliefs, other than those intrinsic to the politically dominant health system of a particular society or culture in a given historical period. CAM includes all such practices and ideas self-defined by their users as preventing or treating illness or promoting health and well-being. Boundaries within CAM, and between the CAM domain and that of the dominant system, are not always sharp or fixed.[3]

The National Center for Complementary and Alternative Medicine (NCCAM) of the National Institutes of Health offers a more descriptive definition:

> Complementary and alternative medicine covers a broad range of healing philosophies, approaches, and therapies. It generally is defined as those treatments and health care practices not taught widely in medical schools, not generally used in hospitals, and not usually reimbursed by medical insurance companies. Many therapies are holistic, which generally means that the health care practitioner considers the whole person, including physical, mental, emotional and spiritual aspects….People use these treatments and therapies in a variety of ways. Therapies are used alone (often referred to as alternative), in combination with other alternative therapies, or in addition to conventional therapies (sometimes referred to as complementary). Some approaches are consistent with physiological principles of Western medicine, while others constitute healing systems with a different origin. While some therapies

are far outside the realm of accepted Western medical theory and practice, others are becoming established in mainstream medicine.[4]

NCCAM now recognizes five major categories of complementary and alternative medicine: alternative medical and traditional indigenous systems (Ayurvedic medicine, curanderismo, traditional oriental medicine, and unconventional Western systems such as homeopathy and naturopathy); mind-body interventions (mind-body systems and methods, biofeedback, guided imagery, meditation, religion, and spirituality); biologically based therapies (herbal medicine, special diet therapies, orthomolecular medicine); manipulative and body-based methods (chiropractic, osteopathy, reflexology); and energy therapies (therapies that focus either on energy fields originating within the body—biofields, or those from other sources—electromagnetic fields (Qi Gong, Reiki, and therapeutic touch). A Statement of the Major Domains of Complementary and Alternative Medicine provides a detailed and analytic summary (Appendix 2).[5]

These definitions clearly differentiate between *alternative* [instead of] and *complementary* [together with] medicine. The use of the term complementary appears to imply that complementary medicine should be just that—complementing conventional or mainstream medicine *only after* an allopathic diagnosis, *only after* being sure that no mainstream treatment is necessary, and performed *only* by practitioners who respect the rules of mainstream medicine.

A third term is now entering into common usage: *integrative* medicine. The essential difference between complementary and integrative medicine is clear—whereas complementary medicine emphasizes the use of unconventional treatments as an adjunct to conventional medicine, integrative medicine seeks to utilize whatever treatment modalities are the most effective, without preference to any one system. The best treatment is selected without any favorable bias given to either system.

A further lack of precision applies to the labeling of the "alternative" to alternative medicine, which is variously called conventional medicine, traditional medicine, orthodox medicine, scientific medicine, Western medicine, and mainstream medicine—all used interchangeably. Mainstream medicine would seem to be preferable in that it is less exclusionary of interconnected and tributary streams of medical practice.

2. EXTENT OF USAGE OF COMPLEMENTARY AND ALTERNATIVE MEDICINE

Alternative medicine has a long history in the U.S. dating back to Thomsonianism, developed at the end of the eighteenth century, which was followed by homeopathy, hydrotherapy, and mesmerism in the nineteenth century. In 1900, it is estimated that nearly 20 percent of all medical practitioners were alternative physicians with more than 10,000 homeopaths, 5,000 eclectics, and another 5,000 practitioners of other alternative systems.

At present, we are witnessing a revival of alternative medicine which constitutes a sharp reversal of the decline that took place during the middle years of the twentieth century and which is motivated in large measure by rising public disaffection with mainstream medical practice. The specific reasons for this resurgence are concisely enumerated by Jonas and Levin[6]:

> Patient alienation from the impersonal and intimidating style of specialized, technological, hospital-based medicine; the dramatic increase during the twentieth century of chronic degenerative diseases, ailments that confound cure but demand caring and cooperative management; awareness of the too-frequent iatrogenic effects of prescription pharmaceuticals; the rise of consumerism and concern for patients' rights and autonomy....and the rising costs of medical care.

Also influential are rejection of paternalism, declining faith in the validity of so-called "breakthroughs" in scientific medicine, and an increased interest in faith and spiritualism. There is widespread public disaffection with mainstream medical practice.

Ten years ago, few consumers were fluent in the language of alternative medicine. Today, large numbers of persons commonly discuss and debate the usage and benefits of echinacea, St. John's wort, food supplements, aromatherapy, Ayurveda, antioxidants, Qigong, acupuncture, homeopathy, touch therapy, reflexology, and the like. Drug stores and health food stores do a brisk business in echinacea for the common cold, ginkgo biloba and huperzine A to enhance memory, tea tree oil to reduce inflammation, ginseng to stimulate the immune system, St. John's wort as an antidepressant, kava as an anxiolytic, black cohosh (Lydia E. Pinkham's Vegetable Compound) for menopausal discomforts, creatine to boost athletic performance, garlic to control cholesterol and prevent heart disease, feverfew for the relief of headaches and migraine,

SAM-e for the relief of arthritis, soy supplements to prevent breast cancer, saw palmetto for relief of prostate problems, and a panoply of products such as DHEA, MSM, selenium, chromium picolinate, coenzyme Q10, pycnogenol, and D-ribose for a host of ailments and conditions.

It is estimated that there was a 380 percent increase in the sale of herbal substances and a 130 percent increase for high-dose vitamin products during the 1990s. Sales of herbal products now approximate $4 billion per year with an annual growth at more than 30 percent despite legislation that bars manufacturers from making specific disease claims for their products, allowing only structure/function claims such as "supports the immune system," or "helps promote urinary tract health." Herbal advertising reached $100 million in 1998. Public attention is also focused on formerly esoteric treatment modalities such as naturopathic medicine, Alexander technique, Bach flower remedies, Feldenkrais, Reiki, shiatsu, Tai Chi, traditional Chinese medicine, chelation therapy, and colonic irrigation.

The rise of interest in alternative medicine in the United States in recent years has been largely consumer- and market-driven. Running counter to the doubts, ruminations, reflections, cautions, disparagement, and negative judgment of the medical community, consumers have enthusiastically embraced alternative medicine. Roy Porter,[7] a noted British medical historian, comments that "The most significant thrust towards the integration of alternative and orthodox practices has come about through people consulting the many tens of thousands of alternative practitioners who are not medically qualified and now operating in Western societies, in parallel with their normal visits to doctors and other health personnel." Resorting to alternative medicine practitioners appears to be in addition to, and not instead of, visits to conventional physicians. Spencer and Jacobs[8] consider this growth of complementary and alternative medicine to be "a paradigm shift in medicine in the United States."

This trend is part of a worldwide movement. It is estimated that one person in ten in the United Kingdom consults a CAM practitioner each year. There are currently more than 5,000 reflexologists, 2,300 osteopaths, and 1,700 acupuncturists in the United Kingdom. The number of complementary practitioners (40,000) exceeds that of family doctors (36,200). In France, one-third of the population uses CAM, with homeopathy being the most popular treatment. By some estimates, no less than 80 percent of all Germans take some form of supplement. In Russia, where alternative medicine was legalized in 1993, the officially recognized methods are reflexology, chiropractic, homeopathy, and a breathing method. In Australia, one-third of the population regularly visits a natural therapist. In Japan, scientific medicine and CAM co-exist, while in Germany and the U.K. the national health system covers many CAM therapies.[9]

The pattern of increasing usage in the U.S. has been well documented by Eisenberg.[10] In 1990, one-third of all Americans used some form of complementary and alternative medicine. Most users were also under the care of traditional medical doctors, 90 percent were self-referred to alternative providers, while less than 40 percent of users discussed their alternative therapies with their doctors. A followup of Eisenberg's 1990 survey[11] showed a rise in CAM usage to 42 percent of the total population in 1997. The number of visits to alternative practitioners jumped 47.3 percent, from 427 million visits in 1990 to 629 million in 1997, thereby exceeding visits to U.S. primary care physicians. Americans spent $21.2 billion for alternative medicine professional services in 1997, with at least $12.2 billion paid out-of-pocket. This exceeds the 1997 out-of-pocket expenditures for all U.S. hospitalizations.

To gain a more current picture of public perception of alternative care, Landmark Healthcare Inc.[12] sponsored in 1999 a telephone survey of a random sample of U.S. households to determine adult attitudes, perceptions, and behavior with respect to alternative care. The survey revealed that 42 percent of respondents used some form of alternative care during the past year, 74 percent used alternative care along with traditional care, 15 percent as a replacement for traditional care, and 11 percent used alternative care along with AND as a replacement for traditional care. Acupuncture, chiropractic, herbal therapy, acupressure, and massage therapy were most often associated with alternative care. Moreover, 40 percent noted that their attitude toward alternative care had become more positive. Thirty-one percent believed that alternative care is very important in selecting a health plan.

It is estimated that 50 percent of all cancer and HIV patients use unconventional medical therapies at some point during the course of their illness. A survey of cancer patients under treatment in Houston at the University of Texas M. D. Anderson Center revealed that 69 percent were using alternative treatments. Usage of CAM in California, according to a Los Angeles Times poll,[13] is approximately double that reported nationwide. Thirty-two percent of people in California are likely to use chiropractic compared with 16 percent nationwide; 30 percent are likely to have used herbal products compared with 17 percent nationwide; and 8 percent are likely to have used acupuncture compared with 2 percent nationwide. The most frequently used therapies in California are chiropractic, herbal medicine, and megavitamin therapy. Most of the large HMOs in California offer acupuncture and chiropractic care. A national survey of HMOs by Landmark Healthcare Inc.[14] indicated that 67 percent offered at least one type of alternative health care, the most common of which were chiropractic and acupuncture.

According to the editorial staff of Natural Health magazine, the ten most influential developments that put alternative medicine on the map during the past decade of the 90s were: (1) the Eisenberg studies; (2) establishment of the NIH Office of Alternative Medicine; (3) the 1994 Dietary Supplements Health and Education Act; (4) FDA classification of acupuncture needles as medical devices; (5) HMO coverage of alternative therapies (e.g., Ornish program); (6) media coverage of St. John's wort; (7) increased popularity of soy; (8) stocking of herbal products by Wal-Mart, Walgreens etc; (9) American Heart Association's endorsement of vitamin E; and (10) publicity on surgeon Memet Oz's use of therapeutic touch.[15]

Oxford Health Plans, an innovative health plan, offers generous coverage of chiropractic, yoga, massage therapy, nutritional counseling, and naturopathy. With more than 2 million members, Oxford was the first to launch a CAM program with a credentialed provider network of more than 2,000 providers. The San Francisco-based Blue Shield of California, with a program called Lifepath, offers its members access to a network of qualified alternative medicine providers. One typical HMO executive comments that "CAM is high-touch, low-tech, low-cost care. So now you're saving money and the public wants it."[16]

Support for complementary and alternative medicine is also forthcoming from private foundations. Examples of this support include the Fetzer Foundation with its funding of Bill Moyers' PBS TV series on Cancer and the Mind; the Laing Foundation in its support of the

University of Maryland acupuncture program; the Rosenthal Foundation's financing of the Columbia University Rosenthal Center; and the Osher Foundation's financial support of the University of California alternative medicine program.

One anonymous, acerbic observer offers a somewhat cynical view of this runaway interest in alternative medicine: "Yuppies lead the charge; messianic proselytizers harangue; profiteers follow the scent of blood; philanthropists make large contributions; media hype drowns out the negatives; and patients spend money that might better go elsewhere. But the more conventional practitioners ridicule alternatives, the more patients distrust conventional physicians."

The current usage of alternative therapies is documented in an extensive study of more than 46,000 readers of *Consumer Reports*.[17] The term "complementary" is given increased meaning by the study's finding that some 60 percent of readers surveyed did report CAM usage to their physicians. Some 35 percent of all respondents had used alternative therapies such as chiropractic, mind-body treatments, and herbals. Overall, 58 percent of conditions were treated with conventional (not complementary) medicine, while 25 percent were treated with both conventional and complementary therapies. Only 9 percent used alternative treatments as the sole treatment. The respondents— "a group of well-educated, information-seeking *Consumer Reports* readers"—rated the therapies that helped them in relation to a total of 43 medical conditions—"helped me feel much better," "helped somewhat," or "helped only a little or not at all." Howard Beckin who served as a consultant in the *Consumer Reports* survey, comments that the data indicate "a sometimes helter-skelter use of alternative products in that thousands of people report using herbal supplements indiscriminately in a way that is both illogical and dangerous... people were using herbal products for things that even the herbal products people wouldn't think they were recommended for."[18]

3. REASONS FOR POPULAR USAGE OF CAM

Many persons resort to CAM in the belief that there are manifold benefits to be gained that are not available from mainstream medicine. Consumers approach CAM with great expectations of a cure, or at least alleviation of

their pain and suffering. The popularity of CAM is also attributable to a powerful inner need for personal attention and compassion that is lacking in modern, biotechnological medical care. The interaction between a doctor and a patient is itself a powerful instrument of healing. Assembly-line medicine, dictated by economic constraints, has led to a deterioration of the physician-patient relationship. The amount of time spent in explanation and personal support has decreased, while the warmth and a healing touch, formerly present, have all but disappeared. Treating the whole person—body, mind, and spirit—is an art that many mainstream doctors have lost the ability to practice. A person paying out-of-pocket is likely to receive more provider time per dollar with an alternative practitioner than with most conventional physicians.

The public perceives alternative medicine not as a peripheral practice, fad, or medical side issue, but rather as a "a genuine public health care need that will not disappear."[19] To some, the most appealing alternative medicine therapies are those that represent complete systems of thought and practice, in which the practices are well-developed, well-articulated, and well-established. These systems include Chinese medicine, Ayurvedic medicine, and curanderismo.[20]

Andrew Weil[21] eloquently expresses the feelings driving many consumers:

> Patients want physicians who have the time to sit down with them and help them understand their problems, who do not push drugs and surgery as the only available therapies, who are conversant with nutritional influences on health, who can answer questions about dietary supplements, who understand mind/body interactions, who look at us as more than physical bodies, and who will not ridicule us for wanting to try Chinese treatment or biofeedback.

Weil points out that while many opponents of CAM continue to write inflammatory rhetoric, consumers are voting with their feet and pocketbooks, and are forcing the medical establishment to consider the value of alternative therapies.

J.A. Astin[22] concludes that many patients use alternative medicine not necessarily out of dissatisfaction with conventional medicine but because alternative medicine is more congruent with their own values, beliefs, and philosophical orientations toward health and life. Dissatisfaction with conventional medicine does not predict use of alternative medicine. Astin points out that variables serving as predictors of usage are more education, poorer health status, a holistic orientation to health, a transformational experience that changed the person's world view, and specific problems including anxiety, backache, and chronic pain. Intractable and refractory medical problems drive chronic sufferers to explore alternatives. Zollman and Vickers[23] comment that, "Qualitative and quantitative studies show that those consulting complementary practitioners usually have longstanding conditions for which conventional medicine has not provided a satisfactory solution, either because it is insufficiently effective or because it causes adverse effects… some 'pick and mix' between complementary and conventional care, claiming that there are certain problems for which their general practitioner has the best approach and others for which a complementary practitioner is more appropriate." About 55-65 percent of those consulting complementary practitioners are female, the greatest number of users are aged 35-60, and users tend to have higher socioeconomic status, and have achieved higher levels of education, than users of conventional care.

Four recognizable patterns of usage of alternative medicine are defined by Edzard Ernst[24]—earnest seekers (who have an intractable health problem for which they try many different forms of treatment); stable users (who either use one type of therapy for most of their health care problems, or who have one main problem for which they use a regular package of one or more complementary therapies); eclectic users (who choose and use different forms of therapy depending on individual problems and circumstances); and on-off users (who discontinue complementary treatment after limited experimentation).

4. SAFETY CONCERNS

Concern with safety does not appear to be paramount to most consumers and patients. It is widely assumed that "natural" is safe so that many persons are still unaware of the absence of regulation in relation to alternative medicine products. This lack of awareness is of concern to many health professionals. Under the 1994 Dietary Supplement Health and Education Act, herbal medicines are classified as supplements and not as drugs and as such are exempted from almost all of the stringent regulations governing pharmaceuticals. Unlike both pharmaceuticals and food additives, supplements do not have to be pre-screened by the FDA, nor do they have

to demonstrate that they are safe before they can be sold. Once on sale, the burden of proof is on the FDA to show that a supplement is dangerous before it can be removed from the market. In view of the absence of validated data regarding safety and efficacy, one researcher argues that Americans are "already engaged in a vast, uncontrolled experiment." Since there is so little information available, physicians are often unable to respond to patients' requests for recommendations and guidance.

What is actually in many of the products sold as dietary supplements is "anybody's guess." The *Los Angeles Times*[25] published an investigative series of articles on herbal products which reported that a quality analysis of 10 brands of St. John's wort revealed that 3 of the 10 brands tested had no more than one-half the potency claimed, while an analysis of 10 ginseng products showed a similar variation in content. Dr. Varro Tyler, a distinguished emeritus professor of pharmacognosy, considers that medicinal herbs in the U.S. are in a "scandalous situation" that has left the public bewildered and confused. Tyler deplores the fact that the market is flooded with "junk products" and warns of the dangers of adding herbs such as St. John's wort to iced tea, soft drinks, and other foods.[26] The public is confused by the tricky wording of the structure/function claims allowed by the FDA, which permits product labeling suggesting that a product "boosts the immune system," "assists in healthy digestion," or "maintains prostate health." Consumers often translate these generalized statements into disease-specific uses.

Of particular concern is the tendency of patients to enter into a parallel course of alternative treatment. Cardiovascular patients should, for example, avoid the use of herbal medicines in that many herbs have anti-clotting properties.[27] Herbal materials such as garlic, ginkgo, kava, and fish oils can interfere with anesthesia administered during surgery. The dangers involved in mixing prescription drugs with herbals are pinpointed by Adriane Fugh-Berman in a recent issue of *Lancet*.[28] Fugh-Berman notes that an estimated one in five Americans is taking an herbal medicine and that 20 percent of these people are also taking prescription medicines. This is of some concern in view of dangerous interactions. It is hazardous, for example, for those taking coumadin or aspirin to use herbs such as ginkgo, garlic, dong quai, or papaya since these herbs can increase thinning of the blood; mixing of St. John's wort with antidepressant medications, such as Prozac or Zoloft, can result in an overload of serotonin; while taking oral or topical corticosteroids and using licorice can increase the effect of the steroids, Aristolochia fangchi is reported to have produced kidney disease, and so on. Fugh-Berman notes that we are just at the beginning of understanding herb-drug and supplement-drug interactions.[29]

There is real cause for concern in that the FDA monitoring system implicated dietary supplements in 2,621 adverse events between 1993 and 1998, with 184 of them resulting in death. The American Association of Poison Control Centers received 6,914 reports on supplements in 1998 alone, including 1,369 cases that required treatment in a health care facility. The 1994 Dietary Supplements Health and Education Act has been disparagingly referred to as The Food Fraud Facilitation Act.[30] The supplement industry not surprisingly is opposed to any FDA attempt to act as "Big Mother" by restricting access to dietary supplements in that such a move would violate the First Amendment and is not in the best interests of consumers.[31] A number of congressional representatives support a move to restrict health claims on dietary supplements.

To assist consumers, the Office of Dietary Supplements at the National Institutes of Health launched in 1999 a new database to provide reliable information on supplements.[32] The International Bibliographic Information on Dietary Supplements (IBIDS) database is intended to assist scientists and the general public in locating credible, scientific literature on dietary supplements. The database is updated quarterly and contains some 350,000 unique scientific citations and abstracts (but no full text). The free Web site (http://dietarysupplements.info.nih.gov) allows consumers to find in one source scientific information on dietary supplements. In addition to maintaining its Web site, the Office of Dietary Supplements, in conjunction with dietitians at the Warren Grant Magnuson Clinical Center, is preparing a series of authoritative fact sheets. The first titles—on Magnesium, Selenium, and Zinc—are already available at www.cc.nih.gov/ccc/supplements. html.

Private enterprise is also endeavoring to fill a regulatory void with a plan to provide assurance of the quality and efficacy of herbal products. Steven Bratman, a physician and alternative medicine author, has tackled the quality control problem through the establishment of ConsumerLab.com, which will evaluate various natural products on the market and place a certifying logo on items that pass their evaluation.[33] ConsumerLab.com's evaluation and certification will make it easier for consumers to identify high-quality products. The testing method used draws upon recognized standards for testing, such as those set forth by the German Commission E Monographs. When an herbal product fails such testing, ConsumerLab.com contacts the manufacturer for a response. If the manufacturer offers a scientifically valid alternative measurement technique, ConsumerLab.com will consider adopting that technique as an option for supplementary testing.

One of the first tests conducted by ConsumerLab.com involved 30 leading brands of Ginkgo biloba products.[34] These products were tested to determine whether or not they possessed proper amounts of appropriate plant chemicals. Nearly one-quarter of the 30 brands tested did not have the expected levels of chemical marker compounds. Even though they failed the testing, all products bore labels claiming standardization of contents. ConsumerLab.com has published the list of products that passed the testing indicating product name, labeled concentration of Ginkgo biloba extract per pill, and the manufacturer and/or distributor. To assist consumers, manufacturers of products that passed ConsumerLab.com's testing will be licensed to display the ConsumerLab.com Seal of Approval. Test results are also available for glucosamine and chondroitin products, saw palmetto, and SAM-e. Such testing to ensure quality is highly useful but whether something works or not is entirely another matter.

5. MAINSTREAM MEDICINE AND CAM

Historically, the movement towards acceptance of alternative medicine has been marked by antagonism and hostility. Disparaging terminology sometimes used to describe alternative medicine includes fringe medicine, folk medicine, medical cultism, and quackery. For decades the medical establishment stridently denounced the proponents of alternative medicine in similar terms such as peddlers of snake oil, fraudulent cures, and quack remedies. Practitioners of alternative medicine were ostracized and even run out of town. Wallace Sampson,[35] a vocal critic of alternative medicine, claims that "even the words 'holistic,' 'alternative,' 'complementary,' 'unconventional,' and 'unorthodox' are invented euphemisms intended to mislead. They are benign terms covering a vast array of practices—most of them unproved, dubious, disproved, absurd, and fraudulent."

Edzard Ernst,[36] Director of the Department of Complementary Medicine at the University of Exeter, cogently comments on the lack of productive discourse:

> The waters are also muddied by the fact that the debate between orthodoxy and non-orthodoxy is typically conducted in the form of a religious war, with 'bunglers and charlatans' locked in battle with 'proponents of cold war, high-tech medicine.' Information available to patients seeking advice almost always comes either from biased proponents of orthodox medicine or from apologists of alternative medicine who promise a cure as the inevitable outcome of treatment.

Clearly, there is a fundamental divide that separates two vastly different historical, philosophical, and theoretical traditions of medical practice. Natural medicine claims a long lineage and has been firmly rooted in many parts of the world for centuries. The arrogance of scientific medicine in dismissing and denigrating this heritage is greatly resented. The present polarization is graphically revealed in opposing statements by Arnold Relman (editor-in-chief emeritus of the *New England Journal of Medicine*) and Andrew Weil (prolific author and director of the University of Arizona Program in Integrative Medicine) in a formal debate held at the University of Arizona.[37]

Relman concisely states the orthodox position:

> Most alternative systems of treatment are based on irrational or fanciful thinking, and false or unproven factual claims. Their theories often violate basic scientific principles and are at odds, not only with each other, but with modern knowledge of the structure and function of the human body as now taught in our medical schools. They could not be woven into the fabric of the medical curriculum without confusion, contradiction, and an undermining of the scientific foundation upon which modern medicine rests....[W]ithout objectively verifiable evidence, there is no reason to believe the claims of alternative medicine.... Modern, science-based medicine is the way of the future. Alternative medicine belongs to the past. It is old wine, albeit sometimes now being served in new bottles, and is unlikely to produce new knowledge or improve future medical care.

Weil responds:

> The vast majority of patients who come to me…are patients who have been through conventional medicine, often many times over, have been tested to death, have tried many conventional therapies, and have found that they haven't worked or have caused harm or both, and it is that which motivates them to look for other kinds of treatment….No informed consumer wants to reject conventional medicine or replace it with unproved therapies. What I and more and more of my colleagues want to do is to broaden the horizons of medical education, research, and practice by integrating ideas and methods not currently taught in medical schools. Everyone I work with would like nothing more than to see good research on botanical remedies and other unconventional treatments. Give us the money and facilities to do the job, and we'll do it!

Stressing the integrative and complementary aspect, Weil insists that:

> If I am in a car accident, don't take me to a herbalist. If I have bacterial pneumonia, give me antibiotics. But when it comes to maximizing the body's natural healing potential, a mix of conventional and alternative procedures seems like the only answer.

Proponents of alternative medicine have pointed out that the scientific method of controlled clinical studies, so dogmatically applied by the gatekeepers of medical orthodoxy, is not well-suited for a holistic, individualized approach to healing. Moreover, many question whether conventional medicine is "scientific" and consider it to be "a dogma of authority and not science." Iain Chalmers, director of the U.K. Cochrane Centre, a vociferous advocate of systematic reviews, holds that

> Critics of complementary medicine seem to operate a double standard, being far more assiduous in their attempts to outlaw unevaluated complementary medical practices than unevaluated orthodox practices…. The double standards might be acceptable if orthodox medicine was based solely on practices which have shown to do more good than harm, and if the mechanism through which their beneficial elements had their effects were more understood, but neither of these conditions apply.[38]

6. TOWARDS INTEGRATION

Organized medicine is making a concerted attempt to sift through alternative medicine to determine what is valuable. In particular, some of the medical research journals have manifested a remarkable interest in CAM. In November 1998, the American Medical Association made the extraordinary decision to devote an entire issue of *Journal of the American Medical Association* (JAMA) (November 11, 1998), with coordinated theme issues of the AMA *Archives* journals, to alternative medicine. This represented a planned and concerted effort by the editors of these scientific journals to present clinically relevant and valid information on alternative therapies.

More than 80 articles and editorials were published on a wide variety of therapies. The *British Medical Journal* (*BMJ*), in a move to review the relevance of complementary therapies to the medical profession in the U.K. published a series of twelve articles by Zollman and Vickers,[39] entitled "ABC of Complementary Medicine," over a three-month period at the end of 1999. The authors state their belief that "many doctors want to be supportive of patients' choices and would welcome further information," and conclude that doctors "have an important role in identifying patients who use complementary medicine, minimizing their risk of harm and, as far as possible, ensuring that their choice of treatment is in their best interests." In addition to describing specific therapies, the problem of integration was addressed in two of the twelve *BMJ* articles —"Complementary Medicine and the Doctor," and "Complementary Medicine and the Patient."[40]

Lingering doubts and skepticism remain. Fontanarosa and Lundberg[41] in a *JAMA* editorial, insist that "There is no alternative medicine. There is only scientifically-proven, evidence-based medicine supported by solid data, or unproven medicine for which there is no scientific evidence." Similarly, Angell and Kassirer[42] warn that, "with the increased interest in alternative medicine, we see a reversion to irrational approaches to medical practice, even while scientific medicine is making some of its most dramatic advances." They argue that, "It is time for the scientific community to stop giving alternative medicine a free ride. There cannot be two kinds of medicine—conventional and alternative. There is only one medicine that has been adequately tested and medicine that has not, medicine that works and medicine that may or may not work."

A report of the Millbank Memorial Fund,[43] "Enhancing the Accountability of Alternative Medicine," maintains that

> Practitioners of alternative medicine therapies should be more receptive to evaluation of their interventions by the best available methods of medical science. Anecdotal evidence and patient testimonials often evoke interest and sympathy from consumers and legislators, but they are not a plausible substitute for rigorous analysis of safety and effectiveness.

The report concluded that protecting patients from being harmed by alternative treatments is a high priority for public policy, private purchasers, health plans, individual professionals and discerning consumers.

As early as 1993, Campion[44] sounded a warning note in a *New England Journal of Medicine* editorial: "The public's romance with unconventional medicine is cause for our profession to worry. This theme was repeated by Fontanarosa and Lundberg;[45] "For alternative medicine therapies that are used by millions of patients every day and that generate billions of dollars in health care expenditures each year, the lack of convincing and compelling evidence on efficacy, safety, and outcomes is unacceptable and deeply troubling." Specific concerns of physicians include the possibility that patients may see unqualified practitioners, risk missed or delayed diagnosis, stop or refuse effective conventional treatment, and experience dangerous adverse effects from treatment.[46] Evidence indicates that only 45 percent of CAM users inform their physicians of their usage. Rather than ignore the widespread use of alternative therapies, it is now urged that conventional practitioners, in view of the dangers inherent in parallel and uncoordinated treatment, should determine whether their patients are using complementary therapies, and if so whether conventional medicine has failed them in some manner. Physicians should end the practice of "Don't ask, Don't tell," and foster openness. Furthermore, physicians should encourage patients to have their complementary providers communicate with them, should monitor their patients' progress, and provide information resources in the form of books, articles, Web sites, and support groups.

In order to support intelligent and informed decision making by their patients, it is essential that physicians understand the purpose of complementary therapies, ascertain the value of such therapies in their treatment, and identify any contraindications, potential interactions, and adverse effects. Any attempt by a medical provider to dismiss CAM as a placebo response or without scientific merit becomes a significant barrier in the achievement of coordination of treatment.

Jonas and Levin[47] offer a short list of questions that should be asked by doctors of their patients regarding the use of complementary therapies: how did you decide to use CAM; what were the goals; why was a particular intervention or treatment chosen; how did you select the alternative provider selected; did the interaction help; and did the intervention result in new problems for you? Likewise, patients might ask questions of their CAM providers relating to efficacy, safety, toxicity, how many treatments are required, reasonable time frame for a fair trial, costs, insurance coverage, and whether the CAM practitioner is willing to communicate with the patient's conventional physician.

A step-by-step approach to shared decision making between providers and patients has been suggested by Eisenberg[48] who argues that conventional providers should ensure that patients recognize and understand their symptoms, and should review with them any potential for harmful interactions. Providers should also plan for a follow-up to review the effectiveness of any CAM treatment.

Learning about CAM concepts and methods is becoming an increasingly important component of both medical school education and clinical practice. Almost two-thirds of U.S. medical schools now offer some form of instruction in CAM. A number of textbooks are aimed at educating mainstream physicians. These books serve several purposes—to educate physicians in the concepts, principles, and methods of a wide variety of alternative treatment modalities, and to illustrate how alternative medicine can be integrated into conventional medical practice.

Recent texts addressing the principles and concepts of complementary and alternative medicine for conventional practitioners care include Jonas and Levin, *Essentials of Complementary and Alternative Medicine* (Lippincott, Williams & Wilkins, 1998); Spencer and Jacobs, *Complementary/Alternative Medicine: An Evidence-Based Approach* (Mosby 1998); Kuhn, *Complementary Therapies for Health Care Providers* (Lippincott, Williams & Wilkins, 1999); Fetrow, *The Complete Guide to Herbal Medicines* (Springhouse, 2000); Fetrow and Avila, *Professional's Handbook of Complementary & Alternative Medicine* (Springhouse 1999); Price and Price, *Aromatherapy for Health Professionals*, 2nd edition (Churchill Livingstone, 1999); Pizzorno and Murray, *Textbook of Natural Medicine* (Churchill Livingstone, 1999); and The American Medical Association recently published *Alternative Medicine: An Objective Assessment* that brings together 74 peer-reviewed papers that were originally published in *JAMA* or the *Archives* journals over the most recent three-year period.

A smaller number of books that focus on how integration can be implemented include Milton and Benjamin, *Complementary & Alternative Therapies: An Implementation Guide to Integrative Health Care* (AHA Press, 1998); Clark, *Integrating Complementary Health Procedures Into Practice* (Springhouse, 1999); *Quick Access Professional Guide to Conditions, Herbs & Supplements* (Integrative Medicine Communications, 2000); Edlin

and Dunford, *Herbal Medicine in Primary Care* (Butterworth, Heinemann, 1999); Novey, *Clinician's Complete Reference to Complementary & Alternative Medicine* (Mosby, 2000); Lavalle, *Natural Therapeutics Pocket Guide* (Lexi-Comp, 2000); and Tiran and Mack, *Complementary Therapies for Pregnancy and Childbirth* (Baillière Tindall/Harcourt, 2000).

A growing number of physicians in clinical practice are expressing interest in exploring the concepts and methods of alternative medicine. Andrew Weil's week-long program in integrative medicine, held twice a year at the Canyon Ranch Health Resort in Tucson, offers instruction and hands-on experience for a cost of $5,670. Harvard Medical School's annual conference on complementary and alternative medicine is well attended. The Harvard program for March 2000—Complementary and Alternative Medicine: Implications for Clinical Practice and State-of-the-Science Symposia—featured a four-day exploration of the efficacy and safety of commonly used CAM therapies and a review of the legal, ethical and financial aspects of CAM practice. The Center for Mind-Body Medicine in Washington DC sponsors conferences and workshops for physicians featuring experts such as Joan Borysenko, Herbert Benson, Bernie Siegel, and Larry Dossey.

Integrative medicine has a friend at court in the United Kingdom. The Prince of Wales launched in 1997 an initiative to plan for integrative care. Four working groups, convened at his suggestion, considered ways of improving collaboration between conventional medicine and CAM practice. The working groups subsequently developed consensus proposals for action in the areas of research, education and training, regulation, and delivery of care.[49]

The enthusiastic espousal of CAM by a small number of innovative mainstream physicians, who are willing to study alternative therapies with the intent of integrating them into their clinical practice, should not lead one to the conclusion that large numbers of conventional practitioners are eager for conversion. Most physicians, trained in the scientific tradition, remain steadfast in opposition or mired in indifference. In this connection, Gillert[50] considers that "Conventional medicine has failed to educate the public about how to derive meaning from the enormous field of medical knowledge to which it is continually, even involuntarily, exposed." Many mainstream physicians are of minimal assistance in providing evaluation and guidance to their patients.

Looking to the future, Stephen E. Straus, Director of the National Center for Complementary and Alternative Medicine (NCCAM) at the National Institutes of Health, believes that "the field of *integrative medicine* will be seen as providing novel insights and tools for human health, and not as a source of tension between and among practitioners of the healing arts and their patients."[51]

7. THE NATIONAL CENTER FOR COMPLEMENTARY AND ALTERNATIVE MEDICINE

The establishment of the Office of Alternative Medicine (OAM) at the National Institutes of Health (NIH) in 1991 was intended to promote a rational dialog and evaluation of complementary and alternative approaches to health care and to disseminate information about these practices to the public and health care providers. This move, opposed by some leading administrators at the National Institutes of Health, has been described as "like setting up an office of deviltry within the Catholic Church."[52] Implicit in the creation of OAM, was the assumption that the widespread use of largely unregulated therapies about which there may be inadequate information might endanger the health of the public. At the same time, scientifically validated information about therapies might demonstrate benefits as well as identify risks. OAM was subsequently elevated to serve as the National Center for Complementary and Alternative Medicine (NCCAM) in 1999 with a budget of $68.4 million for FY2000. It should be noted that other components of NIH also fund research in complementary and alternative medicine. In all, the NIH spends $160 million on CAM research, which is less than one percent of its total research budget.

NCCAM has funded nine specialty research centers at a variety of institutions. These are listed and described in Appendix 5. Centers supported include those at Columbia University, University of Maryland, Oregon Health Sciences University, Palmer Center for Chiropractic, Maharishi University of Management College of Vedic Medicine, and the University of Arizona. The nine NCCAM centers are working in a number of CAM fields of inquiry relating to addictions, aging and women's health, cardiovascular disease, aging in African Americans, chiropractic, craniofacial disorders, pediatrics, and neurological disorders. Each center is responsible for assessing and evaluating research supported in its spe-

cialty area and for developing a prioritized research agenda. Two new botanical research centers on dietary supplements were most recently established at the University of California at Los Angeles (UCLA) and at the University of Illinois at Chicago (UIC). These two centers are jointly sponsored by NCCAM and the NIH Office of Dietary Supplements (ODS).

Current NCCAM-sponsored research also involves an investigation of ginkgo biloba for treating dementia and Alzheimer's disease at four clinical centers; a four-year multi-site clinical trial (in conjunction with the National Institute of Arthritis and Musculoskeletal Diseases, and Skin Diseases), of the dietary supplement glucosamine and chondroitin sulfate as a treatment for osteoarthritis of the knee; a multi-site study of the effectiveness of St. John's wort as an antidepressant; use of herbal medicines in the treatment of liver disease; control of dental pain by acupuncture; and the use of saw palmetto as a treatment for benign prostatic hyperplasia (BPH). NCCAM is also collaborating in the research of other NIH components. The Cancer Advisory Panel for Complementary and Alternative Medicine (CAPCAM), established in 1999, is a joint initiative of NCCAM and the National Cancer Institute (NCI) and serves to advise the NCCAM director about promising CAM approaches for the treatment of cancer patients. The NCI Office of Cancer Complementary & Alternative Medicine has its own Web site—http://occam.nci.nih.gov. NCCAM is also cooperating with the NCI in a 5-year, $1.4 million study of the effectiveness of the unorthodox cancer therapy developed by Dr. Nicholas Gonzalez.

NCCAM operates the National Center for Complementary Medicine Clearinghouse providing a toll-free information line, publications, referrals to other information resources, and health information databases. Information specialists answer a toll-free telephone line (888-644-6226), and provide an automated fax-on-demand service for Clearinghouse publications. Information specialists at the Clearinghouse respond to 2,000 CAM-related requests each month. To date, only a few publications are available, including a quarterly newsletter, *Complementary & Alternative Medicine at the NIH.* NCCAM's Citation Index consists of approximately 180,000 bibliographic citations relating to complementary and alternative medicine derived from the National Library of Medicine's MEDLINE database. The CAM Citation Index is available at NCCAM's Web site— http://nccam.nih.gov. NCCAM also maintains a CAM database, which is part of the Combined Health Information Database. The database contains bibliographic citations (summaries) of books, journal articles, research reports, audiovisuals, and other materials about CAM. The NCCAM Web site averages more than 460,000 hits each month.

To facilitate further integration of conventional and alternative health care practice, NCCAM plans to make awards to foster the incorporation of CAM information into the curricula of medical schools and continuing medical education (CME) programs. NCCAM states that it intends "to work to overcome the reluctance of conventional physicians to consider validated CAM therapies and to assimilate proven ones into practice." Arnold Relman, a leading opponent of alternative medicine, argues against such incorporation and warns that alternative medicine "could not be woven into the fabric of the medical curriculum without confusion, contradiction, and an undermining of the scientific foundation upon which modern medicine rests."[53] NCCAM has also initiated a series of town meetings on CAM, the first of which was held in Boston in March 2000 in conjunction with the Center for Alternative Medicine and Education at Beth Israel Deaconess Medical Center and Harvard Medical School. The series of public forums is intended to focus attention on CAM on the part of health care practitioners. Offering elective courses on complementary and alternative medicine, according to Andrew Weil, does not even begin to address the real issues in that integrative medicine has a much broader vision than the simple addition or substitution of other treatments for those now in fashion in the world of conventional practice.

8. CRITICS OF ALTERNATIVE MEDICINE

Stephen Barrett, MD,[54] Board Chairman of Quackwatch and a long-time foe of alternative medicine, argues that doctors who practice alternative medicine are unscientific, opportunistic frauds, or quacks peddling flawed or junk science, and that federal funding is ill-advised. The NCRHI Newsletter of the National Council for Reliable Health Information (formerly the National Committee Against Health Fraud) runs a continuing campaign against alternative medicine with an unrelenting exposé of fraud and deception. Commenting on NCCAM, the NCRHI Newsletter states: "The NIH Center for Alternative Medicine is giving credibility to sectarian medi-

cine, quackery, and the mavericks and fringe practitioners who promote them."[55] Other targets of NCRHI are Germany's Commission E (obtains clinical reports from practitioners, which are of little value in a country with a strong tradition of romantic vitalism), and the PDR for Herbal Medicine (fails to include brand name particulars with the result that providers cannot evaluate crucial data about herbal efficacy, quality, and safety.[56])

In launching the Scientific Review of Alternative Medicine, the Council for Scientific Medicine noted the lack of readily available, reliable information that impairs people's free choice and increases the risks to their health. The potential harm posed is exacerbated by those "who promote unproven treatments, especially by those who are naive, greedy, or unscrupulous." [www.hcrc.org/sram/defense.html]. In the same vein, the "Alternative Medicine$: The Multi-billion $ Fraud" Web site—[www.glinx.com]— offers information on "Murderous Herbs," "The Ugly Side of Alternative Medicine and Herbals," "Confessions of a Former Iridologist ("I was a lying charlatan"), and "Alternative Medicine and Religious Faith Claims Another Victim." Dr. Victor Herbert of the Mt. Sinai School of Medicine calls NCCAM "a worthless waste of money that was set up to promote fraud."[56]

The quality of the research funded by NCCAM has also come under critical scrutiny. Dr. Marcia Angell, formerly editor of the New England Journal of Medicine, argues that the Center has so far failed to produce any significant articles in peer-reviewed journals. "The proof of the pudding is in the eating. Just show me the papers."[57] But serious work is under way at a number of sites such as at the University of Maryland (acupuncture), Duke University (St. John's wort), University of Pittsburgh (ginkgo biloba and dementia), and M. D. Anderson Cancer Center (shark cartilage as a cancer treatment). Dr. Barrie Cassileth points out that "the research is just coming into maturity. It is bar mitzvah time."[58] Research will also be advanced by the announced collaboration between the University of Pittsburgh's International Traditional Chinese Medicine (TCM) Center and centers and institutes in China to develop scientific and clinical standards for TCM.[59]

The medical establishment has increasingly shifted from outright opposition to alternative therapists to a more accommodating acceptance, incorporating them on a subordinated basis within the orthodox division of labor, in much the same way that other occupational groups, such as physician assistants, nurses practitioners and midwives, have been drawn under the wing of medicine.[60] One trend that is becoming apparent is for alternative medicine clinics to be managed by an M.D., with an assortment of alternative practitioners such as acupuncturists, chiropractors, herbalists, and massage therapists all working under the authority of the medical doctor. There exists a growing number of M.D.s committed to overseeing clinics founded in the spirit and ethos of a holistic approach to health care. It has been suggested that in the future the greatest number of practitioners of alternative medicine will be M.D.s.

9. INNOVATIVE INTEGRATIVE HEALTH CARE

Cooperation between conventional and complementary medicine is still in its infancy. But a growing number of innovative programs involving cutting-edge integration are in development. American WholeHealth operates an integrative medical practice in four cities—Boston, Chicago, Denver, and Washington DC. Each center is intended to combine the strengths of conventional and alternative healing traditions creating a range of therapeutic options. American WholeHealth provides, in addition to family practice and internal medicine, traditional Chinese medicine, chiropractic, Reiki, and other options. Other examples of integrative health care projects are described by Milton and Benjamin[61] as at the Innova Heart Center, Falls Church, Virginia, Columbia-Presbyterian Complementary Care Center in New York City, and the Stanford Complementary Medicine Clinic in California.

California Pacific Medical Center in San Francisco offers community wellness programs in yoga, meditation, t'ai chi, qi gong, and operates a Health and Healing Clinic staffed by board-certified physicians with additional training in complementary therapies. Care provided includes acupuncture, therapeutic touch, meditation, and Reiki. Duke University's Center for Integrative Medicine opened a new holistic outpatient clinic in Spring 2000 to study the effects of prayer, imagery, and touch on patients who are about to undergo angioplasty. Duke employs a team of M.D.s trained in conventional medicine as well as various complementary therapies. The stated goal of the program is "to expand the frontiers of how we practice medicine." In New York City, the Cornell Center for Complementary and

Alternative Medicine was scheduled to open in September 2000 with the goal of incorporating guided imagery, nutrition, music, acupuncture, acupressure, and massage into traditional care.

Oxford Health Plans, a leader in providing access to credentialed complementary and alternative medicine for its members, endeavors "to help take the mystery out of complementary and alternative care." Dr. James Dillard, CAM medical director at Oxford Health Plans, stresses the benefits of integrated care: "By discussing health concerns with a medical doctor and a naturopathic physician at the same time, members can integrate more traditional and complementary care, and feel comfortable with the health care choices they are making."[62]

The American Hospital Association announced in late 1999 a new venture to help its member hospitals tap the lucrative, growing, and mostly private market for alternative health care. The partner in the initiative is the State University of New York at Stony Brook with its University Center for Complementary and Alternative Medicine. The objective of the partnership is to assist hospitals to incorporate alternative medicine into their standard treatment. This initiative by the American Hospital Association is not surprising.[63] "The relentless consumer demand for alternative therapies," Milton and Benjamin[64] point out, "together with the economic collapse of conventional medicine, create a powerful incentive for hospitals, clinics, managed care organizations, and individual practitioners to start integrative practices that attempt to combine standard and alternative modalities of treatment."

The benefits of complementary therapy have been demonstrated for people who have received cancer treatment such as surgery, chemotherapy, and radiotherapy. Alternative therapies that help patients to relax are becoming common additions to traditional cancer treatment. Acupuncture, nutritional supplementation, herbal preparations, and guided imagery are used to alleviate many of the adverse effects of conventional treatment. An NIH Consensus Development Conference on Acupuncture issued in early 1998 a "Consensus Statement on Acupuncture" that concluded that acupuncture is an effective treatment for nausea caused by cancer chemotherapy drugs, surgical anesthesia, pregnancy, and for pain resulting from surgery and a variety of musculoskeletal conditions.[65]

10. ALTERNATIVE MEDICINE AS *TERRA INCOGNITA* FOR PATIENTS AND CONSUMERS

Compared with mainstream medicine, alternative medicine is uncharted territory with few familiar landmarks and much of the landscape yet to be explored. There are few major highways, few maps, and few trusted guides. Consumers are forced to navigate the territory with little confidence and nobody to vouch for their safety in transit. Those who turn to their family physicians for guidance are often disappointed in that most providers have done little themselves to explore what alternative medicine might have to offer.

The contrast with mainstream medicine is stark. In conventional medicine, consumers take for granted the existence of well-known and easily recognizable landmarks. There are schools of medicine, dentistry, pharmacy and other health professions that adhere to known academic standards. Federal agencies such as the Food and Drug Administration, U.S. Department of Agriculture, Health Care Financing Administration, and the Agency for Health Care Research and Quality regulate pharmaceuticals, medical devices, agricultural and food products, nursing homes, and so on. Prestigious hospitals and medical centers have established the highest standards of quality clinical care. Accrediting agencies such as the Joint Commissions on Hospitals and Health Care Organizations (JCAHO) guarantee adherence to minimum standards across the country. State medical boards wield disciplinary authority. Professional associations, such as the American Medical Association, American College of Surgeons, and the American Dental Association, have a long history of public responsibility and service. Think tanks generate reliable research data on which public health policy can be based. Foundations such as Robert Wood Johnson and Hughes Medical Research fund innovative projects calculated to improve health care service and delivery. Watchdog groups with strong advocacy programs like the Public Citizens' Health Research Group are trustworthy and held in high regard. Voluntary health associations, such as the American Cancer Society and the Arthritis Foundation, serve a powerful advocacy, supportive, and educational role nationally and locally. The existence of peer-reviewed professional journals such as the *New England Journal of Medicine*, *JAMA*, and *Lancet* provide a conduit for the dissemination of research findings. Web sites such as Healthfinder, and those of the National Institutes of Health and FDA, offer reliable, current, and accurate information to promote and assist informed consumer decision making.

In contrast, the network of alternative medicine organizations, associations, accrediting agencies, foundations, professional societies, educational institutions, peer-reviewed journals, and watchdog groups is still in its infancy. There is only one federally sponsored CAM information clearinghouse compared with more than 50 federal clearinghouses concerned with various aspects of conventional medicine. Several hundred toll-free information hotlines sponsored by government agencies, professional societies, voluntary health associations and pharmaceutical companies, serve the public around the clock. There are over 1,500 pamphlets, booklets, and brochures on mainstream medical topics but only a handful specifically relating to CAM. Direct-to-consumer advertising of prescription drugs disseminating information to consumers and patients barely exists for herbals since curative claims are prohibited by law. Pointing out the rudimentary and nascent nature of alternative medicine institutions is by no means a value judgment, but is rather a statement of fact that reflects its early stage of development. As the tempo of research, development, and clinical practice increases, this situation will change.

11. AVAILABILITY OF COMPLEMENTARY AND ALTERNATIVE MEDICINE INFORMATION

In mainstream medicine, there is an overwhelming abundance of information reported in professional medical literature and in popular publications. The progression from scientific and technical knowledge generated and communicated though a highly structured and peer-reviewed process to popular medical publications designed for non-professionals follows an orderly course. In scientific medicine, a coterie of science writers and medical editors scan the professional literature continuously to extract and synthesize information of popular interest. Findings published in *JAMA*, *New England Journal of Medicine*, *Lancet*, and the specialty journals are promptly recycled for popular consumption, appearing within weeks in such publications as *Harvard Health Letter*, *Prevention*, or *American Health for Women*. Efforts are directed towards identifying, selecting, extracting, digesting, compacting, interpreting, and simplifying technical information for public perusal in a variety of newsletters that provide the reader with explanations and expert interpretation and recommendations on topics frequently fraught with uncertainty and conflicting opinions. Press releases from *JAMA* and *New England Journal of Medicine* to medical writers and television newsrooms facilitate this translation from professional to popular discourse.

In contrast, there is a severely limited amount of high-quality, empirical, and evidence-based research currently being undertaken in complementary and alternative medicine. This limited body of research means that there is little professional literature to be digested and reported. In the absence of a solid research underpinning, most of the writing is characterized by enthusiastic espousal and advocacy of one or more alternative therapies. The most popular book topics in 2000 concern herbal medicine, homeopathy, acupuncture, reflexology, acupuncture, Chinese medicine, Ayurveda, and naturopathy. Many of these books make little attempt to present a balanced or critical appraisal. The quality of the content will doubtless improve, however, as the knowledge base of alternative medicine solidifies.

There are several outstanding popular books that attempt to answer the basic questions confronting consumers—what are the most effective therapies; are they safe; what is the scientific evidence; and for which medical conditions are they most appropriate? These include Kenneth Pelletier's *The Best Alternative Medicine: What Works, What Does Not?* (Simon & Schuster, 2000); Steven Bratman's *The Alternative Medicine Sourcebook: A Realistic Evaluation of Healing Methods*, 2nd edition (Lowell House, 1999); and his *The Alternative Medicine Ratings Guide: An Expert Panel Ranks the Best Treatments for Over 80 Conditions* (Prima, 1998). Several publications have attempted to measure the quality and strength of the evidence currently existing as to the safety and efficacy of alternative treatments and medicinal plants. The *Natural Pharmacist Series* of Prima Publishing, edited by Steven Bratman and David Kroll, evaluates the evidence that exists for alternative therapies, while Robert McCaleb's *The Encyclopedia of Popular Herbs: Your Complete Guide to the Leading Medicinal Plants* (Prima, 1999) assesses the strength of the scientific evidence by means of a five-star rating scale that takes into account variables such as the amount of research, type of research, history of use, and safety record of herbs commonly used.

The number of CAM books published continues to grow. At present, nearly 30 percent of all popular medical books published relate to the broad field of alternative medicine, having risen from about 22 percent in

1998. The sixth edition of the *Consumer Health Information Source Book* (Oryx Press, 2000) reviews 650 popular health books. Of that total, 155 (23.8 percent) are related to CAM. The 1999 *Library Journal* Consumer Health Supplement listed 144 CAM books from a total of 590 consumer health books (24.4 percent). Majors comprehensive *Consumer Health and Complementary Health Books Catalog 2000* lists 611 popular books on consumer health and 165 professional books relating to complementary medicine. Projecting into the future, it is quite likely that the number of alternative medicine books will equal those relating to conventional medicine by the year 2003. A small number of publishers account for much of the growth in book publication. These prolific and innovative publishers include Avery, Ulysses, Prima, Keats, Rodale, Kensington, Element, Dorling Kindersley, Storey, Element, and Wiley. Reviews of some 50 recent Avery books are included in Section 9. The annual production of complementary and alternative medicine books is more than 400.

A search for "alternative medicine" on amazon.com yielded 1,362 titles, while the same search on barnesandnoble.com produced 1,754 titles. *Redwing Reviews*, the catalog of the Redwing Book Company,[66] lists more than 2,000 books, audios, videos and CD-ROMs under headings such as Eastern Healing Arts, Essential Oils and Aromatherapy, and Classical Chinese Medicine.

The small number of popular CAM magazines and newsletters consist of explanations of current alternative practice with little attention paid to efficacy or safety. The major focus is on alternative rather than complementary medicine. The prevailing tone of the popular literature is impregnated with crusading zeal, untempered advocacy, and uncritical acceptance. The textual matter is sprinkled with an abundance of personal narratives, case histories, and anecdotal evidence of cures. Most publications contain an extensive assortment of advertisements promoting natural health products and services. Popular advocates for alternative medicine such as Andrew Weil, Deepak Chopra, Gary Null, and Larry Dossey, contribute regularly to the popular magazines and newsletters. Weil also publishes his own newsletter.

Public access to CAM has been facilitated by the establishment of the Center for Complementary and Alternative Medicine Clearinghouse and by the move of the National Library of Medicine (NLM) to increase the number of alternative medicine journals indexed in

MEDLINE. Approximately 1,500 articles on CAM are published annually in the journals regularly covered by MEDLINE. According to Donald Lindberg, Director of NLM, 74 alternative medicine journals are now being indexed in MEDLINE, compared with 38 journals indexed for ophthalmology, and 38 for orthopedics. Alternative medicine journals currently indexed include *Alternative Therapies in Health and Medicine*, *Chinese Medical Journal*, *Journal of Manipulative and Physiological Therapeutics*, and *Journal of Traditional Chinese Medicine*. Articles on various alternative therapies are also published in the mainstream journals already regularly indexed. To facilitate searching, there are 25 MESH headings in MEDLINE relating to alternative medicine, such Acupuncture, Moxibustion, and Therapeutic Touch.

A study of the number of MEDLINE-listed articles during the period January 1966 to December 1996 by Barnes[67] reported that the number of articles indexed as alternative medicine formed a very small percentage (0.4 percent) of the total number of articles. The paucity of published papers may result from publication bias on the part of mainstream journals but can be more likely attributed to the predilection of authors to submit their papers to the newer, specialty complementary journals not yet indexed by MEDLINE.

A useful directory of databases covering clinical and scientific research relating to alternative medicine treatments and background is available from the Richard and Hinda Rosenthal Center for Complementary and Alternative Medicine. This international directory includes major databases specific to CAM, therapy or modality-specific bibliographic databases, and researcher/research project databases. (http://cpmcnet.columbia.edu/dept/rosenthal/Databases.html). The National Library of Medicine offers a valuable guide to searching for dietary supplements, medicinal plants, and other complementary and alternative medicines together with links to relevant Web sites—(www.nlm.nih.gov/services/dietsup.html).

The number of Web sites continues to grow. A conservative estimate indicates that there are several thousand alternative medicine Web sites. While some are sponsored by organizations, others are maintained by pharmaceutical suppliers, online drugstores, clinics, practitioners, and alternative medicine professional associations. Others are less reputable providing, for example, the sale of laetrile, vitamin B17, and other misbranded and unapproved drugs. Yet other sites peddle miracle cures for obesity.

Obtaining information on complementary and alternative medicine on the Internet has never been easier. The problem relates more to quality than quantity. Typically, searchers rely on a number of excellent gateways that serve as portals to a wide range of selected Web sites. Gateway sites that serve as a convenient and reliable point of entry include:

- McMaster University's Alternative Medicine— Health Care Information Resources. www.hsl.mcmaster.ca/tomflem/altmed.html
- The Alternative Medicine Home Page. Falk Library, University of Pittsburgh. www.pitt.edu/~cbw/altm.html
- Healthfinder. Alternative Medicine. www.healthfinder.gov
- Ask NOAH About Alternative (Complementary) Medicine. www.noah.cuny.edu/alternative/alternative.html

In addition, there are a number of sites that offer both entrée to other sites and access to their own proprietary content. These content-rich sites include:

- About.com Guide to Alternative Medicine— http://altmedicine.about.com
- Mayo Clinic HealthOasis www.mayohealth.org
- WebMDHealth—http://my.webmd.com
- Yahoo-Health-Alternative Medicine—http://dir.yahoo.com/Health/Alternative_Medicine

Tom Flemming in Section 8 provides a comprehensive listing and guidance in using the Internet

12. CONSUMER EMPOWERMENT

Complementary and alternative medicine constitutes the new frontier in medical consumerism. It is the ultimate in self-help and empowerment in that it provides more responsibility and freedom of choice to the individual. Empowerment also shifts the burden of health care decision-making to the patient. "Turning to a CAM practitioner," according to Spencer and Jacobs[68] "is a predictable and overt expression of empowerment—the ability to choose one's healing paradigm despite what the physician might suggest." As the enthusiasm for CAM grows, however, there is an impelling need for consumers and patients to be aware of the potential for harm posed by the unmonitored use of alternative therapies. Consumers considering the use of alternative medicine therapies should be well aware of both the benefits and the risks. Specifically, consumers need to know about the safety and effectiveness of the therapy or treatment, training and qualifications of the provider, and the quality of service delivery. NCCAM points out that specific information about an alternative and complementary therapy's safety and effectiveness may be less readily available than information about conventional medical treatments. NCCAM recommends that health consumers should search the literature, ask the practitioner about specific medical research that may or may not support safety and effectiveness of a treatment or therapy, examine the practitioner's qualifications, check with state medical boards and other regulatory agencies, talk to other patients and with the practitioner in person, and visit the practitioner's office, clinic, or hospital. Other factors to be considered are the amount of time the practitioner spends with a patient, the condition of the office or clinic, costs, and possible insurance coverage. Of utmost importance, patients should discuss all issues concerning treatments and therapies with their health care provider, whether a physician or a CAM practitioner. "Competent health care management requires knowledge of both conventional and alternative therapies for the practitioner to have a complete picture of your treatment plan." (Appendix 4. "Considering Complementary and Alternative Therapies?")

A number of questions should be addressed by patients to their alternative providers:

- Is the [alternative medicine] provider's belief in the effectiveness of the therapy based upon clinical experience with similar patients? If so, is it possible to speak to such a patient?
- Of what will the therapy consist? What is the recommended frequency of therapy?
- How many weeks will it be necessary before it is possible to decide whether the therapy is, or is not, beneficial?
- What is the cost per session, with or without medication, and the estimated total cost for the specified time period? Is third party reimbursement available?
- Are there potential side effects? What are these?
- Is the provider willing to communicate diagnostic findings, therapeutic plans, and follow-up data with the patient's primary care provider or sub-specialist? Are there any limitations placed on this communication?[69]

This laundry list of qualifications, precautions, and reservations places much responsibility on the consumer who is confronted with the difficult task of gathering information, evaluating the significance of what is so often inconclusive if not nebulous information, contacting and questioning an alternative practitioner, and maintaining an information bridge between the alternative and mainstream practitioner. Although there are books on the evaluation of alternative therapies, these obviously do not assess the value of such therapies for a specific individual and condition.

In the same manner that many books and magazine articles lack critical perspective, the press is also a major vector for the spread of misinformation. Television reporting of alternative medicine often verges on the gullible acceptance of dubious claims and unsubstantiated personal testimony.

13. THE FUTURE

A number of scenarios have been suggested that point towards integration and complementarity rather than insularity and rejection. There can be little doubt that the investment in research, albeit miniscule compared with the funding of research in conventional medicine, will result in the recognition of new and promising approaches to the treatment of disease. The adoption of such techniques and their integration into traditional medical practice depends, however, upon the willingness of conventional practitioners to adopt new procedures that are alien to the style of practice in which they were trained. Scientific medicine at the present time dominates medical beliefs and practices, power, finances, and research funding and complementary medicine has "lived in the shadows of science as a professional outcast." Morrell[70] considers that many doctors are more answerable to science than to their patients. Patients demand safe and natural complementary medicine. Clinicians who ignore their patients will suffer the same fate as dinosaurs.

Medical therapies can no longer be based solely on one methodology in that no single modality can serve as an effective treatment for all people in all circumstances. All treatment options must be considered. Dr. Mehmet Oz, a cardiovascular surgeon, who directs the New York Presbyterian Hospital's Complementary Care Center, believes that alternative medicine is "not about donning a saffron-colored robe and chanting Hare

Krishna," but is rather about offering patients the option of having therapies such as hypnosis, yoga, meditation, and massage in combination with conventional surgery. Oz plays tapes of Turkish Sufi music as part of pre-surgical preparation and during surgery to help patients stay relaxed and not feel pain.

Towards this end, Nash[71] argues that:

Integrative medicine will bring the best knowledge of traditional and non-traditional medicine into a common space where the patient's welfare becomes paramount. By exploring all options with the patient and remembering the prime principle of biomedical ethics—respect for patient autonomy—we will usher into being an exciting new era of what we might call Integrative or Outcomes Medicine.

Evidence exists that indicates the growing credibility and acceptance of complementary medicine. Vickers[72] discerns recent substantive shifts in the scientific base and organizational structure of CAM. These shifts would indicate that complementary medicine is becoming more integrated. Vickers cites a number of signs pointing to integration:

The quality of applied research in complementary medicine is growing rapidly and the quality is improving

There is good evidence supporting the use of some complementary medicine treatments

Guidelines and consensus statements issued by conventional medical organizations have recommended some complementary medicine treatments

Complementary medicine is increasingly practiced in conventional medical settings, particularly acupuncture for pain, and massage, music therapy, and relaxation techniques for mild anxiety and depression

Osteopaths and chiropractors recently became the first complementary medicine practitioners in the United Kingdom to be regulated

There is a more open attitude to complementary medicine among conventional health professionals, partly explained by the rise of evidence-based medicine.

In the political arena, the public's embrace of complementary medicine has not escaped attention. Acknowledgment of this powerful force can be seen in the appointment in April 2000 of the White House Commission on complementary and Alternative Medicine Policy.[73] The Commission, chaired by James S. Gordon M.D., comprises 13 members representing a wide variety of interests and constituencies. The principal mission of the commission is to prepare a report to the president on "legislative and administrative recommendations for assuring that public policy maximizes the benefits to Americans of complementary and alternative medicine." The commission is charged with the task of producing recommendations that address the following key issues:

- education and training of health care practitioners in complementary and alternative medicine
- coordinated research to increase knowledge about complementary and alternative medicine
- provision to health care professionals of reliable and useful information about complementary and alternative medicine that can be made readily accessible and understandable to the general public
- guidance for appropriate access to and delivery of complementary and alternative medicine

Both NCCAM and the mandate of the White House Commission underscore the need to identify whether the manifold, untested alternative practices so widely embraced by the American public are safe and effective. This is a matter of public health policy. The rate at which integration is taking place is also a matter of concern to many who believe that consumer acceptance and use of alternative therapies are progressing much faster than the "plodding, bureaucratic way most providers are trying to integrate these therapies into their mix of services." NCCAM and the White House Commission will doubtless speed this process through the creation of policy guidelines on the training of conventional providers, coordination of research into alternative practices and products, and how best to disseminate information to providers and patients. NCCAM has summarized the goal in terms of a "Need To Investigate, Train, Communicate, and Integrate."

It has been suggested that CAM is splitting into two camps—physicians and non-academic healers providing CAM irrespective of evidence and proof of efficacy; and those scientists who study efficacy in isolation from patients and alternative medicine practice. This dichotomy between clinicians and researchers is not peculiar to alternative medicine. A more apparent dichotomy is represented by the divergence between physicians and health care professionals trained by mainstream medicine and those who received their qualifications and training outside of traditional medicine. This split is personified by individuals such as Andrew Weil,

Edzard Ernst, and David Eisenberg with formal M.D. training and those alternative medicine practitioners with degree qualifications in naturopathy, herbal medicine, traditional Chinese medicine, and so on.

Present interest in CAM appears to be focused on the theme of "What Works; What Doesn't." This is the thrust of recent books by Pelletier and Fugh-Berman, and in continuing education conferences such as "Alternative Medicine—Shattering Myths, Forging Realities," held by American Health Consultants in May 2000, which featured separate sessions devoted to what works for allergies, arthritis, hyperlipidemia, and so on. The May 2000 issue of *Consumer Reports* presented the findings of a survey of 46,000 readers as to what alternative health practices work for the treatment of 43 medical conditions.

Clearly, integration places an extraordinary responsibility on individuals who must find their way through a morass of conflicting, inconclusive, fragmented, opinionated, and undocumented information in order to assess whether an alternative treatment will be beneficial or detrimental to their health. To achieve complementary and truly integrative care, patients must act as intelligent and diplomatic intermediaries between their conventional health provider and their chosen alternative practitioner. This involves a delicate bridging role and is fraught with problems of communication and trust. Typical dilemmas faced by patients would involve the necessity of discussing with a psychiatrist a decision to take St. John's wort in conjunction with Zoloft, or informing a vascular medicine specialist of the use of horse chestnut and butcher's broom in the treatment of varicose veins. To assist consumers in quantifying the reliability of CAM information, the National Center for Complementary and Alternative Medicine has defined four levels of confidence reflecting the amount of rigorous research existing on a given therapy, herb, or supplement.[74] The four levels are based on the amount of published, rigorous, clinical research conducted or sponsored by NCCAM, other Institutes or Centers of the NIH, and other biomedical research institutions in the United States, or internationally. A top score of 3 designates "Extensive Research"—the existence of numerous high-quality scientific studies including clinical trials and research published in peer-reviewed journals; a score of 2 reflects "Some Research"—some good quality, scientific studies have been published in peer-reviewed journals; a score of 1 indicates "Limited Research"—a small number of scientific studies have been done but few have

been published in peer-reviewed journals; while a score of 0 represents "No Research"—no scientific studies have been done and no information is available.

Consumers should necessarily use caution in taking herbal products in conjunction with prescription medications without checking with a pharmacist or other reliable source. Typical examples of "complementogenic" disease resulting from improper combinations include difficulty in controlling hypertension due to ginseng, severe headaches caused by evening primrose oil, and myopathy caused by creatine.[75]

If consumer acceptance and usage of CAM therapies is naïve and uninformed, the fault lies not in public gullibility but rather in the comparative lack of quality information for judicious decision making. Within the context of public health, mainstream medicine and the federal government have a clear responsibility to invest in research and to inform and educate the public.

REFERENCES

1. Catherine Zollman and Andrew Vickers. "ABC of Alternative Medicine: What Is Complementary Medicine?" *BMJ* 319 (September 11, 1999): 693.

National Institutes of Health. *Alternative Medicine: Expanding the Horizons. A Report to the National Institutes of Health on Alternative Medicine Systems and Practices in the United States.* Washington DC: U.S. Government Printing Office, 1992.

National Center for Complementary and Alternative Medicine. *Draft Five-Year Strategic Plan.* May 2000. 30pp. Web site: http://nccam.nih.gov/nccam/strategic.

2. David M. Eisenberg, R.C. Kessler, C. Foster, F.E. Norlock, D.R. Calkins, and T.L. Delbanco. "Unconventional Medicine in the United States: Prevalence, Costs, and Patterns of Use." *New England Journal of Medicine* 328 (1993): 246-252.

3. Quoted by Catherine Zollman and Andrew Vickers, "ABC of Alternative Medicine: What is Complementary Medicine? *BMJ* 319 (September 11, 1999): 693.

4. National Center for Complementary and Alternative Medicine. *Frequently Asked Questions.* October 1998. (See Appendix 3.)

5. National Center for Complementary and Alternative Medicine. *Classification of CAM Practices.* Updated March 1, 2000. Web site: www.nccam.nih.gov.

National Center for Complementary and Alternative Medicine. *Draft Five-Year Strategic Plan,* May 2000, p. 7. Web site: http://nccam.nih.gov/nccam/strategic.

6. Wayne B. Jonas and Jeffrey S. Levin. *Essentials of Complementary and Alternative Medicine.* Philadelphia: Lippincott Williams & Wilkins, 1999.

7. Roy Porter. *Medicine, A History of Healing: Ancient Traditions to Modern Practices*. New York: Marlowe & Company, 1998, 208.

8. John W. Spencer and Joseph J. Jacobs. *Complementary/ Alternative Medicine: An Evidence-Based Approach*. St. Louis: Mosby, 1999.

9. Milbank Memorial Fund. *Enhancing the Accountability of Alternative Medicine*. New York: Milbank Memorial Fund, January 1998. Web site: www.milbank.org/mraltmed.html.

10. David M. Eisenberg, R.C. Kessler, C. Foster, F.E. Norlock, D.R. Calkins, and T.L. Delbanco. "Unconventional Medicine in the United States: Prevalence, Costs, and Patterns of Use." *New England Journal of Medicine* 328 (1993): 246-252.

11. David M. Eisenberg, Roger B. Davis, Susan L. Ettner, Scott Appel, Sonja Wilkey, Maria Van Rompay, and Ronald C. Kessler. "Trends in Alternative Medicine Use in the United States, 1990-1997." *JAMA* 280(19): 1569-75.

12. Landmark Healthcare, Inc. *The 1998 Landmark Report I on Public Perceptions of Alternative Care*. Sacramento, CA: Landmark Healthcare Inc., 1998. Web site: www. landmarkhealthcare.com/98tlrI.htm.

13. Terence Monmaney and Shari Rosen. "Alternative Medicine: The 18-Billion Dollar Experiment." *Los Angeles Times*, August 30, 1998-September 2, 1998 (Series of 4 articles).

14. Landmark Healthcare, Inc. *The 1999 Landmark Report II on HMOs and Alternative Care*. Sacramento, CA: Landmark Healthcare, Inc., 1999. Web site: www.landmarkhealthcare. com/ research.htm.

15. "NCRHI Bulletin Board." *NCRHI Newsletter* 23, no. 1 (January/February 2000). Quoting from *National Health* [no date or pages cited].

16. Laura Daily. "More HMO's Covering Alternative Treatments and Complementary Care." *Physicians Financial News* 17, no. 9 (1999): S1, S6. Web site: www.medscape.com/ PFNPublish.

17. "Alternative Medicine Survey: What's Good for What Ails You." *Consumer Reports*, May 2000, 17-25.

18. Quoted by Rita Beamish. "Alternatives Find a Place." *OnHealth with WebMD*, April 13, 2000. Web site: http:// onhealth.webmd.com/alternative/in-depth/item/ item%2C88167_1_1.asp.

19. Ronald A. Chez, Wayne B. Jonas, and David Eisenberg. "The Physician and Complementary and Alternative Medicine." In *Essentials of Complementary and Alternative Medicine* by Wayne B. Jonas and Jeffrey S. Levin. Philadelphia: Lippincott Williams & Wilkins, 1998, 31.

20. Daniel Redwood. "Interview with Marc Micozzi." *HealthWorld Online*, 1995. Web site: www.healthy.net/library/ interviews/redwood/micozzi.htm.

21. Andrew Weil. "Perspective on Medicine: Healthy Alternate to Health Care." *HerbalGram* 46 (Spring 1999): 1.54. Reprinted from the *Los Angeles Times*, October 13, 1998.

22. J. A. Astin. "Why Patients Use Alternative Medicine: Results of a National Study." *JAMA* 279(19): 1548-53.

23. Catherine Zollman and Andrew Vickers. "ABC of Alternative Medicine: Users and Practitioners of Complementary Medicine?" *BMJ* 319 (September 25, 1999): 836-838.

24. Edzard Ernst, ed. *The Complete Book of Symptoms & Treatment: Your Comprehensive Guide to the Safety and Effectiveness of Alternative and Complementary Medicine for Common Ailments*. Boston: Element Books, 1998, xv.

25. Terence Monmaney. "Remedy's U.S. Sales Zoom, but Quality Control Lags: St. John's wort—Regulatory Vacuum Leaves Doubt About Potency, Effects of Herbs Used for Depression." *Los Angeles Times*, August 31, 1998. Web site: www.latimes.com/NEWS/REPORTS.

26. Varro Tyler. "The Truth About Herb/Drug Interactions." *Prevention*. 52 (3): 129.

Denise Grady. "Scientists Say Herbs Need More Regulation." *New York Times*, March 7, 2000.

27. "Heart Effects of Herbal Medicine." *Harvard Heart Letter* 10(6): 3-4.

28. Adriane Fugh-Berman. "Herb-Drug Interactions." *Lancet* 355, no. 9198 (January 8, 2000): 134-138.

29. Adriane Fugh-Berman and Lucinda G. Miller. "Herbal Medicinals: Selected Clinical Considerations, Focusing on Known or Potential Drug-Herb Interactions." *Archives of Internal Medicine* 159, no. 16 (September 13, 1999): 1957.

30. Guy Gugliotta. "Health Concerns Grow Over Herbal Aids." *Washington Post*, March 19, 2000. Web site: www.washingtonpost.com; See also, June H. McDermott and Thomas M. Motyka. "Expert Column: Assessing the Quality of Botanical Products." *MedScape*, January 28, 2000. Web site: www.medscape.com.

31. "The FDA as 'Big Mother'—Alternative Medicine Political Issues." *Alternative Medicine.com*, September 18, 2000. Web site: www.alternative medicine.com.

32. National Institutes of Helath, Office of Dietary Supplements. *NIH Office of Dietary Supplements Announces New Database of Scientific Literature on Dietary Supplements*, December 31, 1998. Web site: http://odp.od.nih.gov/ods/news.

33. Steven Bratman. "Assessing the Quality of Herbal Supplements." *The Natural Pharmacist*, February 29, 2000. Web site: www.tnp.com.

34. ConsumerLab.com. *Product Reviews*. Web site: www.consumerlab.com/results.

35. "Alternative Medicine Under the Microscope." *Natural Health* 27, no. 5 (September-October 1998): 116. *See also* Wallace Sampson and Lewis Vaughn (eds.) *Science Meets*

Alternative Medicine: What the Evidence Says About Unconventional Treatments. Amherst, NY: Prometheus Books, 2000.

36. Edzard Ernst, ed. *The Complete Book of Symptoms & Treatments.* Boston, MA: Element Books, 1998, xv.

37. Arnold Relman and Andrew Weil. "Is Integrative Medicine the Medicine of the Future?" *Archives of Internal Medicine* 159, no. 18 (October 11, 1999): 2122.

38. Quoted by Hilary Bower. "Double Standards Exist in Judging Traditional and Unorthodox Medicine." *BMJ* 316 (June 6, 1998): 1694.

39. Andrew Vickers and Catherine Zollman. "ABC of Complementary Medicine. Clinical Review." *BMJ* 319 (September-December 1999) (Series of 12 articles).

40. Catherine Zollman and Andrew Vickers. "ABC of Alternative Medicine: Complementary Medicine and the Patient." *BMJ* 319 (December 4, 1999): 1486-1489; Catherine Zollman and Andrew Vickers. "ABC of Alternative Medicine: Complementary Medicine and the Doctor." *BMJ* 319 (December 11, 1999): 1558-1561.

41. P.B. Fontanarosa and George Lundberg. "Alternative Medicine Meets Science." *JAMA* 280, no. 18 (November 11, 1998): 1618-1619.

42. Marcia Angell and Jerome Kassirer. "Alternative Medicine—The Risks of Untested and Unregulated Remedies." *New England Journal of* Medicine 339, no. 12 (September 17, 1998): 839.

43. Milbank Memorial Fund. "Enhancing the Accountability of Alternative Medicine." New York: Milbank Memorial Fund, January 1998. Web site: www.milbank.org/mraltmed.html.

44. Edward W. Campion. "Why Unconventional Medicine?" *New England Journal of Medicine* 328, no. 4 (January 28, 1993): 282-283.

45. P. B. Fontanarosa and George Lundberg. "Alternative Medicine Meets Science." *JAMA* 280, no. 18 (11 November 1998): 1618-1619.

46. Catherine Zollman and Andrew Vickers. "ABC of Alternative Medicine. Complementary Medicine and the Patient." *BMJ* 319 (December 4, 1999): 1486-1489.

47. Wayne B. Jonas and Jeffrey S. Levin. *Essentials of Complementary and Alternative Medicine.* Philadelphia: Lippincott Williams & Wilkins, 1999.

48. David M. Eisenberg. "Advising Patients Who Seek Alternative Medical Therapies." *Annals of Internal Medicine* 127, no. 1 (July 1, 1997): 61-69.

49. J.R. Coates and others. "Integrated Healthcare: A Way Forward for the Next Five Years? A Discussion Document from the Prince of Wales' Initiative on Integrated Medicine." *Journal of Alternative and Complementary Medicine: Research on Paradigm, Practice, and Policy* 4, no. 2 (1998): 209-247.

50. George A. Gellert. Letter to the Editor. *New England Journal of Medicine* 329, no. 16 (October 14, 1993): 1203.

51. Statement by Stephen E. Straus, M.D., Director, National Center for Complementary and Alternative Medicine before the House Appropriations Subcommittee on Labor. President's Budget Request for the NCCAM, March 2, 2000. Web site: www.nccam.nih.gov.

52. Sheryl Gay Stolberg. "Alternative Care Gains a Foothold." *New York Times*, January 31, 2000.

53. Steve Bunk. "Is Integrative Medicine the Future: Relman-Weil Debate Focuses on Scientific Evidence Issues." *The Scientist* 13, no. 10 (May 10, 1999): 1.

54. See Stephen Barrett's four Web sites: Quackwatch: www.quackwatch.com; Chirobase: www.chirobase.org; MLM Watch: www.mlmwatch.org; and Nutriwatch: www.nutriwatch.org.

55. National Council for Reliable Health Information. *National Council for Reliable Health Information (CRHI) Newsletter* 22, no. 3 (May-June 1999).

56. Sheryl Gay Stolberg. "Alternative Care Gains a Foothold." *New York Times*, January 31, 2000.

57. Marcia Angell and Jerome Kassirer. "Alternative Medicine—The Risks of Untested and Unregulated Remedies." *New England Journal of* Medicine 339, no. 12 (September 17, 1998): 1840.

58. Sheryl Gay Stolberg. "Alternative Care Gains a Foothold." *New York Times*, January 31, 2000.

59. Leonard Wisneski. *The Integrative Medicine Consult* 2, no. 4 (April 2000): 40.

60. Roy Porter. *Medicine, A History of Healing: Ancient Traditions to Modern Practices.* New York: Marlowe & Company, 1998, 212.

61. Doris Milton and Samuel Benjamin. *Complementary & Alternative Therapies: An Implementation Guide to Integrative Health Care.* Chicago: Health Forum/American Hospital Association, 1998.

62. James Dillard. "It's Natural, But Is It Safe?" *OnHealth.com,* March 17, 2000. Web site: http://onhealth.com.

63. Sidney Stevens. "Hospitals Exploring Alternative Therapies." *Physicians Financial News* 17, no. 14 (October 15, 1999): 1. Web site: www.medscape.com/PFNPublish.

64. Doris Milton and Samuel Benjamin. *Complementary & Alternative Therapies: An Implementation Guide to Integrative Health Care.* Chicago: Health Forum/American Hospital Association, 1998.

65. "Acupuncture." *NIH Consensus Statement* 15, no. 5 (November 3-5, 1997): 34pp.

66. *Redwing Reviews.* Brookline, MA: Redwing Book Company. Quarterly.

67. Joanne Barnes, Neil C. Abbot, Elaine F. Harkness, and Edzard Ernst. "Articles on Complementary Medicine in the Mainstream Medical Literature." *Archives of Internal Medicine* 159 (August 9, 1999): 1721.

68. John W. Spencer and Joseph J. Jacobs. *Complementary/ Alternative Medicine: An Evidence-Based Approach.* St. Louis: Mosby, 1999, 412.

69. David M. Eisenberg. "Advising Patients Who Seek Alternative Medical Therapies." *Annals of Internal Medicine* 127, no. 1 (July 1, 1997): 61-69.

70. Peter Morrell. "Are Medical Dinosaurs Heading for Extinction?" *BMJ* 320, no. 7242 (April 22, 2000): 1145.

71. Robert A. Nash. "The Biomedical Ethics of Alternative, Complementary, and Integrative Medicine." *Alternative Therapies in Health and Medicine* 5, no. 5 (September 1999): 94.

72. Andrew Vickers. "Recent Advances: Complementary Medicine." (Clinical Review). *BMJ:* (September 16, 2000): 683-686.

73. Office of the Press Secretary. *Executive Order: White House Commission on Complementary and Alternative Medicine Policy,* March 8, 2000.

74. This rating scale is used in "Hepatitis C: Treatment Alternatives." The National Center for Complementary and Alternative Medicine Clearinghouse, Publication No. Z-04, May 2000.

75. Anne M. Pettigrew. "'Complementogenic' Disease May Be Increasing." Letter to the Editor. *BMJ* 320 (May 13, 2000): 1341.

SECTION 2

The Best of Complementary and Alternative Medicine Information Resources

This section lists 61 outstanding information resources that are highly valuable and useful to patients and consumers. Included are the best books, popular magazines and newsletters, online and CD-ROM databases, Internet sites, personal health software, and supportive professional books, journals and newsletters. Resources were judged with respect to a number of criteria—authority, credibility, comprehensiveness, readability, ease of use, and identification of further sources of information. In addition, those sources that discussed complementarity and integration were favored over those that dismissed the value of, or need for, conventional health care.

BEST BOOKS

**** Outstanding

Gordon, James S. and Sharon Curtin. *Comprehensive Cancer Care: Integrating Alternative, Complementary, and Conventional Therapies.* Perseus Publishing, 2000.

Horstman, Judith. *The Arthritis Foundation's Guide to Alternative Therapies.* Arthritis Foundation, 1999.

Ornish, Dean. *Love & Survival: The Scientific Basis for the Healing Power of Intimacy.* HarperCollins, 1998.

Pelletier, Kenneth R. *The Best Alternative Medicine: What Works? What Does Not?* Simon & Schuster, 1999.

Shealy, C. Norman. *The Complete Encyclopedia of Alternative Healing Therapies.* Element Books, 1999.

Sifton, David (ed). *The PDR Family Guide to Natural Medicines and Healing Therapies.* Three Rivers Press, 1999.

*** Excellent

Cassileth, Barrie. *The Alternative Medicine Handbook: The Complete Reference Guide to Alternative and Complementary Therapies.* Norton, 1998.

Fetrow, Charles W. and Juan R. Avila. *The Complete Guide to Herbal Medicines.* Springhouse, 1999.

Mortimore, Denise. *The Complete Illustrated Guide to Nutritional Healing.* Element Books, 1998.

Warrier, Gopi and Deepika Gunawant. *The Complete Illustrated Guide to Ayurveda The Ancient Indian Healing Tradition.* Element Books, 1997.

** Very Good

Feinstein, Alice (ed). *Better Homes and Gardens Smart Choices in Alternative Medicine.* Better Homes and Gardens Books, 1999.

Marti, James E. and Heather Burton. *Holistic Pregnancy and Childbirth.* Wiley, 1999.

McCaleb, Robert, Evelyn Leigh, and Krista Morien. *The Encyclopedia of Popular Herbs: Your Complete Guide to the Leading Medicinal Plants.* Prima Health, 1999.

Quick Access Consumer Guide to Conditions, Herbs & Supplements. Integrative Medicine Communications, 2000.

*Good

Bratman, Steven. *The Alternative Medicine Ratings Guide.* Prima, 1998.

Dillard, James and Terra Ziparyn. *Alternative Medicine for Dummies*. IDG Books Worldwide, 1998.

George, Stephen C.. *The Doctors Book of Herbal Home Remedies: Cure Yourself With Nature's Most Powerful Healing Agents*. Rodale, 1999.

Lawless, Julia. *The Complete Illustrated Guide to Aromatherapy: A Practical Approach to the Use of Essential Oils for Health and Well-Being*. Element Books, 1997.

Oxenford, Rosalind. *Reflexology: Simple Techniques to Relieve Stress and Enhance Your Mind*. Lorenz Books, 1997.

Papas, Andreas. *The Vitamin E. Factor: The Miraculous Antioxidant for the Prevention and Treatment of Heart Disease, Cancer, and Aging*. HarperPerennial, 1999.

Simon, David. *Return to Wholeness, Embracing Body, Mind, and Spirit in the Face of Cancer*. Wiley, 1999.

Thase, Michael E. and Elizabeth E. Loredo. *St. John's Wort: Nature's Mood Booster*. Avon, 1998.

Book Series

*** *Excellent*

The Natural Pharmacist TNP.com Series. Steven Bratman and David Kroll. (Series Editors). Prima Health, 1999.

- Barton, Anna and others. *Natural Treatments for Cold and Flu*. 161pp. 1999.
- Dentali, Steven. *Natural Treatments to Improve Memory*. 123pp. 1999.
- Head, Kathi. *Natural Treatments for Diabetes*. 157pp. 1999.
- Hobbs, Ron and others. *Natural Treatments for Arthritis*. 162pp. 1999.
- Ingels, Darin. *Natural Treatments for High Cholesterol*. 137pp. 1999.
- Snow, Joanne Marie. *Natural Treatments for Menopause*. 157pp. 1999.

** *Very Good*

Avery's FAQs (Frequently Asked Questions) All About Series

- Avery Press. $2.99 for each of 24 volumes.
- Berkson, Burt. *All About B Vitamins*. Avery, 1999. 96pp.
- Cass, Hyla. *All About Herbs*. Avery, 1999. 96pp.
- Cass, Hyla. *All About St. John's Wort*. Avery, 1999. 96pp.
- Challem, Jack. *All About Caretenoids: Beta-Carotene, Leutein & Lycopene*. Avery, 1999. 96pp.

- Challem, Jack. *All About Vitamin E*. Avery, 1999. 96pp.
- Challem, Jack. *All About Vitamins*. Avery, 1999. 96pp.
- Clouatre, Dallas. *All About Grape Seed Extract*. Avery, 1999. 96pp.
- Clouatre, Dallas. *All About SAM-e*. Avery, 1999. 96pp.
- Dennison, Margaret. *All About MSM*. Avery, 1999. 96pp.
- Dolby, Victoria. *All About Green Tea*. Avery, 1999. 96pp.
- Dolby, Victoria. *All About Soy Isoflavones and Women's Health*. Avery, 1999. 96pp.
- Evans, Gary. *All About Chromium Picolinate*. Avery, 1999. 96pp.
- Felix, Clara. *All About Omega-3 Oils*. Avery, 1999. 96pp.
- Fulder, Stephen. *All About Garlic*. Avery, 1999. 96pp.
- Fulder, Stephen. *All About Ginseng*. Avery, 1999. 96pp.
- Janson, Michael. *All About Saw Palmetto and Prostate Health*. Avery, 1999. 96pp.
- Mindell, Earl. *All About Kava*. Avery, 1999. 96pp.
- Murray, Frank. *All About Menopause*. Avery, 1999. 96pp.
- Passwater, Richard. *All About Antioxidants*. Avery, 1999. 96pp.
- Passwater, Richard. *All About Pycnogenol*. Avery, 1999. 96pp.
- Passwater, Richard. *All About Selenium*. Avery, 1999. 96pp
- Sahelian, Ray. *All About Coenzyme Q10*. Avery, 1999. 96pp.
- Sahelian, Ray. *All About Creatine*. Avery, 1999. 96pp.
- Sahelian, Ray. *All About DHEA*. Avery, 1999. 96pp.
- Sahelian, Ray. *All About Glucosamine & Chondroitin*. Avery, 1999. 96pp.
- Simontacchi, Carol. *All About Chitosan*. Avery, 1999. 96pp.
- Smith, Tracy. *All About Ginkgo Biloba*. Avery, 1999. 96pp.
- Tuttle, Dave and Ray Sahelian. *All About Creatine*. Avery, 1999. 96pp.

- Vukovic, Laurel. *All About Echinacea & Goldenseal.* Avery, 1999. 96pp.
- Watson, Cynthia M. *All About Alpha-Lipoic Acid.* Avery, 1999. 96pp.

BEST POPULAR MAGAZINES

Alternative Medicine. Future Medicine Publishing. $20, bimonthly.

HerbalGram. American Botanical Council. $29, quarterly.

Natural Health. Weider Publications. $24, 9 issues.

Prevention Magazine. Rodale Press. $17.88, monthly.

BEST POPULAR NEWSLETTERS

Alternatives. Mountain Home Publishing. $69, monthly.

Dr. Andrew Weil's Self Healing. Thorne Communications. $16, monthly.

NCRHI Newsletter: Quality in the Health Care Marketplace. National Council for Reliable Health Information. $30, Bimonthly.

WholeHealthMD Advisor. WholeHealth.com LLC. $24, monthly.

BEST PROFESSIONAL BOOKS

Blumenthal, Mark. *Herbal Medicine: Expanded Commission E Monographs:* American Botanical Council. Integrative Medical Communications, 2000. $49.95.

Dossey, Larry. *Reinventing Medicine: Beyond Mind-Body to a New Era of Healing.* HarperCollins, 1999. $24.

Jonas, Wayne B. and Jeffrey S. Levin. *Essentials of Complementary and Alternative Medicine.* Lippincott, 1998. $35.

Kuhn, Merrily A.. *Complementary Therapies for Health Care Providers.* Lippincott, 1999. $19.95.

Milton, Doris and Samuel Benjamin. *Complementary and Alternative Therapies: An Implementation Guide to Integrative Health Care.* American Hospital Association, 1998. $35.

Novey, Donald W.. *Clinician's Complete Reference to Complementary and Alternative Medicine.* Mosby, 2000. $49.

The PDR for Herbal Medicines. 2nd edition. Medical Economics, 2000.

Pizzorno, Joseph E. and Michael T. Murray. *Textbook of Natural Medicine.* 2 vols. Churchill Livingstone. 1999. $195.

Zollman, Catherine and Andrew Vickers. *ABC of Complementary Medicine.* BMJ Publishing Group, 2000. $29.95.

BEST PROFESSIONAL JOURNALS

Alternative and Complementary Therapies: A Bimonthly Publication for Health Care Professionals. Mary Ann Liebert Publishers. $69, bimonthly.

Alternative Therapies in Health and Medicine. InnoVision Communications. $59, monthly.

Complementary Therapies in Medicine. Harcourt. $93, quarterly.

Journal of Alternative and Complementary Medicine: Research on Paradigm, Practice and Policy. Mary Ann Liebert Publishers. $93, bimonthly.

BEST PROFESSIONAL NEWSLETTERS

Alternative Medicine Alert. American Health Consultants. $219, monthly.

Complementary Medicine for the Physician. Saunders. $87, 10 issues.

The Integrative Medicine Consult. Integrative Medicine Communications. $189, monthly.

BEST WEB SITES*

About.com: Alternative Medicine (http://altmedicine.about.com/health/altmedicine/)

American Chiropractic Association Online (http://www.ACAToday.com/)

Ask Dr. Weil (http://www.pathfinder.com/drweil/)

Chiropractic in Canada (http://www.ccachiro.org/)

International Vegetarian Union (http://www.ivu.org/)

The Natural Pharmacist (http://www.tnp.com/home.asp)

OneBody.com (http://www.onebody.com/index.jhtml)

onhealth Alternative Herbal Index (http://onhealth.com/alternative/resource/herbs/index.asp)

The Vegetarian Society of the United Kingdom (http://www.vegsoc.org/)

WholeHealthMD.com (http://www.WholeHealthMD. com)

BEST CD-ROMS

Alt-Health Watch. ccplanet.com, and available online through EbscoHOST.

Ibis Integrated BodyMind Information System. Integrated Medical Arts.

Natural Products Explorer. Facts and Comparisons.

---

*Picked by Tom Flemming, head of public services, McMaster University Health Science Library, Hamilton, Ontario, Canada.

SECTION 3

Complementary and Alternative Medicine Resource Organizations

The following organizations offer a mix of information, referrals, counseling, and educational services relating to complementary and alternative medicine. These organizations represent the major stakeholders in CAM and include educational institutions, academic and professional associations, health care practitioners, educators, accrediting bodies, clinics, NIH component institutes and centers, other government agencies, academies, research centers, certification boards, and nonprofit research institutions and foundations. The research centers currently supported by the National Center for Complementary and Alternative Medicine of NIH are also included.

Every effort has been made to obtain and verify current mailing addresses, telephone and fax numbers, e-mail addresses, and Web sites. All organizations were contacted in May-June 2000.

Academy for Five Element Acupuncture
1170-A East Hallandale Beach Boulevard
Hallandale, FL 33009
954-456-6336
954-456-3944 Fax
e-mail: afea@compuserve.com

Academy for Guided Imagery
P.O. Box 2070
Mill Valley, CA 94942
800-726-2070
Web site: www.interactiveimagery.com

Academy of Chinese Culture and Health Sciences
1601 Clay Street
Oakland, CA 94612
510-763-7787
510-834-8646 Fax
e-mail: acchs@best.com
Web site: www.acchs.edu

Academy of Chinese Healing Arts
505 South Orange Avenue
Sarasota, FL 34236
941-955-4450
e-mail: acha@gte.net
Web site: www.acha.net

American Academy of Neural Therapy
410 East Denny Way
Seattle, WA 98122
206-749-9967
206-723-1367 Fax
Web site: www.neuraltherapy.com

Academy of Oriental Medicine
2700 West Anderson Lane,
Austin, TX 78757
512-454-1188
512-454-7001 Fax
e-mail: acuaoma@aol.com
Web site: www.aoma.edu

Academy of Psychosomatic Medicine
5824 North Magnolia
Chicago, IL 60660
773-784-2025
773-784-1304 Fax
e-mail: ApsychMed@aol.com
Web site: www.apm.org

Academy of Scientific Hypnotherapy
P.O. Box12041
San Diego, CA 92112
619-427-6225

Accreditation Commission for Acupuncture and Oriental Medicine
1010 Wayne Avenue
Silver Spring, MD 20910
301-608-9680
301-608-9576 Fax
e-mail: 73352.2467@compuserve.com

Acupressure Institute
1533 Shattuck Street
Berkeley, CA 94709
800-442-2232
510-845-1059 Fax

Acupressure-Acupuncture Institute
10506 North Kendall Drive
Miami, FL 33176
305-595-9500
305-595-2622 Fax
e-mail: aai@acupuncture.pair.com
Web site: www.aai.acupuncture.pair.com

Alchemy Institute of Healing Arts
2310 Warwick Drive
Santa Rosa, CA 95405
800-950-4984
707-579-4984
Web site: www.alchemyinstitute.com

Alexander Technique International
1692 Massachusetts Avenue
Cambridge, MA 02138
617-497-2242
412-497-2615 Fax
e-mail: ttatint@aol.com

Alternative Health Benefit Services Inc
P.O. Box 6279
Thousand Oaks, CA 91359-6279

818-226-9829
818-226-9820 Fax
e-mail: HealthyIns@AOL.com
Web site: AlternativeInsurance.com

Alternative Medical Association
7909 SE Stark Street
Portland, OR 97215

Alternative Medicine Foundation
5411 W. Cedar Lane #205-A
Bethesda, MD 20814
301-581-0116
888-258-4420
e-mail: amfi@AMFoundation.org
Web site: www.amfoundation.org

American Academy of Environmental Medicine
7701 E. Kellogg #625
Wichita, KS 67201
316-684-5500
316-684-5709 Fax
e-mail: aaem@swbell.net
Web site: www.aaem.com

American Academy of Guided Imagery
P.O. Box 2070
Mill Valley, CA 94942
800-726-2070

American Academy of Medical Acupuncture
5820 Wilshire Bvd #500
Los Angeles, CA 90036
323-937-5514
800-521-2262
323-937-0959 Fax
e-mail: webmaster@medical acupuncture.org
Web site: www.medicalacupuncture.com

American Academy of Osteopathy
3500 DePauw Boulevard #1080
Indianapolis, IN 46268
317-879-1881
317-879-0563 Fax
e-mail: aaomm@aol.com
Web site: www.academyofosteopathy.org

American Alliance of Aromatherapy
P.O. Box 309
Depoe Bay, OR 37341
800-809-9850

American Apitherapy Society
P.O. Box 54
Hartland Four Corners, VT 05049

American Association for Music Therapy
1 Station Plaza
Ossining, NY 10562

American Association for Teachers of Oriental Medicine
P.O. Box 9563
Austin, TX 78766
512-451-2866
e-mail: acuaoma@aol.org
Web site: www.aatom.org

American Association for Therapeutic Humor
222 South Meramec #303
St. Louis, MO 63105
314-963-6232
Web site: www.aath.org

American Association of Acupuncture and Bio-Energetic Medicine
2512 Manoa Road
Honolulu, HI 96822
808-946-2069
808-946-0378 Fax

American Association of Acupuncture and Oriental Medicine
4101 Lake Boone Trail
Raleigh, NC 27607
919-787-5181

American Association of Alternative Healing
1122 Walnut Glen Court
Chico, CA 95926
530-345-8622
Web site: www.cris.com/aaah.com

American Association of Ayurvedic Sciences
2115 112th Avenue NE
Bellevue, WA 98004
425-453-8022
Web site: www.ayurvedicscience.com

American Association of Drugless Practitioners (AADP)
708 Madelaine Drive
Gilmer, TX 75644-3140
903-843-6401
888-764-AADP

e-mail: info@aadp.net
Web site www.aadp.net

American Association of Naturopathic Physicians
601 Valley Street #105
Seattle, WA 98109-4229
206-298-0126
206-298-0129 Fax
e-mail: 74602.3715@compuserve.com
Web site: www.naturopathic.org

American Association of Oriental Medicine
433 Front Street
Catasauqua, PA 18032
610-433-2448
610-264-2768 Fax
e-mail: aaom1@aol.com
Web site: www.aaom.org

American Association of Professional Hypnotherapists
P.O. Box 29
Boones Mill, VA 24065

American Biologics/Bradford Research Institute
1180 Walnut Avenue
Chula Vista, CA 91911
800-227-4458
619-429-8200
619-429-8200 Fax
e-mail: hospital@americanbiologics.com
Web site: www.americanbiologics.com

American Board of Chelation Therapy
1407-B North Wells
Chicago, IL 60610
800-356-2228
312-787-2228

American Board of Holistic Medicine
P.O. Box 5388
Lynnwood, WA 98043
425-741-2996
425-745-8040 Fax
e-mail: blh@halcyon.com

American Board of Homeotherapeutics
801 North Fairfax Street #306
Alexandria, VA 22314
703-548-7790
703-548-7792 Fax
e-mail: nchinfo@igc.org

American Board of Psychological Hypnosis
5410 Connecticut Avenue NW #112
Washington DC 20015
e-mail: hjwain@erols.com

American Bodywork and Massage Professionals
28677 Buffalo Park Road
Evergreen, CO 80439-7347
303-674-8478
800-458-2267
303-674-0859 Fax
e-mail: expectmore@abmp.com
Web site: www.abmp.com

American Botanical Council
P.O. Box 144345
Austin, TX 78714-4345
512-926-4900
512-926-2345 Fax
e-mail: abc@herbalgram.org
Web site: www.herbalgram.org

American Center for the Alexander Technique
39 West 14th Street
New York, NY 10011
212-633-2229
Web site: www.alexandertech.com

American Chiropractic Association
1701 Clarendon Boulevard
Arlington, VA 22209
703-276-8800
703-243-2593 Fax
e-mail: AmerChiro@aol.com
Web site: www.amerchiro.org

American Chronic Pain Association
P.O. Box 850
Rocklin, CA 95788

American College of Acupuncture & Oriental Medicine
9100 Park West Drive
Houston, TX 77063
713-780-9777
713-781-5781 Fax
Web site: www.acaom.edu

American College for Advancement of Medicine
23121 Verdugo Drive #204
Laguna Hills, CA 92653
949-583-7666

949-455-9679 Fax
e-mail: acam@acam.org
Web site: www.acam.org

American College of Traditional Chinese Medicine
455 Arkansas Street
San Francisco, CA 94107
415-282-7600
415-282-0856 Fax
e-mail: lhuang@actcm.org
Web site: www.actcm.org

American Council of Hypnotists Examiners
700 South Central Avenue
Glendale, CA 91204
818-242-5378
Web site: www.sonic.net/hypno/ache.html

American Cranio Sacral Therapy Association
11211 Prosperity Farms Road D-325
Palm Beach Gardens, FL 33410-3487
800-311-9204
Web site: www.iahe.com

American Dance Therapy Association
2000 Centure Plaza 3108
Columbia, MD 21044-3263
410-997-4040
410-997-4048 Fax
e-mail: info@adta.org
Web site: adta.org

American Dianthus Society
P.O. Box 22232
Santa Fe, NM 87502-2232
505-438-7038

American Dietetic Association
216 West Jackson Boulevard
Chicago, IL 60606
312-899-0040
312-899-1712 Fax
Web site: www.eatright.org

American Federation for Traditional Chinese Medicine
P.O. Box 330267
San Francisco, CA 94133
415-392-7002
415-392-7003 Fax
e-mail: aftcm@earthlink.net

American Foundation of Traditional Chinese Medicine
505 Beach Street
San Francisco, CA 94133
415-392-7002
415-392-7003 Fax

American Guild of Hypnotherapists
2200 Veterans Boulevard
Kenner, CA 70062
504-468-3223
504-468-3213 Fax

American Herbalists Guild
P.O. Box 70
Roosevelt, UT 84066
435-722-8434
435-722-8452 Fax
e-mail: office@earthlink.net
Web site: www.healthy.net

American Holistic Health Association
P.O. Box 17400
Anaheim, CA 92817-7400
714-779-6152
e-mail: ahha@healthy.net
Web site: www.ahha.org

American Holistic Medical Association
6728 Old McLean Drive
McLean, VA 22101
703-556-9728
703-556-8729 Fax
e-mail: ahma@degnon.org
Web site: www.holisticmedicine.org

American Holistic Nurses Association
P.O. Box 2130
Flagstaff, AZ 86003
800-278-2462
520-526-2752 Fax
Web site: www.ahna.org

American Holistic Veterinary Medical Association
2218 Old Emmorton Road
Bel Air, MD 21015
410-569-0795
410-569-2346 Fax
e-mail: ahvma@compuserve.com
Web site: www.altvetmed.com

American Institute for Mental Imagery
351 East 84th Street #10D
New York, NY 10028
212-988-7750

American Institute of Homeopathy
801 North Fairfax Street #306
Alexandria, VA 22314
703-548-7790
703-548-7792 Fax

American Institute of Hypnotherapy
16842 Von Karman Avenue #475
Irvine, CA 92714
714-261-6400
800-872-9996
e-mail: aih@hypnosis.com/abh

American Institute of Massage Therapy
2156 Newport Boulevard
Costa Mesa, CA 92627
949-642-0735
949-642-1729 Fax

American Institute of Reflexology
606 E. Magnolia Boulevard #B
Burbank, CA 91501
818-841-7741

American Institute of Vedic Studies
P.O. Box 8357
Santa Fe, NM 87504-8357
505-983-9385
e-mail: vedainst@aol.com
Web site: www.vedanet.com

American Massage Therapy Association
820 Davis Street #100
Evanston, IL 60201-4444
847-864-0123
847-864-1178 Fax
e-mail: info@inet.amtamassage.org
Web site: www.amtamassage.org

American Meditation Institute
P.O. Box 430
Averill Park, NY 12018
518-674-8714
e-mail: postmaster@americanmeditation.org
Web site: www.americanmeditation.org

American Music Therapy Association
8455 Colesville Road #1000

Silver Spring, MD 20910
301-589-3300
301-589-5175 Fax
e-mail: info@musictherapy.org
Web site: www.musictherapy.org

American Naturopathic Medical Association
P.O. Box 96273
Las Vegas, NV 89193
702-897-7053
Web site: www.anma.net

American Oriental Bodywork Therapy Association
1010 Haddonfield-Berlin Road #408
Voorhees, NJ 08043
609-782-1616
609-782-1653 Fax
e-mail: aobta@prodigy.net
Web site: www.healthy.net/aobta

American Osteopathic Association
142 East Ontario Street
Chicago, Il 60611
312-202-8000
800-621-1773
312-202-8200 Fax
Web site: www.aoa-net.org

American Pacific University
College of Clinical Hypnotherapy and Esoteric Studies
615 Pi'ikoi Street #501
Honolulu, HI 96814-4142
e-mail: info@apu.org
Web site: www.apu.org

American Polarity Therapy Association
2888 Bluff Street #149
Boulder, CO 80301
303-545-2080
303-545-2161 Fax
e-mail: satvahq@aol.com
Web site: www.PolarityTherapy.org

American Preventive Medical Association
P.O. Box 458
9912 Georgetown Pike
Great Falls, VA 22066
800-230-2762
703-759-6711
e-mail: apma@healthy.net

American Reflexology Certification Board
P.O. Box 620607
Littleton, CO 80162
303-933-6921
303-904-0460 Fax

American School of Ayurvedic Sciences
10025 N.E. 4th
Bellevue, WA 89004

American Society of Alternative Therapists
P.O. Box 703
Rockport, MA 01966
978-281-4400
e-mail: asat@asat.org
Web site: www.asat.org

American Society for the Alexander Technique
401 East Market Street
Charlottesville, VA 22902
800-473-0620
e-mail: alexandertech@earthlink.net
Web site: www.alexandertech.org

American Society of Clinical Hypnosis
33 West Grand Avenue #402
Chicago, IL 60610
312-645-9810
312-645-9818 Fax

American Society of Clinical Nutrition
9650 Rockville Pike
Bethesda, MD 20814
301-530-7038
301-571-8303 Fax
e-mail: secretar@ascn.faseb.org
Web site: www.faseb.org/ascn

American Society of Pharmacognosy
P.O. Box 9558
Downer's Grove, IL 60515
708-971-6417
708-971-6097 Fax

American Yoga Association
513 South Orange Avenue
Sarasota, FL 34236
941-953-5859
Web site: http://aol.com/AmYogaAssn/AYA/
home.html

Association for Advancement of Behavioral Therapy
305 7th Avenue
New York, NY 10001
212-647-1890
212-647-1865 Fax
Web site: www.aabt.org

Association for Applied Psychophysiology and Biofeedback
10200 West 44th Street #304
Wheat Ridge, CO 80033-2840
303-422-8436
303-422-8894 Fax
e-mail: aabp@resourcenter.com
Web site: www.aabp.org

Association for Integrative Medicine
Box 1
Mont Clare, PA 19453
610-933-8145
e-mail: aim@IntergrativeMedicine.org
Web site: www.integrativemedicine.org

Association for Network Chiropractic
444 North Main Street
Longmont, CO 80501
303-678-8101
303-678-8089 Fax
e-mail: amcoffice@aol.com
Web site: www.networkchiropractic.org

Association of Chiropractic Colleges
4424 Montgomery Avenue
Bethesda, MD 20814
301-652-5006
800-284-1062
301-913-9146 Fax
e-mail: obryonco@aol.com
Web site: www.chirocolleges.org

Association of Holistic Healing Centers
109 Holly Crescent #201
Virginia Beach, VA 23451

Association of Music and Imagery
901 Ruby Street
Blaine, WA 98230
360-332-9357

Atlantic Institute of Oriental Medicine
1057 SE 17th Street

Fort Lauderdale, FL 33316
954-463-3888
954-463-3878 Fax
e-mail: atom3@ix.netcom.com
Web site: www.khang.com/atom

Ayurvedic Institute
11311 Menaul NE
Albuquerque, NM 87112
505-291-9698
505-294-7572 Fax
Web site: www.ayurveda.com

Baltimore School of Massage
6401 Dogwood Road
Baltimore, MD 21207
410-944-8855
e-mail: registrar@bhhc.com
Web site: www.bsom.com

Barbara Brennan School of Healing
P.O. Box 2005
East Hampton, NY 11937
631-329-0951
631-324-0298 Fax
e-mail: bbshoffice@barbarabrennan.com
Web site: www.barbarabrennan.com

Bastyr University
14500 Juanita Drive NE
Kenmore, WA 98028
425-823-1300
425-823-6222 Fax
Web site: www.bastyr.edu

Bio-Electro Magnetics Institute
2490 West Moana Lane
Reno NV 89509
775-827-9099

Biofeedback Certification Institute of America
10200 West 44th Avenue #310
Wheat Ridge, CO 80033-2840
303-420-2902
303-422-8894 Fax
e-mail: bcia@resourcenter.com

Blazing Star Herbal School
P.O. Box 6
Shelburne Falls, MA 01370
413-625-6875

Blue Iris School of Herbal Studies
P.O. Box 10914
Eugene, OR 97440
541-744-1013
Web site: www.herbalism.net/coletteg

Boiron Research Foundation
6 Campus Boulevard
Newton Square, PA 19073
610-325-0918
800-BOIRON-1

Bonnie Prudden Institute for Physical Fitness and Myotherapy Pain Erasure Clinic
7800 East Speedway
Tucson, AZ 85710
602-529-3979
800-221-4634
Web site: www.bonnieprudden.com

Boulder College of Massage Therapy
6255 Longhow Drive
Boulder, CO 80301
800-442-5131
303-530-2100

The Breema Center
6076 Claremont Avenue
Oakland, CA 94618
510-428-0937
510-428-9235 Fax
Web site: www.breema.com

British Institute of Homeopathy and Complementary Medicine
520 Washington Boulevard #423
Marina Del Rey, CA 90292
800-498-6323
800-495-8277 Fax

British Medical Acupuncture Society
Newton House
Newton Lane
Whitley, Warrington
Cheshire WA4 JA
United Kingdom
44-1925-730-727
e-mail: bmasadmin@aol.com
Web site: www.medical-acupuncture.co.uk

The Buffalo Trust
P.O. Box 89

Jemez Springs, NM 87025-0089
505-829-3635
505-829-3450 Fax
e-mail: natachee@aol.com

Burzynski Research Institute
9432 Old Katy Road
Houston, TX 77055
Web site: http://catalog.com/bri/bri.htm

California Institute of Integral Studies
1453 Mission Street
San Francisco, CA 94103
415-575-6100
Web site: www.ciis.edu

California School of Traditional Hispanic Herbalism
2801 Lincoln Avenue
Richmond, CA 93804
510-233-5837
Web site: www.HispanicHerbs.com

California State Oriental Medical Association
2710 X Street #2A
Sacramento, CA 95818
Web site: www.caaom.org

Canadian Association of Ayurvedic Medicine
P.O. Box 749, Station B .
Ottawa, ON KIP 5P8,
Canada

Canadian Naturopathic Association
4174 Dundas Street West
Etobicoke, ON M8X 1X3
Canada
416-496-8633

Cancer Hyperthermia Holistic Center
Valley Cancer Institute
12099 West Washington Boulevard #304
Los Angeles, CA 90066
310-398-0013
310-398-4470 Fax
Web site: www.vci.org

Center for Addiction and Alternative Medicine Research
University of Minnesota Medical School
914 South Eighth Street #D917
Minneapolis, MN 55404
612-347-7670

612-337-7367 Fax
Web site: www.mmrfweb.org/caamrpages/
    caamrcover.html

Center for Alternative Medicine Pain Research and Evaluation
University of Maryland School of Medicine
Division of Complementary Medicine
2200 North Forest Park
Baltimore, MD 21207
410-448-6361
Web site: http://207.123.250.14

Center for Alternative Medicine Research
Beth Israel Hospital Deaconess Medical Center
330 Brookline Avenue
Boston, MA 02215
Web site: www.bidmc.harvard.edu/medicine/camr/
    index.html

Center for Alternative Medicine Research in Asthma and Immunology
3150B Meyer Hall
University of California, Davis
Davis, CA 95616
916-752-6575
916-752-1297 Fax
e-mail: camra@ucdavis.edu
Web site: http://www-camra.ucdavis.edu

Center for Alternative Research in Cancer
University of Texas at Houston Science Center
P.O. Box 20186
Houston, TX 77225
Web site: www.sph.uth.tmc.edu/utcam

Center for Attitudinal Healing
33 Buchanan
Sausalito, CA 94965
415-331-6161

Center for Complementary and Alternative Medicine
State University of New York at Stony Brook
33 Research Way
E. Setauket, NY 11789
516-444-0685
516-444-4990 Fax

Center for Complementary and Alternative Medicine Research in CVD
CAM Research Center for Cardiovascular Diseases
University of Michigan Taubman Health Care Center

Box 0344
Ann Arbor, MI 48109
734-936-4984
734-764-2255 Fax

Center for Environmental Therapeutics
P.O. Box 532
Georgetown, CO 80444

Center for Enzyme Therapy
507 A Avenue
Lake Oswego, OR 97034
888-635-4413
Web site: www.enzyme-therapy.com

Center for Holistic Urology
Department of Urology at Columbia-Presbyterian
    Medical Center
16 East 60th Street
New York, NY 10022
212-305-0347

Center for Meditation and Healing
Columbia Presbyterian/Eastside
16 East 60th Street #400
New York, NY 10021
212-326-8435
212-326-8590 Fax
e-mail: loizzoj@cpmail-nz.cis.columbia.edu

Center for Mind-Body Medicine
5225 Connecticut Avenue NW #414
Washington DC 20015
202-966-7338
202-966-2589 Fax
e-mail: cmbm@mindspring.com
Web site: www.cmbm.org

Center for Mindfulness in Medicine, Health Care and Society
Stress Reduction Clinic
University of Massachusetts Memorial Health Care
55 Lake Avenue North
Worcester, MA 01655
508-856-2656
508-856-1977 Fax
e-mail: jon.kabat@banyan@ummed.edu

Center for Research in Complementary and Alternative Medicine for Stroke and Neurological Disorders
Kessler Institute for Rehabilitation
1199 Pleasant Valley Way

West Orange, NJ 07052
973-243-6972
201-243-6984 Fax
Web site: www.umdnj.edu/altmdweb/web.html

Center for Spirituality and Healing
University of Minnesota School of Medicine
420 Delaware Street SE
Minneapolis, MN 55404
612-624-9439
Web site: www.csh.umn.edu

Center for Stress, Pain, and Wellness Management
315 West 36th Street
Wilmington, DE 19802
302-654-1840

Center for the Study of Complementary and Alternative Therapies
University of Virginia
McLeod Hall, Suite 5006
Charlottesville, VA 22903-3395
804-924-0113
804-982-1809 Fax
Web site: www.med.Virgina.edu/nursing/centers/alt-ther.html

Chopra Center for Wellbeing
7630 Fay Street
La Jolla, CA 92037
888-424-6772
619-551-7788
858-551-7811 Fax
e-mail: info@chopra.com
Web site: www.chorpa.com

Clayton School of Natural Health
2140-HQ 11th Avenue South
Birmingham, AL 35205
800-659-8274

College of Maharishi Vedic Medicine
1603 North Fourth Street
Fairfield, IA 52556
515-472-8477
515-472-1179 Fax
Web site: www.mum.edu/CMVM

College of Traditional Chinese Medicine
200 7th Avenue
Santa Cruz, CA 95062
831-476-9424
Web site: www.fivebranches.edu

Colorado School of Traditional Chinese Medicine
1441 York Street #202
Denver, CO 80206
303-329-6355

Commission on Massage Therapy Accreditation
820 Davis Street #100
Evanston, IL 60201
847-864-0123
847-864-1178 Fax
Web site: www.comta.org

Complementary-Alternative Medical Association (CAMA)
P.O. Box 373478
Decatur, GA 30037
404-284-7592
e-mail: cama@mindspring.com
web site: www.health.net/cama

Complementary and Alternative Medicine Program
730 Welch Road
Palo Alto, CA 94304-1583
Web site: http://scrdp.stanford.edu/camps.html

Consortial Center for Chiropractic Research
Palmer Center for Chiropractic Research
741 Brady Street
Davenport, IA 52803
e-mail: info@c3r.org
Web site: www.palmer.edu

Council for Homeopathic Certification
P.O. Box 460190
San Francisco, CA 94146
415-789-7677
415-695-8220 Fax
Web site: www.homeopathycouncil.org

Council of Colleges of Acupuncture and Oriental Medicine
1010 Wayne Avenue #1270
Silver Spring, MD 20910
301-608-9175
301-608-9576 Fax
Web site: www.ccaom.org

Council on Chiropractic Education
7975 North Hayden Road
Scottsdale, AZ 85258
602-443-8877
602-443-7333 Fax
e-mail: cceoffice@aol.com

Council on Homeopathic Education
801 North Fairfax Street #306
Alexandria, VA 22314-1757
212-560-7136

Council on Naturopathic Medical Education
P.O. Box 11426
Eugene, OR 97440-3626
541-484-6028
e-mail: crest@clipper.net
Web site: www.cnme.org

Cranial Academy
8202 Clearvista Parkway # 9D
Indianapolis, IN 46256
317-594-0411
317-594-9299 Fax
e-mail: CranAcad@aol.com

Dallas Institute of Acupuncture and Oriental Medicine
1807B Wilshire Boulevard
Santa Monica, CA 90403
310-453-8300
310-829-3838 Fax
e-mail: dsl@emperors.edu

Department of Botanical Medicine
Bastyr University
14500 Juanita Drive NE
Bothell, WA 98011-4966
425-823-1300
425-823-6222 Fax
e-mail: botmed@bastyr.edu
Web site: www.bastyr.edu/academic/botmed

Desert Institute of the Healing Arts
639 N 6th Street
Tucson, AZ 85705
520-882-0899
800-733-8089
Web site: www.diha.com

Dine College
P.O. Box 731
Tuba City, AZ 86045
520-283-6321
520-283-4590
e-mail: nccce@crystal.ncc.cc.nm.us

Dinsha Health Society
1399 Orchard Road
Vineland. NJ 08360
609-692-4686

Dongguk-Royal University
440 South Shatto Place
Los Angeles, CA 90020
213-487-0527
800-303-1800
e-mail: dru@pdc.net
Web site: www.dru.edu

East-West School of Herbology
P.O. Box 712
Santa Cruz, CA 95061
800-717-5010
e-mail: herbcourse@planetherbs.com

Esalen Institute
Highway One
Big Sur, CA 93920
831-667-3000
831-667-2724 Fax

Feldenkrais Guild
P.O. Box 489
524 Ellsworth Street West
Albany, OR 97321-0143
e-mail: feldengld@peak.org
Web site www.feldenkreis.com

Fetzer Institute
9292 West KL Avenue
Kalamazoo, MI 49009-9398
616-375-2000
616-372-2163 Fax
Web site: www.fetzer.org

Five Branches Institute
College and Clinic of Traditional Chinese Medicine
200 Seventh Avenue. #115
Santa Cruz, CA 95062
831-476-9424
831-476-8928 Fax
e-mail: tcm@fivebranches.edu
Web site: www.fivebranches.edu

Florida Institute of Traditional Chinese Medicine
5335 66th Street North
St. Petersburg, FL 33709
727-546-6565
727-547-0703 Fax
e-mail: fitcm@gte.net
Web site: www.fitcm.com

Flower Essence Society
P.O. Box 459

Nevada City, CA 95959
800-736-9222
530-265-0584 Fax
e-mail: mail@flowersociety.org
Web site: www.flowersociety.org

Foundation for Chiropractic Education and Research

704 East Fourth Street
Des Moines, IA 50309
515-282-7118
515-282-3347 Fax
e-mail: fcernow@aol.com
Web site: www.fcer.org

Foundation for Shamanic Studies

P.O. Box 1939
Mill Valley, CA 94942
415-380-8282
e-mail: info@shaminsm.org

Foundation for the Advancement of Innovative Medicine

485 Kinderkarmack Road
Oradell, NJ 07649
877-634-3246
201-634-1871 Fax
e-mail: info@faim.org
Web site: www.faim.org

Gerson Institute and Cancer Curing Society

Max Gerson Memorial Cancer Center
P.O. Box 430
Bonita, CA 91908
619-585-7610
800-759-2966
Web site: www.gerson.org

Guild for Structural Integration

P.O. Box 1559
Boulder, CO 80306
800-447-0150
303-447-0122
Web site: www.rolfguild.org

Hahnemann College of Homeopathy

1152 Solano Avenue Suite B
Albany, CA 94706
510-524-3117
510-526-4262 Fax

Healing Touch International

12477 West Cedar Drive #202
Lakewood, CO 80228
303-989-7982
e-mail: HTIheal@aol.com
Web site: www.healingtouch.net

Hellerwork International

406 Berry Street
Mount Shasta, CA 96067
800-392-3900
530-926-6839 Fax
hellerwork@hellerwork.com
Web site: www.hellerwork.com

Herb and Botanical Alliance

5916 Duerer Street
P.O. Box 93
Egg Harbor, NJ 08215-0093
609-965-0337
609-965-4488 Fax

Herb Research Foundation

1007 Pearl Street # 200
Boulder, CO 80302
303-449-2265
303-449-7849 Fax
e-mail: info@herbs.org
Web site: www.herbs.org

Herb Society of America

9019 Kirtland-Chardon Road
Kirtland, OH 44094
440-256-0514
440-256-0541 Fax
e-mail: herbsociety@aol.com
Web site: www.herbsociety.org

Himalayan International Institute of Yoga Science and Philosophy of the USA

RR1 Box 400
Honesdale, PA 18431
570-253-5551
800-822-4547
570-253-9078 Fax
Web site: www.himalayaninstitute.org

Holistic Dental Association

3905 Richmond Square
Oklahoma City, OK 73118
405-840-5600
405-843-0417 Fax

Homeopathic Academy of Naturopathic Physicians
P.O. Box 69565
Portland, OR 97201

Homeopathic Educational Services
2124 Kittredge Street
Berkeley, CA 94704
510-649-0294
Web site: www.homeopathic.com

Insight Meditation Society
1230 Pleasant Street
Barre, MA 01005
978-355-4378
978-355-6398 Fax
Web site: www.dharma.org

Institute for Traditional Medicine and Preventive Health Care
2017 S.E. Hawthorne
Portland, OR 97214
503-233-4907
503-233-1017 Fax
e-mail: itm@itmonline.org
Web site: www.itmonline.org

Institute of Chinese Herbology
5459 Shafter Avenue
Oakland, CA 94618
510-428-2061
800-736-0182
510-420-1039 Fax
e-mail: ich@slip.net
Web site: www.ich-herbland.com

Institute of Noetic Sciences
475 Gate Five Road #300
Sausalito, CA 94965-9090
415-331-5650
415-331-5673 Fax

Integrated Visual Healing
655 Lewelling Boulevard #214
San Leandro, CA 94579
510-357-0477

Integrative Medicine Center
Memorial Sloan-Kettering
303 East 65th Street
New York, NY 10021
212-639-8629
Web site: www.mskcc.org

International Academy of Classical Homeopathy
P.O. Box 242
Gardiner, NY 12525
877-973-6339
e-mail: homeopath4@aol.com

International Academy of Nutrition and Preventive Medicine
P.O. Box 18433
Asheville, NC 28814-0433
704-258-3243

International Aromatherapy and Herb Association
3541 West Acapulco Lane
Phoenix, AZ 85053
602-938-4439
e-mail: jeffreys@aztec.asa.edu

International Association of Infant Massage
5660 Clinton Street #2
Elma, NY 14059
800-248-5432

International Association of Interactive Imagery
P.O. Box 124
Villa Grande, CA 95486
e-mail: IAII@iaii.org
Web site: www.iaii.org

International Association of Massage Therapy
3000 Connecticut Avenue NW #308
Washington, DC 20008

International Association of Reiki Professionals
P.O. Box 481
Winchester, MA 01890
781-729-3530
781-721-7306 Fax
e-mail: info@iarp.org
Web site: www.iarp.org

International Association of Yoga Therapists
Yoga Research and Education Center
P.O. Box 1386
Lower Lake, CA 95457
707-928-9898
707-928-4738 Fax
e-mail: mail@yrec.org
Web site: www.yrec.org

International Ayurvedic Institute
11 Elm Street
Worcester, MA 01609

508-755-3744
508-770-0618 Fax
Web site: www.gis.net/~AYURVEDA

International Chiropractors Association
1110 North Glebe Road #1000
Arlington, VA 22201-5722
703-528-5000
800-423-4690
703-528-5023 Fax
Web site: www.chiropractic.org

International College of Advanced Longevity Medicine
1407-B North Wells Street
Chicago, IL 60610
888-855-5050
708-579-3097 Fax
Web site: www.longevityplus.net

International College of Applied Kinesiology
6405 Metcalf Avenue #503
Shawnee Mission, KS 66202
913-384-5336
913-384-5112 Fax
Web site www.icakusa.com

International College of Traditional Chinese Medicine of Vancouver
1508 West Broadway #201
Vancouver, BC V6J 1W8
Canada
Web site: www.tcmcollege.com

International Foundation of Bio-Magnetics
3705 Waialae Avenue #200
Honolulu, HI 96816
808-737-2114
808-737-2114 Fax
Web site: http://planet-hawaii.com/bio-magnetics

International Herb Association
P.O. Box 317
Mundelein, IL 60060
847-949-4372
847-949-5896 Fax

International Institute of Chinese Medicine
P.O. Box 4991
Santa Fe, NM 87502
505-473-5233
800-377-4561

505-473-9279 Fax
e-mail: panda@thuntek.net
Web site: www.thuntek.net/iicm

International Institute of Reflexology
P.O. Box 12462
St. Petersburg, FL 33733-2642
727-343-4811
727-381-2807 Fax
e-mail: ftreflex@concentric.net
Web site: www.reflexology-usa.net

International Macrobiotic Shiatsu Society
1122 M Street,
Eureka, CA 95501

International Massage Association
92 Main Street
P.O. Box 421
Warrenton, VA 20188-0421
540-351-0800
540-351-0186 Fax
Web site: www.imagroup.com

International Myotherapy Association
4330 East Havasu Road
Tucson, AZ 85718
800-221-4634
e-mail: info@bonnieprudden.com

International Oxidative Medicine Association
P.O. Box 891954
Oklahoma City, OK 73189
405-634-1310
405-634-7320 Fax

International Rolf Institute
205 Canyon Boulevard
Boulder, CO 80302
303-449-5903
303-449-5978 Fax
Web site: www.rolf.org

International School of Magnetic Therapy
121 Counter Street #902
Kingston, ON K7K 6C7
613-541-1703 Fax
Web site: www.shyft.com/magnet

International School of Shiatsu
10 South Clinton Street
Doylestown, PA 18901
215-340-9918
e-mail: info@shiatsubo.com
Web site: www.shiatsubo.com

International Society for Orthomolecular Medicine
16 Florence Avenue
Toronto, ON M2N 1E9
Canada
416-733-2117
Web site: www.orthomed.org/isom/isom.htm

International Society for the Study of Subtle Energies and Energy Medicine
11005 Ralston Road #100D
Arvada, CO 80004
303-425-4625
Web site: www.issseem.org

Jin Shin Do Foundation for Body/Mind Acupressure
1084G San Miguel Canyon Road
Watsonville, CA 95076
831-763-7702
831-763-1551 Fax

Kushi Institute
Cancer and Diet Information
P.O. Box 7
Becket, MA 01223
800-975-8744
413-623-5741
413-623-8827 Fax
e-mail: Kushi@macrobiotics.org
Web site: www.macrobiotics.org/cancerdiet.html

Leshan Healing
315 East 68th Street Box 9G
New York, NY 10021

Macrobiotics Foundation
George Ohsawa Macrobiotics Foundation
1999 Myers Street
Oroville, CA 95966
530-533-7702

Maharishi University of Management
1000 North 4th Street
Fairfield, IA 52557
515-472-7000
515-472-1179 Fax
Web site: www.mum.edu/CMVM

Meiji College of Oriental Medicine
2550 Shattuck Avenue
Berkeley, CA 94704
510-666-8248

510-666-0111 Fax
e-mail: meiji@pacbell.net

Mercy College Graduate Program in Acupuncture and Oriental Medicine
555 Broadway
Dobbs Ferry NY 10522
914-674-7401
914-674-7374 Fax
e-mail: acu@mercynet.edu
Web site: www.Mercynet.edu

Midwest College of Oriental Medicine
6226 Bankers Road
Racine, WI 53403
262-554-2010
262-554-7475 Fax
e-mail: info@acupuncture.edu
Web site: www.acupuncture.edu

Mind/Body Institute
Department of Medicine
Beth Israel Deaconess Medical Center
110 Francis Street
Boston, MA 02215
617-632-9530
617-632-7383 Fax
e-mail: Mind/body_Medical_Institute@bidmc.
   harvard.edu
Web site: www.med.harvard.edu/programs/mindbody

Mind/Body Medical Unit
Memorial Hermann Healthcare System
7500 Beechnut #321
Houston, TX 77074
713-776-5020
Web site: www.mhhs.org

Minnesota Institute of Acupuncture and Herbal Studies
2501 West 84th Street
Bloomington, MN 55431
612-888-4777
612-887-1398 Fax
e-mail: miahs@nwhealth.edu
Web site: www.nwhealth.edu

The Moss Reports
144 St. John's Place
Brooklyn, NY 11217
718-636-0186
Web site: www.ralphmoss.com

National Acupuncture and Oriental Medical Alliance
14637 Starr Road SE
Olalla, WA 98359
253-851-6896
253-851-6883 Fax
Web site: www.acuall.org

National Acupuncture Detoxification Association
P.O. Box 1927
Vancouver, WA 98668-1927
888-765-6232
805-969-6051 Fax

National Acupuncture Foundation
P.O. Box 2271
Gig Harbor, WA 98335-4271
253-851-6538
253-851-6538 Fax

National Association for Chiropractic Medicine
15427 Baybrook Drive
Houston, TX 77062
281-280-8262
Web site: www.chiromed.org

National Association for Holistic Aromatherapy
836 Hanley Ind. Court
St. Louis, MO 63144
888-ASK-NAHA
314-963-4454 Fax
e-mail: info@naha.org
Web site: www.naha.org

National Association for Music Therapy
8455 Colesville Road #1000
Silver Spring, MD 20910
302-589-3300
301-589-5175 Fax
e-mail: info@musictherapy.org
Web site: www.musictherapy.org

National Association for Poetry Therapy
5505 Connecticut Avenue NW
Washington, DC 20015
202-966-2536
Web site: www.poetrytherapy.org

National Association of Nurse Massage Therapists
1720 Willow Creek Circle
Eugene, OR 97402

National Board for Certified Clinical Hypnotherapists
8750 Goergia Avenue #142E
Silver Spring, MD 20901
301-608-0123
800-449-8144

National Board of Chiropractic Examiners
901 54th Avenue
Greeley, CO 80634
970-356-9100
970-356-6134 Fax
e-mail: nbce@nbce.org
Web site: www.nbce.org

National Center for Complementary and Alternative Medicine Clearinghouse
Building 31
National Institutes of Health
Bethesda, MD 20892
888-644-6226
Web site: http://nccam.nih.gov

National Center for Homeopathy
801 North Fairfax Street #306
Alexandria, VA 22314
703-548-7790
703-548-7792 Fax
e-mail: nchinfo@igc.org
Web site: www.homeopathic.org

National Certification Board for Therapeutic Massage and Bodywork
8201 Greensboro Drive #300
McLean, VA 22102
703-610-9015
800-296-0664
703-610-9005 Fax
Web site: www.ncbtmb.com

National Certification Commission for Acupuncture and Oriental Medicine
11 Canal Center Plaza #300
Alexandria, VA 22314
703-548-9004
703-548-9079 Fax
Web site: www.nccaom.org

National College of Naturopathic Medicine
049 SW Porter
Portland, OR 97201
503-499-4343

503-499-0022 Fax
e-mail: admissions@ncnm.edu
Web site: www.ncnm.edu

National College of Oriental Medicine
71000 Lake Ellenor Drive
Orlando, FL 32809-5721
407-888-8689
407-888-8211 Fax
e-mail: info@acupunctureschool.com
Web site: www.acupunctureschool.com

National Council for Reliable Health Information
[Formerly National Council Against Health Fraud]
300 East Pink Hill
Independence, MO 64057
816-228-4595
816-228-4995 Fax
Web site: www.ncahf.org

National Holistic Institute
5900 Hollis Street
Emeryville, CA 94608
510-547-6442
510-547-6621 Fax
e-mail: nhi@nhimassage.com

National Institute of Ayurvedic Medicine
584 Milltown Road
Brewster, NY 10509
914-278-8700
Web site: www.niam.com

National Institute of Craniosacral Studies
7827 North Armenia Avenue
Tampa, FL 33604
813-933-6335

National Oils Research Association
894H Route 52
Beacon, NY 12508
914-838-4340
e-mail: norassoc@aol.com

National Qigong (Chi Kung) Association
P.O. Box 20218
Boulder Springs, CO 80308
888-218-7788
Web site: www.nqa.org

National Society of Hypnotherapists
2175 NW 86th Street
Des Moines, IA 50325
515-270-2280

New England School of Acupuncture
40 Belmont Street
Watertown, MA 02472
617-926-1788
617-924-4167 Fax
Web site: www.nesa.edu

New York College for Wholistic Health Education and Research
6801 Jericho Turnpike
Syosset, NY 11791-4415
516-364-0808
516-364-0989 Fax
e-mail: nycinfo@nycollege.edu
Web site: www.nycollege.edu

North American Society of Homeopaths
1122 East Pike Street
Seattle, WA
206-720-7000
e-mail: nash@homeopathy.org
Web site:www.homeopathy.org

North American Society of Teachers of the Alexander Technique
310 Hennepin Avenue #10
Minneapolis, MN 55408
800-473-0620
e-mail: nastat@ix.netcom.com
Web site: www.alexandertech.com

North American Vegetarian Society
P.O. Box 72
Dolgeville, NY 13329
518-568-7970

Northeast School of Botanical Medicine
P.O. Box 6626
Ithaca, NY 14851
607-539-7172
e-mail: 7Song@lightlink.com
Web site: www.7song.com

Northwest Institute of Acupuncture and Oriental Medicine
701 North 34th Street
Seattle, WA 98103-880
206-633-2419
206-633-5578 Fax
e-mail: folks@niaom.edu
Web site: www.niaom.edu

NPLEX (Naturopathic Physicians Licensing Examination)
P.O. Box 69657
Portland, OR 97201
503-250-9141
e-mail: 73422.3360@compuserve.com

Nurse Healers—Professional Associates International
11250 Roger Bacon Drive
Reston, VA 20190
703-234-4149
703-435-4390 Fax
e-mail: nhpa@nursecominc.com
Web site: www.therapeutic-touch.org

Omega Institute for Holistic Studies
2009 Renaissance Boulevard #100
King of Prussia, PA 19406
888-581-0214
Web site: www.EarthMed.com

Oregon College of Oriental Medicine
10525 SE Cherry Blossom Drive
Portland, OR 97216
503-253-3443
505-253-2701 Fax
e-mail: lpowell@teleport.com
Web site: www.ocom.edu

Pacific College of Oriental Medicine
915 Broadway
New York, NY 10010
212-982-3456
800-729-3468

Pacific College of Oriental Medicine
7445 Mission Valley Road #105
San Diego, CA 92108
619-574-6909
619-574-6641 Fax
800-729-0941
e-mail: jmiller@ormed.edu
Web site: www.ormed.edu

Pacific Institute of Aromatherapy
P.O. Box 6723
San Rafael, CA 94903
415-479-9121
415-479-0119 Fax

Pediatric Center for Complementary and Alternative Medicine
University of Arizona Health Sciences Center
Department of Pediatrics
1501 North Campbell Avenue
Tucson, AZ 85724-5073
520-626-5170
520-626-3636 Fax

Preventive Medicine Association
13911 Ridgedale Drive
Minnetonka, MN55305
612-593-9458
612-593-0097 Fax

Psychosynthesis International
P.O. Box 136
Whittier, CA 90608-0136
652-696-7484 Fax
e-mail: psin@earthlink.net

Qigong Institute
East-West Academy of Healing Arts
450 Sutter Street
San Francisco, CA 94108
415-788-2227
415-788-2242 Fax
Web site: www.eastwestqi.com

Qigong Research and Practice Center
P.O. Box 1727
Nederland, CO 80466
303-258-0971
Web site: www.qigonghealing.com

Qi Gong Research Society
3804 Church Road
Mt. Laurel, NJ 08054
856-234-3056
856-727-1233 Fax
Web site: www.qigongresearchsociety.com

Radix Institute
3212 Monte Vista NE
Albuquerque, NM 87106-2120
888-77-RADIX
e-mail: information@radix.org
Web site: www.radix.org

Reflexology Association of America
4012 S. Rainbow Boulevard
Box K585
Las Vegas, NV 89103-2059
702-871-9522

The Reiki Alliance
P.O. Box 41
Cataldo, IN 83810
208-783-3535
208-783-4848 Fax
e-mail: Reikialliance@compuserve.com

Reiki Outreach International
P.O. Box 609
Fair Oaks, CA 95628

Rocky Mountain Center for Botanical Studies
P.O. Box 19254
Boulder, CO 80308
303-442-6861

Rolf Institute of Structural Integration
205 Canyon Boulevard
Boulder, CO 80306
303-449-5903
800-530-8875
e-mail: Rolfinst@aol.com
Web site: www.rolf.org

Rosen Method Professional Association
P.O. Box 11144
Berkeley, CA 94712
510-644-4166
800-893-2622
Web site: www.mcn.org/B/rosen

Richard and Hinda Rosenthal Center for Complementary and Alternative Medicine Research in Women's Health
Columbia University
630 West 168th Street
New York, NY 10032
212-543-9536
Web site: http://cmpnet.columbia.edu/dept/rosenthal

Rubenfeld Synergy Center
45 West 60th Street
New York NY 10023
212-254-5100
212-254-1174 Fax

Sage Mountain Retreat Center and Botanical Sanctuary
P.O. Box 420
East Barre, VT 05649
802-479-9825
802-476-3722 Fax
Web site: www.sagemountain.com

Samra University of Oriental Medicine
3000 South Robertson Road
Los Angeles, CA 90034
310-202-6444
310-202-6007 Fax
e-mail: admissions@samra.edu
Web site: www.samra.edu

Santa Barbara College of Oriental Medicine
1919 State Street
Santa Barbara, CA 93101
805-898-1180
805-682-1864 Fax
e-mail: admissions @sbcom.edu
Web site: www.sbcom.edu

School for Body-Mind Centering
189 Pondview Drive
Amhest, MA 01002
413-256-8615
413-256-8239 Fax
Web site: www.bodymindcentering.com

Seattle Institute of Oriental Medicine
916 NE 65th Street
Seattle, WA 98115
206-517-4541
206-526-1932 Fax
e-mail: info@siom.com
Web site: www.siom.com

Shambhala International
1084 Tower Road
Halifax, NS B3H 2Y5
Canada
902-420-1118
902-423-2750 Fax
e-mail: info@shambhala.org
Web site: www.shambhala.org

Society for Acupuncture Research
6900 Wisconsin Avenue #700
Bethesda, MD 20815
301-571-0624
301-961-5340 Fax

Society for Clinical and Experimental Hypnosis
2201 Header Road #1
Pullman, WA 99163
509-332-7555
509-332-5907 Fax
e-mail: sceh@pullman.com
Web site: http://sunsite.utk.edu/IJCEH/scehframe.htm

Society for Light Treatment and Biological Rhythms
10200 West 44th Avenue #304
Wheat Ridge, CO 80033
Web site: www.websciences.org/sltbr

Society of Behavioral Medicine
7611 Elmwood Avenue #2012
Middleton, WI 53562
608-827-7267
808-831-5122 Fax
e-mail: sbm@tmahq.com
Web site: www.sbmweb.org

Society of Orthomolecular Health-Medicine
2698 Pacific Avenue
San Francisco, CA 94115

Soma Institute of Neuromuscular Integration
730 Klink Street
Buckley, WA 98321
360-829-1025

Somatidian Orthobiology
920 Milf Street
Rock Forest, QC J1N 3B6
Canada
819-564-0492
Web site: www.cerbe.com

Sound Healers Association
P.O. Box 2240
Boulder, CO 80306
303-443-8181

Southwest Acupuncture College
2960 Rodeo Park Drive West
Santa Fe, NM 97505
505-438-8884
505-438-8883 Fax
Web site: www.swacupuncture.com

Southwest College of Naturopathic Medicine and Health Sciences
2140 East Broadway Road
Tempe, AZ 85282
602-858-9100
602-858-9116 Fax
Web site: www.scnm.edu

Soy Protein Council
1255 23rd Street NW #850
Washington, DC 20037

202-467-6610
Web site: www.spcouncil.org

Swedish Institute: School of Acupuncture and Oriental Medicine
226 W. 26th Street
New York, NY 10001
212-924-5900
212-924-7600 Fax
Web site: www.swedishinstitute.com

Tai Hsuan Foundation College of Acupuncture and Herbal Medicine
2600 South King Street
Honolulu, HI 96826
800-942-4788
808-947-1152 Fax
e-mail: taihsuan@acupuncture-hi.com
Web site: www.acupuncture-hi.com

Tao and Zen Research Center
5910 Amboy Road
Staten Island, NY 10309
718-967-4624
718-356-1922 Fax

Taoist T'ai Chi Society of USA
1060 Bannock Street
Denver, CO 80204
303-623-5163
303-623-7908 Fax

Texas College of Traditional Chinese Medicine
4005 Manchaca Road
Austin, TX 78704
512-444-8082
512-444-6345 Fax
e-mail: texastcm@texastcm.edu
Web site: www.texastcm.edu

Tibet House
22 West 15th Street
New York, NY 10011
212-807-0563
212-807-0565 Fax
e-mail: mail@tibethouse.org
Web site: www.tibethouse.org

Touch for Health Association
11262 Washington Boulevard
Culver City, CA 90230
800-466-8342
Web site: www.tfh.org

Traditional Acupuncture Institute
American City Building
10227 Wincopin Circle
Columbia, MD 21004-3422
301-596-6006
410-964-3544 Fax
e-mail: admissions@tai.edu
Web site: www.tai.edu

Traditional Chinese Medical College of Hawaii
P.O. Box 2288
Kamuela, HI 96743
808-885-7886
e-mail: chinese@ilhawaii.com
Web site: www.ilhawaii.net/~chinese

The Trager Institute
21 Locust Avenue
Mill Valley, CA 94941
415-388-2688
415-388-2710 Fax

Tri-State Institute of Traditional Chinese Acupuncture
80 8th Avenue
New York, NY 10011
212-242-2255
212-242-2920 Fax
e-mail: tsitca@aol.com

University of Bridgeport College of Naturopathic Medicine
60 Lafayette Street
Bridgeport, CT 06601
203-576-4108
e-mail: natmed@cse.bridgeport.edu
Web site: www.bridgeport.edu/naturopathy

Upledger Institute
11211 Prosperity Farms Road D-325
Palm Beach Gardens, FL 33410-3487
e-mail: upledger@upledger.com
Web site: www.upledger.com

Vedic Sciences Institute
P.O. Box 2537
Jupiter, FL 33468-2537

Vegetarian Resource Group
P.O. Box 1463
Baltimore, MD 21203
410-366-8343
Web site: www.vrg.org

World Federation of Chiropractic
3080 Yonge Street #5065
Toronto ON M4N 3N1
Canada
416-484-9978
416-484-9665 Fax
e-mail: worldfed@sympatica.ca
Web site: www.wfc.org

World School of Massage and Advanced Healing
401 42nd Avenue
San Francisco, CA 94121
415-221-2533

Yo San University of Traditional Chinese Medicine
1314 Second Street
Santa Monica, CA 90401
310-917-2202
310-917-2203 Fax
e-mail: info@yosan.edu
Web site: www.yosan.edu

Yoga Research and Education Center
P.O. Box 1386
Lower Lake, CA 95457
707-928-9898
e-mail: yogaesrch@aol.com
Web site: www.yrec.org

Yoga Research Foundation
6111 SW 74th Avenue
Miami, FL 33143
305-666-2006

Zero Balancing Association
P.O. Box 1727
Capitola, CA 95010
831-476-0665
Web site: www.zerobalancing.com

The following publications are useful in identifying and locating organizations:

Gotkin, Janet and Kate Page. *HealthInform's Resource Guide to Alternative Health.* Montrose, NY: HealthInform, 2000.

Greeley, Hugh P. and Anne M. Banas. *The Directory of Complementary & Alternative Medicine.* Marblehead, MA: Opus Communications, 2000.

Rappaport, Karen. *Directory of Schools for Alternative & Complementary Health Care.* 2nd edition. Phoenix, AZ: Oryx Press, 1999.

SECTION 4

Complementary and Alternative Medicine Magazines and Newsletters

The number of magazines and newsletters continues to grow. Most of these publications are devoted to self-health practices and to an explanation of what alternative medicine has to offer. The emphasis is on non-invasive, non-toxic, and natural approaches, including herbal cures, antioxidants, nutritional therapies, meditation, yoga, homeopathic preparations, and alternative therapies such as reflexology and aromatherapy. The writing is often characterized by an almost total lack of critical commentary. Little attention is paid to the complementary or integrative approach that is currently favored in the professional literature. Moreover, scant guidance is given on the potential dangers of combining conventional and complementary therapies.

The periodical literature differs significantly from the magazines, journals and newsletters concerned with mainstream medicine. Whereas popular mainstream publications rest on the solid rock of professional (research) literature that presents current scientific knowledge, the alternative literature in many instances reports hearsay, anecdotal evidence, and testimonials together with elementary explanation of alternative therapies. There is no counterpart to the mainstream consumer health newsletters that digest, interpret, and elucidate what are often the fragmentary and contradictory findings published in scientific medical journals. Research in complementary and alternative medicine is still in its infancy and until a larger body of research

information is reported in the professional literature, there will continue to be a deficit of validated and relevant popular publications.

Recommended publications are denoted by an asterisk.

MAGAZINES

Alive: Canadian Journal of Health and Nutrition. Canadian Health Reform Products Ltd. 7436 Fraser Park Drive, Burnaby, BC. V5H 3X1, Canada. $34, monthly.

> A glossy magazine that is mainly distributed through Canadian health food stores. Focuses on alternative healing methods such as naturopathy, nutrition, nutritional supplements, and exercise. Predictably loaded with advertisements for natural products.

*Alternative Medicine: The Voice of Health. Future Medicine Publishing. 21 Main Street, Tiburon, CA 94920. $20, bimonthly.

> A highly attractive and readable publication that, according to the publisher, can contribute to the retardation of aging, reduction of stress, and control of arthritis, panic disorder, asthma, prostate enlargement, and other ailments. Regular features include "Sexual Health," "Health and Spirituality," "The Healing Grocery," Alternative Medicine Digest," "The Alternative Bookshelf," and in-depth book reviews.

Contains lively correspondence, and "On the Edge" with Burton Goldberg.

Alternative Medicine Digest. Future Publishing Company. P.O. Box 10205, Riverton, NJ 08706 . $20, monthly.

Self-labeled as "the voice of alternative medicine," this magazine highlights "what's new and effective in alternative medicine." Contains feature articles and news notes on a variety of topics — treatment of cancer and stroke, natural pharmacy, aromatherapy, and holistic medicine. Emphasizes freedom of choice in medicine.

The Canadian Journal of Herbalism. Ontario Herbalists Association. 11 Winthrop Place, Stoney Creek, ON L8G 3M3, Canada. $30 Canadian with membership, quarterly.

Recent issues have discussed herb salves and ointments, holistic herbal approaches to diseases, recent books on herbs and natural healing, the problem of standardizing herbal extracts, together with abstracts of recent research articles.

Country Living's Healthy Living. Hearst Communications. P.O. Box 7467, Red Oak, IA 51591-2467. $12, bimonthly.

Reflects a natural and alternative approach to health concerns of women — battling Irritable Bowel Syndrome, precautions in taking antibiotics, "down home remedies," Dr. Weil's Wisdom, herbal skin care, aromatherapy, and healthy nutrition.

Fitness: Mind-Body-Spirit for Women. G+J USA Publishing. P.O. Box 5309, Harlan, IA 51593-2809. $13.97, monthly.

A glossy publication that focuses on self-health care, physical fitness, and beauty care for women. Attention is paid to vitamins, exercise, weight control, and mind and spirit.

Healing Retreats & Spas Magazine. 24 East Cota #101. Santa Barbara, CA 93101. $19.95, bimonthly.

This magazine is a fascinating cross between an upscale travel magazine and an alternative fitness publication — how to meditate and achieve fitness in luxurious and exotic locales such as Baden-Baden, Palm Beach, and Beverly Hot Springs. The textual material is greatly enhanced through the use of stunning color photographs.

Health Naturally: Canada's Self-Health Care Magazine. Box 580. Parry Sound, ON P2A 2X5, Canada. $30, bimonthly.

A popular, full-color magazine with articles on, for example, vegan diets, how to beat fibromyalgia and chronic fatigue, the holistic approach to health, yoga, healing herbs, and colonic irrigation. Contains simple articles that are both informative and readable.

The Herb Companion. Herb Companion Press. P.O. Box 7714, Red Oak, IA 51591-0714. $24, bimonthly.

Contains profiles of herbs, how to grow herbs, essential oils, coffee substitutes (Faux-joe), use of herbs in cooking, aromatherapy, and herbs for health (thyme, horehound, licorice, slippery elm etc).

The Herbal Connection. Herb Growing and Marketing Network. P.O. Box 245, Silver Springs, PA 17575-0245. Price on request, bimonthly.

Offers an insightful look into the world of the herbal industry. Provides lists of resources, publications, Web sites, together with news notes. This is a good source to locate suppliers of herbal teas/beverages, fresh and dried herbs, ginseng, St. John's wort, and the like.

The Herb Quarterly. Long Mountain Press. 223 San Anselmo Avenue, San Anselmo, CA 94960. $24, quarterly.

Features interesting articles on topics such as herbs and cancer, herbal cuisine, saw palmetto for prostate cancer, homegrown healing south of the border (curanderismo), and witch's pharmacopeia. A Herbal HealthWatch is contributed by Michael Castleman.

Herbs for Health. Herb Companion Press. P.O. Box 7711, Red Oak, IA 51591-2711. $19.95, bimonthly.

This is a Rodale publication. Predictably, one finds an attractive assortment of feature stories on topics such as anti-aging herbs, natural treatment of menopausal symptoms, holistic healing pre- and post-surgery, and plants and cancer. An attractive, full-color publication with contributions by well-known authors such as Dana Ullman, Steven Foster, and Earl Mindell.

*HerbalGram. American Botanical Council. P.O. Box 144345, Austin, TX 78714-4345. $29, quarterly.

This is an excellent, highly credible publication of the prestigious American Botanical Council with well-researched articles on herbal medicines. Summaries of current research, book reviews, herbs in clinical practice, and conference proceedings are included in each issue. In sum, an informative and authoritative publication produced by the publisher of *The Complete German Commission E Monographs.*

Journal of Longevity. Health Quest Publications. 316 California Avenue, Reno, NV 89509. $39.95, monthly.

A publication that reflects a natural approach to sexual problems, urinary discomforts, memory loss, hepatitis, prostate enlargement, arthritis, and other ailments. The remedies prescribed involve herbal medicines, antioxidants, nutritional supplements, and minerals.

Life Extension Magazine. Life Extension Foundation. P.O. Box 229120, Hollywood, FL 33022. $40, monthly.

A magazine that advances the case that life extension can be enhanced through the use of nutritional modification, phytonutrients, amino acids, antioxidants, SAM-e ("methyl magic"), MSM, and vitamins. A particularly valuable feature is the inclusion of a large number of medical updates and abstracts of research reports and journal articles. There is also in-depth discussion of current developments from around the world.

Macrobiotics Today. George Ohsawa Macrobiotic Foundation. 1999 Myers Street, Oroville, CA 95966. $20, bimonthly.

Covers the theory and practice of macrobiotics as established by George Ohsawa — Macro (big) and Biotic (life). Attention is paid to macrobiotic cooking, healing, and shiatsu. The basic emphasis is on understanding the working of ying and yang in day-to-day living, especially in the daily preparation and consumption of food.

Massage & Bodywork. Associated Bodywork & Massage Professionals. 1271 Sugarbush Drive, Evergreen, CO 80439-9766. $26, bimonthly.

A bimonthly publication that contains popular articles on topics such as massage and sex (a crude stereotype), benefits of holistic massage, light massage for cancer patients, insurance coverage, and neuromuscular reprogramming. Also covers cranial sacral therapy, Polarity therapy, Reiki, and therapeutic touch. Effective use is made of color diagrams and photographs.

Natural Health. Weider Publications. P.O. Box 37474, Boone, IA 50037-0474. $24, 9 issues per year.

News and notes on a wide variety of subjects such as acupuncture, alternative therapies and asthma, best organic oils, flower essences, use of Reiki to treat acute and chronic pain, and home remedies. One issue offered

an educational guide for consumers in selecting the right alternative medicine doctor. A unique feature is an index in each issue to all conditions and treatments mentioned in the text.

Natural Living Today. P.O. Box 3000, Denville, NJ 07834-9262. $14.95, bimonthly

This is a magazine targeted towards younger, educated women with feature stories relating to yoga, homeopathy, iridology, and optimal health together with in-depth interviews with alternative medicine movers and shakers such as Deepak Chopra.

New Age. P.O. Box 1949, Marion, OH 43306-2049. $14.95, bimonthly.

An annual subscription also includes *Body & Soul: The Annual Guide to Holistic Living* (published in December), and *Guide to Holistic Health* (published in June). The broad coverage of the three magazines includes news of alternative medicine, herbs and supplements, fitness, nutrition, mind and spirit, and articles by Dean Ornish, Stephen Sinatra, and Deepak Chopra.

NewLife Magazine. Serenity Health Organization. 218 West 72nd Street, New York, NY 10023. $25, bimonthly.

While this magazine contains some well-written articles on topics such as traditional Chinese medicine, Qi gong, and acupuncture, the bulk of the content consists of a showcase providing profiles of practitioners of Chinese medicine, holistic dentists, chiropractors, Reiki masters, Rolfers, and clinics, mainly in the New York City area.

*Prevention Magazine. P.O. Box 7305, Red Oak, IA 51591-2305. $17.88, monthly.

With a circulation of millions, *Prevention* features articles and news on alternative medicine and self-health care. Major areas of interest are nutrition, healing, regeneration, weight control, fitness and exercise, and natural remedies for a wide range of ailments and medical conditions. Regular features include Supplement News, Alternative Medicine News, Herb News, and Home Remedies. *Prevention* provides a large amount of interesting and useful information embedded in pages of seemingly endless advertisements for vitamin and nutritional products.

Qi: The Journal of Traditional Eastern Health & Fitness. Insight Graphics Inc. Box 18476, Anaheim Hills, CA 92817. $18.95, quarterly.

News notes and feature stories related to Qi (energy) that follows a pathway along meridians that the Chinese refer to as Jing Luo. Covers medical Qi gong therapy, Feng Shui, and T'ai Chi.

T'Ai Chi. Wayfarer Publications. 2601 Silver Ridge Avenue, Los Angeles, CA 90039. $20, bimonthly.

A bimonthly publication that covers T'ai chi, Qi gong, and meditation positions. Content includes multiple photographs, diagrams, and a good listing of T'ai chi resources.

Vegetarian Journal. Vegetarian Resource Group. P.O. Box 1463, Baltimore, MD 21203. $20, bimonthly.

Highlights tips on cooking, where to buy non-animal products, and where to eat vegan. Typical content provides practical information on meatless meals for working people, vegan menu items at fast food and family-style restaurants, how to avoid animal fats, and diabetes with a vegetarian diet.

Vegetarian Times. P.O. Box 420166, Palm Coast, FL 32142-9107. $29.95, monthly.

Offers excellent coverage of most aspects of vegetarianism including diet and menus, vegan recipes, environmental issues, and animal rights. The publication also contains multiple menus and practical tips.

Yoga International. Himalayan International Institute. RR 1 Box 407, Honesdale, PA 18431-9960. $18, bimonthly.

Focuses more on the philosophy of yoga rather than on the practice of yoga. One section is devoted to Yoga Therapy. An Annual Health Issue is published in March/April.

Yoga Journal. California Yoga Teachers Association. P.O. Box 12008, Berkeley, CA 94712-3008. $19.97, bimonthly.

News and articles from the world of yoga from a theoretical, practical, and spiritual point of view with feature articles on self-care and natural living. Also contains in-depth articles exploring multiple aspects of yoga together with good book and media reviews.

NEWSLETTERS

*Alternatives: For the Health Conscious Individual. Mountain Home Publishing. 1201 Seven Locks Road, Rockville, MD 20854. $69.95, monthly.

The editor, Dr. David G. Williams, is a strong and vocal proponent of alternative medicine. His highly personalized newsletter has an emphasis on natural cures, use of herbs and medicinal plants, shark cartilage

therapy, role of trace metals in maintaining health, the benefits of chitosan, and "News to Use From Around the World. Informative!

Cancer Forum. F.A.C.T. (Foundation for the Advancement of Cancer Therapy) Ltd. Box 1242, Old Chelsea Station, New York, NY 10113. Free, quarterly.

A newsletter that "supports and encourages biological cancer research, nutritional science investigation, and dissemination of information about non-toxic treatment for cancer victims." Reflects strong advocacy of alternative medicine and natural therapies in the treatment of cancer.

HealthInform: Essential Information On Alternative Health Care. HealthInform. 31 Albany Post Road, Montrose, NY 10548. $60, 11 times a year.

This is a monthly alerting tool on alternative and complementary medicine, "designed specifically to deliver timely, vital, fact-based, need-to-know information to researchers, healthcare professionals, and informed consumers." Combines detailed summaries of research articles, lists of resources (books, journals, organizations), and interviews.

Healthnotes Newsletter. 1505 SE Gideon, Suite 200, Portland, OR 97202. $24, monthly.

This newsletter is available by subscription and is also distributed as a free item by many health food stores. The content focuses on herbal remedies and supplements, with short articles on ginkgo, chromium, soy, black cohosh, arginine, and so on. The text is well documented with references to the professional literature.

Homeopathy Today. National Center for Homeopathy. 801 Fairfax Street, Suite 306, Alexandria, VA 22314. Included in membership fee of $40, monthly except for a combined July/August issue.

This newsletter, a publication of the National Center for Homeopathy, features short articles on homeopathic theory and practice, news notes, book reviews, summaries of conference proceedings, and Highlights from Homeopathy in the News (abstracts of articles in newspapers, journals, and other publications). An excellent window for viewing the world of homeopathy.

*NCRHI Newsletter: Quality in the Health Care Marketplace. National Council for Reliable Health Information, Inc. P.O. Box 1276, Loma Linda, CA 92354-1276. $20 for individuals, $30 for professionals, $18 for libraries; bimonthly.

Short news notes on health care fraud and quackery, exposing natural healing, "snake-oil cures," false claims, unproved remedies, unscientific "research," hucksters, and deceptive advertising. Particular attention is paid to rebutting the claims of leading advocates of chiropractic, chelation therapy, and other forms of alternative medicine. Characterized by strong advocacy. Excellent reading!

Nutrition Forum. Prometheus Books, 59 John Glenn Drive, Amherst, NY 14228-2197. $35 individuals, $50 for institutions; bimonthly.

A crusading publication that contains in-depth articles that target a wide assortment of quackery and health fraud practices. Reflects a blanket condemnation of alternative medicine, including homeopathy, chiropractic, naturopathy, and acupuncture. Alternative medicine is equated with health care fraud and quackery. A "Web Watch" feature authored by Stephen Barrett rates the factual accuracy and usefulness of Internet sites containing nutrition and health information. Provocative and stimulating. This publication ceased to be published in September 2000.

WholeHealthMD Advisor: The New Approach to Healing. P.O Box 366, Canal Street Station, New York, NY 10015-0366. $24, monthly.

This publication was formerly entitled *Alternative Medicine Advisor*. The change of title to "Whole Health "connotes an open, holistic approach to healing, one that bridges the gap between conventional medicine and alternative therapies." Regular features include What Works and What Doesn't, Ask Our Experts, the Healing Kitchen, Additional Therapies, and Global Research Reports. An attractive and informative publication. Back articles and further information are available through its Web site at *www.wholehealthmd.com*

Dr. Andrew Weil's Self Healing. P.O. Box 787, Mount Morris, IL 61054. $16, monthly.

The newsletter of alternative medicine's leading guru and advocate. Contains readable digests of current information on biofeedback, acupuncture, herbal medicine, homeopathy, therapeutic touch, visualization, and more. Although Andrew Weil is not your typical doctor, his newsletter is somewhat humdrum and bland.

SECTION 5

Pamphlet Materials

Compared with the number of pamphlets available for conventional medicine, those relating to complementary and alternative medicine are sparse in number. However, as the tempo of research picks up, and as a result of increased interest on the part of federal agencies, the number will doubtless increase in the future.

American Academy of Family Physicians

Herbal Health Products — What You Should Know. March 1, 1999. www.aafp.org/healthinfo

American Botanical Council

HerbalGram

Botanical Booklet Series
  One dollar for each title. Complete set of 14 titles (Echinacea, Siberian Ginseng, Asian Ginseng, Ginkgo, Milk Thistle, Peppermint, Chamomile, American Ginseng, Goldenseal, Feverfew, Garlic, Valerian, St. John's Wort, Black Cohosh,, Common Herbs: An Introductory Guide.), $11.50.

Herb Reference Guide

American Cancer Society

Biofeedback: A Complementary Therapy for Treating Chronic Pain, Insomnia. (ACS News Today). February 2000. www.2.cancer.org/zine/dsp

Columbia University

Directory of Databases. 1999. http:/cpmcnet. columbia.edu/dept/rosenthal

Choosing Complementary and Alternative Medicine: Questions to Consider. 1997. http:/cpmcnet. columbia.edu/dept/rosenthal

Complementary and Alternative Medicine Clinical Trials. 1997. http://cpmcnet.columbia.edu/dept/rosenthal

How Other Medical Systems View Cancer. 1997. http:/cpmcnet.columbia.edu/dept/rosenthal

Federal Trade Commission

Fraudulent Health Claims: Don't Be Fooled. June 1999. www.ftc.gov

Promotions for Kids' Dietary Supplements Leave Sour Taste. May 2000. www.ftc.gov

Food and Drug Administration

Overview of Dietary Supplements. April 1999. http://vm.cfsan.fda.gov

National Cancer Institute

Cancell: Cancer Facts. December 1999. http://cancernet.nci.nih.gov/cgi-b

Cartilage [PDQ]. Complementary and Alternative Medicine. July 1999. http://cancernet.nci.gov/cam/cartilage.htm

Gerson Therapy: Cancer Facts. December 1999. http://cancernet.nci.gov/cgi-b

Immuno-Augmentative Therapy: Cancer Facts. October 1999. http://cancernet.nci.gov/cgi-b

Hydrazine Sulfate [PDQ]. Complementary and Alternative Medicine. July 1999. http://cancernet.nci.gov/cam/hydrazine.htm

Laetrile. September 1999. http://cancernet.nci.gov/cgi-b

Preguntas y Respuestas sobre la Medicina Complementaria en el Tratamiento del Cáncer. http://cis.nci.nih.gov/fact (Spanish version of next item listed).

Questions and Answers About Complementary and Alternative Medicine in Cancer Treatment. July 1999. http://cancernet.nci.gov/cgi-b

National Center for Complementary and Alternative Medicine Clearinghouse

Acupuncture Information and Resources Package. Publication Z01. April 1999.

St. John's Wort. Publication Z02. April 1999.

National Diabetes Information Clearinghouse

Alternative Therapies for Diabetes. May 1999. www.niddk.nih.gov/health/diabetes/summary

National Institutes of Health

Office of Dietary Supplements, Clinical Nutrition Service

Magnesium. March 2000. www.cc.nih.gov/ccc/supplements

Selenium. March 2000. www.cc.nih.gov/ccc/supplements

Zinc. March 2000. www.cc.nih.gov/ccc/supplements

Oxford Health Plans

Alternative Medicine Program

Questions to Ask Your Doctor Before You Agree to Treatment

Talking to Your Doctor About Alternative Medicine

Richard & Hinda Rosenthal Center for Complementary and Alternative Medicine

Directory of Databases. 1999. http:/cpmcnet.columbia.edu/dept/rosenthal

Choosing Complementary and Alternative Medicine: Questions to Consider. 1997. http:/cpmcnet.columbia.edu/dept/rosenthal

Complementary and Alternative Medicine Clinical Trials. 1997. http:/cpmcnet.columbia.edu/dept/rosenthal

How Other Medical Systems View Cancer. 1997. http:/cpmcnet.columbia.edu/dept/rosenthal

University of Texas-Houston

Health Science Center
Center for Complementary and Alternative Medicine Research in Cancer (UT-CAM)

Reviews of Therapies:

Herbal/Plant Therapies: Aloe, Cat's Claw, Coriolus Versicolor (mushroom), Essiac, Garlic, Green Tea, Hoxsey, Mistletoe, Saw Palmetto, Traditional Chinese Medicine

Biologic/Organic Therapies: Cartilage, Coenzyme Q10, Coley Toxins, Govallo Embryo Therapy, Homeopathy, Immune Augmentation Therapy, Melatonin, Modified Citrus Pectin, MTH-68, Selenium

Clinical/Pharmacologic Therapies: 714-X, Antineoplastons, Hydrazine Sulfate

Special Regimens: Gerson, Livingston-Wheeler, Macrobiotics, Revici Guided Chemotherapy

All available at www.sph.uth.tmc.edu/utcam/therapy.htm

Section 6

Professional Literature

PROFESSIONAL BOOKS

For those consumers who wish to explore the multiple facets of complementary and alternative medicine indepth, there are a number of valuable professional publications that vary in technical detail and complexity. The following is a select listing dealing with the principles and concepts of CAM; specific therapies such as acupuncture, massage, and herbal medicine; and strategies for achieving integrated clinical practice. Many texts were originally published in the United Kingdom by such publishers as Churchill Livingstone and Butterworth/Heinemann. Outstanding texts are denoted by an asterisk.

Introductory Texts on Alternative Medicine

Beck, Mark F. *Milady's Theory and Practice of Therapeutic Massage,* 3rd edition. Albany, NY: Milady Publishing, 1999. 750pp. $53.95.

Massage therapy has a wide range of application and treatment goals—muscular and general relaxation, stress reduction, pain management, recovery from injury, and body awareness. Although primarily a textbook on massage therapy, this book has much to offer consumers by way of explanation of human anatomy and physiology; the benefits, indications, and contraindications of massage; how massage is performed; typical applications; and what to expect. A useful purchase for a consumer health reference collection.

Birch, Stephen J., and Robert L. Felt. *Understanding Acupuncture.* Edinburgh: Churchill Livingstone, 1999. 335pp. $39.

One reviewer of this book noted that it brings together the many disciplines necessary to achieve a deeper understanding of acupuncture and attempts to bridge this ancient medicine with modern science. The authors describe in detail the history and theoretical basis of acupuncture, cultural factors, available scientific evidence, how it works and how acupuncture is practiced, needle techniques, treatment, and case histories. Emphasis is placed on correct diagnosis, patient assessment, and treatment. Several hundred references document the text. Valuable appendix material lists resources and questions. The authors admirably succeed in presenting a large amount of accumulated data and in "relating the theoretical basis of acupuncture to the tenets of modern medicine and science."

*Blumenthal, Mark, and others. *The Complete German Commission E Monographs: Therapeutic Guide to Herbal Medicines.* Developed by a Specialist Expert Committee of the German Federal Institute for Drugs and Medical Devices. Austin, TX: American Botanical Council, 1998. 685pp. $165.

In Germany, 70 percent of the physicians in general practice prescribe thousands of registered herbal remedies in the amount of about $1.7 billion in annual sales. In 1978, Commission E was founded to evaluate the safety and effectiveness of such phytomedicines. Taken as a whole, the monographs prepared by the commission represent the most accurate information available in the world as to the safety and efficacy of herbs and phytomedicines. A total of 380 monographs are published in this book. Each monograph includes the name and composition of the drug, pharmacological properties, and clinical data such as usage, contraindications, side effects, interactions with other drugs, dosage, and mode of administration. A "Therapeutic Index" section provides a guide to therapeutic use of Commission E herbs as to uses, indications, side effects, interactions of herbs with conventional drugs, and duration of use. Both positive and negative assessments are included. This is a monumental reference work that provides the basic scientific evidence for the safety and efficacy of major herbs.

*Blumenthal, Mark, and others. *Herbal Medicine: Expanded Commission E Monographs: The American Botanical Council.* Newton, MA: Integrative Medicine Communications, 2000. 519pp. $49.95.

This is a compilation of herb monographs based on those created by a special expert committee of the German Federal Institute for Drugs and Medical Devices. The Commission's monographs were intended primarily as package inserts for herbal preparations sold as drugs in German pharmacies. As such, they lacked references and further elaboration. In this expanded edition, Blumenthal and colleagues include updated and detailed information on botany, history, composition, safety, and therapeutic use. Attention is focused on the more than 100 herbs commonly sold in the United States. Each monograph contains a color photograph, common name, Latin name, pharmacopeial name, overview, description, chemistry and pharmacology, and uses that have been approved by Commission E. Contraindications, side effects, dosage, and administration are also indicated with extensive references. Valuable appendixes list top-selling herbs in the United States; herb sales in the United States by retail outlet; top-selling drugs in Germany; clinical studies conducted on top-selling German phytomedicines, and the most frequently prescribed and researched phytomedicine brands in Germany and their U.S. brand counterparts. A most valuable and authoritative compilation that provides ready access to the clinical research on herbal products. The authors conclude that the Commission E process provides an excellent model of regulatory reform for the United States.

Chirali, Ilkay Zihni. *Traditional Chinese Medicine: Cupping Therapy.* London, UK: Churchill Livingstone/ Harcourt Brace, 1999. 214pp. $39. paper.

Cupping is a therapy that regulates the flow of Qi and blood. It helps draw out and eliminate pathogenic factors such as wind, cold, damp and heat. Cupping also moves Qi and blood and opens the pores of the skin, thus precipitating the removal of pathogens through the skin itself. This therapy has been used in China for thousands of years. Chirali, an acupuncturist and practitioner of Chinese medicine, describes the history of cupping, the benefits, how it is done, and the therapies that benefit from cupping—such as chiropractic, Alexander technique, Shiatsu, and reflexology. Good black and white photographs and diagrams illustrate the text. The author states that he is working to revive an almost lost art.

Clark, Carolyn Chambers (editor). *Encyclopedia of Complementary Health Practice.* New York: Springer, 1999. 638pp. $64. paper.

The intention of the editor is clear: "the primary audience for this encyclopedia is the educated inquirer who needs a brief, authoritative introduction to key topics and issues of complementary health care approaches." The *Encyclopedia* is divided into six parts: Part One, "Contemporary Issues in Complementary Health Practices," includes economic and practice concerns, education and research issues, and historical perspectives; Part Two, "Conditions," deals with how complementary medicine approaches major medical conditions and disorders; Part Three, "Influential Substances," includes constituents such as herbs that are powerful or effective, either in a negative or positive way; Part Four, "Practices and Treatments," describes complementary treatments and disciplines such as auriculotherapy and dance/movement therapy; Part Five is a "Contributors Directory"; while Part Six is a "Resource Directory." There are 68 pages of references. Each entry ranges from one to four pages in length and identifies the contributor. Cross-references are also supplied for related explanations. The entries would be more useful if related references were appended to each entry rather than accumulated at the end of the book. Highly useful for the rapid lookup of definitions and summary explanation.

DerMarderosian, Ara (editor). *Guide to Popular Natural Products: Facts and Comparisons.* St. Louis, MO: Facts and Comparisons, 1999. 288pp. $29.95. paper.

This guide to popular phytomedicines and dietary supplements contains more than 100 monographs on natural products categorized by scientific name, common name, patient information (short synopsis of uses, drug interactions, and side effects), history, pharmacology and toxicology, and pertinent medical and scientific references. High quality photographs of the major botanicals are also provided for their natural beauty and for reference purposes. This compact manual offers a concise up-to-date reference guide for advising patients about natural products. Appendix material lists potential herb-drug interactions, herbal diuretics, poison control centers, and sources of natural product information.

Diemer, Deedre. *The ABCs of Chakra Therapy: A Workbook.* York Beach, ME: Samuel Weiser, 1998. 174pp. $12.95. paper.

The basis of Chakras is that the body is an ever-changing energy system that is affected by and affects the energy around you. The magnetic energy field shaped like an egg that surrounds the body is called an "aura." This is created by the energy of the Chakras. Chakras resemble a spinning disc about the size of a silver dollar that opens and closes like the lens of a camera and act as energy centers that receive and send information on life force energy. Each of the several Chakras corresponds with particular body organs and emotional and psychological patterns. Physical illness and disease appear in the etheric body (energy system) prior to manifesting in the physical body. Diemer discusses the mental, emotional, and health issues associated with each Chakra and provides a self-diagnostic questionnaire to assist the reader in discovering where energies may be blocked. After determining where the blocks to healing are located, one can then proceed to therapies for opening and balancing the Chakras. Finally, Diemer details techniques for clearing your energy field. These techniques include color therapy, aromatherapy, reflexology, and yoga. Clearly written and easy to understand.

*Dossey, Larry. *Reinventing Medicine: Beyond Mind-Body to a New Era of Healing.* San Francisco: HarperCollins, 1999. 270pp. $24.

Dossey, one of the pioneers of mind/body medicine, defines three medical eras in which health, healing, and the nature of the mind have been differentiated. Era I was mechanical or physical medicine—drugs, surgery, radiation, and so on. Era II, mind/body medicine, grew out of psychosomatic medicine following WWII. The two perspectives of Era I and Era II exist side-by-side— for heart disease, stress management is used *with*

medications and coronary artery bypass graft, not as replacements for them. Era III is nonlocal medicine in which mind is not completely localized to points in space (brains or bodies) or time. In this manner, mind has the freedom to roam freely in space and time. The medical implications reveal that healing can be achieved at a distance by directing loving and compassionate thought, intentions, and prayers to others. Era III healing means that "we are in it together," and that no one's illness is a purely individual matter. Dossey believes that "nonlocality is one of the most important discoveries that humans have ever made." This is a fascinating and brilliant exposition of the case for nonlocality describing how we experience nonlocality thoughts, dreams, and prayer. One particularly insightful chapter shows how to put nonlocality to use in healing.

Emmons, Michael L., and Janet Emmons. *Meditative Therapy: Facilitating Inner Directed Healing.* Atascadero, CA: Impact Publishers, 1999. 213pp. $27.95. paper.

Meditative therapy represents a synthesis of two powerful healing disciplines—meditation and psychotherapy. The fusion of the ancient practice of mindful meditation with modern psychology results, according to the authors in a natural, holistic therapeutic process. The "Inner Source" is the natural healing resources within every person. This "Inner Source" can be accessed, and holistic healing facilitated, through meditation therapy. Separate chapters deal with the process of meditation therapy, therapeutic experiences, meditation therapy outcomes, enhancing therapy, and "Cleaning Cobwebs from My Mind." A professional book that also serves to provide a clear explanation of meditative therapy to the lay reader.

Ernst, Edzard, and Adrian White. *Acupuncture: A Scientific Appraisal.* Oxford, UK: Butterworth/ Heinemann, 1999. 162pp. $40. paper.

This concise volume, edited by two British researchers, consists of six contributed chapters that summarize the scientific evidence for acupuncture from a number of perspectives such as history, current practice, efficacy, methods of treatment, neurophysiology, and adverse effects. One chapter, authored by Ernst, analyzes the clinical effectiveness of acupuncture in the treatment of dental pain, low back pain, neck pain, osteoarthritis, stroke, smoking cessation, and weight loss. The major conclusion reached is that compelling evidence exists showing that acupuncture is efficacious only in the treatment of back pain, nausea, and dental pain. This is a concise summary of current scientific research of value to health care providers and those consumers who wish to examine the effectiveness and safety of acupuncture.

Ernst, Edzard (editor). *Herbal Medicine: A Concise Overview for Professionals.* Oxford, UK: Butterworth Heinemann, 2000. 120pp. $36. paper.

A number of the leading experts in phytomedicine worldwide summarize the present state-of-the-art in plant-based therapy. Eight contributed chapters discuss the history of phytomedicine, how plants work, adverse effects, problems of quality and regulation, and future research. This is a concise, evidence-based look at herbal medicine from the viewpoint of efficacy and safety. The book is an excellent introduction to herbal medicine edited by Edzard Ernst, Director of the Department of Complementary Medicine at the University of Exeter, UK.

Fetrow, Charles W., and Juan R. Avila. *Professional's Handbook of Complementary & Alternative Medicines.* Springhouse, PA: Springhouse, 1998. 762pp. $39.95. paper.

The authors set out to create a clinically sound reference book about complementary and alternative medicine that answers questions raised by professionals—such as, what is hawthorn and what do I tell my patient taking it, how does mugwort work, and does oleander contain ingredients that may produce an allergic response in my patients? The bulk of the book consists of detailed summaries of nearly 300 of the most commonly used herbal agents. Each monograph contains generic name, synonyms, common forms, source, chemical composition, actions, reported usage, dosage, adverse reactions, interactions and contraindications, and precautions. A short list of select references is appended to each entry. Sidebars are used to highlight Research Findings. Although intended primarily as a reference book for health care professionals, this book is readily understandable by consumers. A concise, and informative, compendium.

Fontanarosa, Phil B. (editor). *Alternative Medicine: An Objective Assessment.* Chicago: American Medical Association, 2000. 605pp. $75.

This book was unfavorably reviewed by *Library Journal* as a "muddled attempt from the American Medical Association [that] might as easily been entitled 'The AMA Bends Over Backwards To Please Everybody.'" However, this flippant dismissal fails to take into account the burgeoning interest in alternative medicine manifested by physician-readers of *JAMA* and the AMA specialty journals. The AMA has made a very creditable effort to weigh the evidence by assembling 74 articles

on various aspects of complementary and alternative medicine that were published in *JAMA* and the AMA specialty journals, mainly in 1998. All articles make a serious attempt to evaluate the scientific evidence relating to, for example, mind-body medicine, herbal therapies, homeopathy, acupuncture, and the like. A number of articles deal with cultural/social aspects, prevalence of use, and perspectives of integration. While the volume offers more questions than answers, it serves a useful purpose in blazing a path through a thicket of anecdotal reports, unproven therapies, and unfounded opinions.

Jellin, Jeff M; Forrest Batz; and Kathy Hitchens. *Natural Medicines Comprehensive Database,* Also available as a Web product. Stockton, CA: Therapeutic Research Faculty, 2000. 1310pp. $92.

The database, available in print and online, is intended to provide practitioners with a comprehensive collection of data and a consensus of available scientific information on natural medicines. The database, compiled by a team of pharmacists, researchers, dietitians, and pharmacologists, contains a listing for almost all natural medicines sold in the U.S. In all, 964 natural medicines are subjected to scientific scrutiny. Fifteen categories of information are supplied for each product. These categories include name, brand name, "also known as," scientific name, "people use this product for," dosages, adverse reactions, references, and so on. The category dealing with Safety rates each product as Likely Safe, Possibly Safe, Possibly Unsafe, Likely Unsafe, or Unsafe. Only 15 percent of the natural products are rated as safe and 11 percent as effective or likely effective. The database is available on the Web at http://www.naturaldatabase.com with interactive capability.

*Jonas, Wayne B., and Jeffrey S. Levin. *Essentials of Complementary and Alternative Medicine.* Philadelphia: Lippincott, Williams & Wilkins, 1998. 605pp. $35.

This is a multi-authored and current book designed to be a companion volume to a forthcoming textbook of *Complementary and Alternative Medicine* (CAM). Jonas and Levin bring together 30 chapters that detail the social and scientific foundations of CAM. The authors draw upon 30 contributors with expertise in diverse areas to ensure balanced and comprehensive coverage. Part One of the book includes five chapters outlining the history and utilization patterns of CAM; Part Two contains five chapters reviewing the safety of herbal and animal products, dietary and nutrient products, and homeopathy; while Part Three has 20 chapters providing overviews of various therapies such as osteopathy, spiritual healing, biofeedback therapy, and naturopathic medicine. Each overview covers history, principal concepts, patient assessment, diagnostic procedures, indications and contraindications, and so on. A comprehensive, authoritative, well-documented and highly useful reference resource. Jonas is a former director of the NIH Office of Alternative Medicine; Levin is a senior research fellow at the National Institute for Healthcare Research.

Kaptchuk, Ted. *The Web Has No Weaver: Understanding Chinese Medicine.* Lincolnwood, IL: Contemporary Books, 1998. 500pp. $18.95. paper.

This is the 2nd edition of a book that first appeared in 1982. Kaptchuk, with a degree in Oriental Medicine from the Macau Institute of Chinese Medicine and currently a professor of medicine at Harvard, has updated his earlier work after nearly two decades of experience, study, and reflection. He admirably succeeds in his task of translating what is admittedly esoteric into readily understandable text. An introductory chapter—Medicine East and West: Two Ways of Seeing, Two Ways of Thinking—describes and contrasts the Western and Eastern approaches. This introduction is followed by chapters on Fundamental Textures (Qi, blood, essence, spirit, and fluids), The Meridians, Origins of Disharmony, Eight Principal Patterns: The Faces of Ying and Yan, and Chinese Medicine as an Art. The text is a mind-bending exploration of Chinese medicine that, in the words of Andrew Weil, "merges the insight of a Taoist sage with the skepticism of a modern, inquiring scientist."

*Kuhn, Merrily A. *Complementary Therapies for Health Care Providers.* Philadelphia: Lippincott, Williams & Wilkins, 1999. 381pp. $19.95. paper.

This is an outstanding pocket-sized reference book that discusses 100 complementary therapies, provides detailed monographs regarding 33 of the most commonly used herbs, details holistic nutrition (including 20 different diets claimed to treat cancer and other medical conditions), and provides detailed monographs on 31 phytochemicals such as indoles, isoflavonoids, and carotenoids. The subject content closely follows the earlier categorization of complementary and alternative medicine developed by the National Institutes of Health, which consists of seven specific fields of practice—herbal medicine, dietary and nutritional approaches, mind/body or behavioral interventions, alternative systems of medical practice, manual healing methods, bioelectromagnetics, pharmacologic, and biologic treatments. A consistent format used for each complementary therapy provides a description, history,

what the therapy can treat or improve, what happens during a visit to a practitioner, the risks involved with the therapy and the training that is required of a practitioner. An up-to-date bibliography and list of references is provided at the end of each therapy or herb described together with resources and Web sites. An analytical introductory chapter discusses the role of complementary therapies. The interface between traditional and complementary therapies is analyzed in a short chapter entitled Responsibility of Health Care Providers Whose Patients are Participating in Complementary Therapies. One of the best books on complementary medicine to date, and of value to both health care professionals and consumers.

LaValle, James B., and others. *Natural Therapeutics Pocket Guide.* Hudson, OH: Lexi-Comp Inc., 2000. 680pp. $37.95. paper.

This compact volume is intended as "a handy reference that will offer the health care provider a logical first step for suggesting natural therapeutics as a part of health management." Part One offers the provider introductory information on natural medicine with respect to herbs, nutrition, homeopathy, and glandular extracts. Part Two, the core of the book, deals with more than 80 common conditions with lifestyle recommendations, decision trees, and a table of common natural products used to support each condition. Part Three contains individual monographs for each herb, vitamin, mineral, amino acid, nutraceutical, and glandular extract discussed. Each monograph details dosage ranges, reported uses, description of its pharmacology, and any warnings, toxicities or contraindications related to its use. Part Four has a number of useful charts such as a Homeopathic Quick Reference Chart for Common Complaints and a Nutrient Depletion and Cancer Chemotherapy Chart. Part Five contains a glossary of natural medicine terms. A handy guide packed with concise and useful information.

PDR for Herbal Medicines, 2nd edition. Montvale, NJ: Medical Economics, 2000. 858pp. $59.95.

The PDR states that it "is pleased to bring you the closest available analog to FDA-approved labeling—the findings of the German Regulatory Authority's watchdog agency, commonly called Commission E." That agency has conducted an intensive assessment of the peer-reviewed literature on some 300 common botanicals, weighing the quality of clinical evidence and identifying the uses for which herbs can be reasonably considered as effective. This new, enhanced, and expanded second edition contains detailed information on over 700 botanicals with respect to botanical overview, actions and pharmacology, indications and usage, contraindications, precautions, adverse reactions, dosages and over-dosages, and backup literature. For herbs not considered by the German Commission E, the results of an exhaustive literature review form the basis for the additional monographs. Daily dosage information is supplied for unprocessed herbs and commercially available products. Monographs are listed alphabetically and are indexed by name, therapeutic category, indications, and side effects. An Herb Identification Guide supplies color photographs of some 400 most widely used herbs. More comprehensive and detailed but less readable than Steven Foster and Varro Tyler's *Tyler's Honest Herbal* (4th edition. Haworth Herbal Press, 1998).

*Pizzorno, Joseph E., and Michael T. Murray (editors). *Textbook of Natural Medicine*, 2nd edition. Edinburgh: Churchill Livingstone, 1999. 1620pp. $195.

Pizzorno (president of Bastyr University) and Murray (faculty member at Bastyr), with contributions from multiple authors, outline in two massive volumes the scientific support for the philosophical and therapeutic foundation of natural medicine (naturopathy). Six sections cover the philosophy of natural medicine; supplementary diagnostic procedures (those not usually taught in conventional medical schools); therapeutic modalities; syndromes (underlying issues relevant to many diseases); pharmacology of natural medicine (pharmacognosy, pharmacy); and specific health problems — an in-depth natural approach to over 70 specific diseases and conditions. The text contains 10,000 citations to the peer-reviewed research literature. Of particular interest to lay persons are the two introductory chapters relating to the philosophy, clinical application, and history of naturopathic medicine, or naturopathy (a generally used term that began with its founder, Benjamin Lust in 1902).

Spencer, John W., and Joseph J. Jacobs. *Complementary/Alternative Medicine: An Evidence-Based Approach*. St. Louis: Mosby, 1999. 442pp. $39.95. paper.

This is a most comprehensive compilation of research data arranged primarily by clinical treatment outcomes in relation to major disease categories such as asthma and allergies, cardiovascular disease, diabetes mellitus, cancer, neurologic disorders, psychiatric illness, and so on. A review in the *New England Journal of Medicine* (10 June 1999) complains that "the book can be tedious and reads like an annotated bibliography" with a minimum of interpretation. However, despite the massive weight of the references supplied (each chapter appends several hundred references), this book offers a useful summary of the application of complementary and alternative medicine for major diseases such as cancer and neurologic disorders. Difficult reading but useful as a reference resource.

Stedman's Alternative Medicine Words. Philadelphia: Lippincott Williams & Wilkins, 2000. 476pp. $36.95. paper.

This is a small and highly valuable reference tool for "the wordsmiths of the health care professions"— the medical transcriptionists, medical and copy editors, health information management personnel, medical librarians, and court reporters. The compilation consists of more than 40,000 entries, fully cross-referenced, encompassing all facets of alternative medicine. The arrangement permits the user to view all the terms that contain a particular descriptor. Ginseng, for example, is in 21 entries including ginseng abuse syndrome, radix ginseng, and Panax ginseng. Abbreviations are separately defined and cross-referenced. Appendices list acupuncture and acupressure meridians and points, chakras, common enzymes, treatments by indication, scientific and common names of herbs, and common phytochemicals. An excellent, authoritative lexicographic resource.

Swayne, Jeremy (editor). *International Dictionary of Homeopathy*. London : Churchill Livingstone, 2000. 251pp. $29.95.

This compact dictionary, compiled by an international team of experts, stems from an initiative of the Homeopathic Medicine Research Group, an expert group supported by the European Commission. The purpose of the dictionary is "to define, inform, and clarify" and to give the reader an understanding of the language of homeopathy and its most important concepts. Concise definitions are provided for terms associated with 22 categories such as disease processes, healing processes, materia medica, and symptomatology. Extensive cross-referencing exists between entries while terms with their own entries are given in bold type. Synonyms are listed immediately after a main entry. The etymology of terms is supplied on a selective basis. Many entries include a section on Comment intended to give the concept a wider perspective. A useful and inexpensive reference work that helps to bridge the conceptual and philosophical differences between homeopathy and mainstream medical thought.

*Zollman, Catherine, and Andrew Vickers. *ABC of Complementary Medicine*. London, UK: BMJ Books, 2000. 50pp. $26.95.

This slender volume assembles the text of a series of twelve articles published in the *BMJ* at the end of 1999. The authors have "attempted to capture something of the essence of complementary medicine as a whole, and to explore the respects to which it is similar to and different from conventional medical practice." Separate chapter titles include "What Is Complementary Medicine?" "Users and Practitioners of Complementary Medicine," and "Complementary Medicine in Conventional Practice," in addition to those devoted to acupuncture, herbal medicine, and the like. Two final chapters explore "Complementary Medicine and the Patient," and "Complementary Medicine and the Doctor." Each chapter contains definitions, color photographs, suggested further readings, and key references. Although intended primarily to educate doctors who have "never received any formal education in the field," this concise volume is also a splendid reference resource for consumers. Zollman is a British GP; Vickers, a research methodologist, is now at Memorial Sloan-Kettering in New York City. Highly recommended for professional and popular use.

Books on Implementing Integrative Medicine

Clark, Carolyn Chambers. *Integrating Complementary Health Procedures Into Practice.* New York: Springer, 1999. 286pp. $42.95.

Clark, a nurse educator and holistic practitioner, is also editor-in-chief of the *Encyclopedia of Complementary Health Practice* (Springer, 1999). In this book, her intent is "to provide health care practitioners with specific ways to integrate complementary health procedures into their practice," to make judicious client referrals to complementary practitioners, or to monitor their clients' complementary treatment. Clark believes that allopathic health care practitioners should stay informed of the burgeoning field of complementary practice. Part One of her book deals with general principles of integration—reasons for integrating complementary procedures, overcoming resistance, elements of the practitioner/client relationship, guidelines for choosing the right therapy, evaluating results, costs, and insurance coverage. Part Two focuses on specific therapies—nutrition, herbs, and essential oils; healing systems; and mind/body approaches. Each practice described includes information on concepts, directions for use, cautions, and application of use. Comparable to Merrily A. Kuhn's *Complementary Therapies for Health Care Providers* (Lippincott, Williams & Wilkins, 1999) but not as well organized, less detailed, and with fewer resources listed for each of the therapies described. Clark does however

provide a clear exposition, spanning nearly 60 pages, of how to integrate complementary procedures.

Eldin, Sue, and Andrew Dunford. *Herbal Medicine in Primary Care.* Oxford, UK: Butterworth/Heinemann, 1999. 180pp. $37.50. paper.

A book that "does not set out to provide yet another detailed text on herbal medicine," but rather "aims to present succinctly those aspects of herbal medicine that are of particular relevance to health care professionals in that they may be able to inform accurately those patients who increasingly request this form of 'alternative' treatment." Although focused on the practice of herbal medicine within the context of the British National Health Service, Eldin (an herbal practitioner) and Dunford (a GP) show how herbal medicine can live "very comfortably" alongside orthodox medical practice. After describing the nature and history of herbal medicine, the authors show how herbal medicine can exist within an allopathic health care center with respect to consultation, focus on diet, and medications and methods. A lucid book that suggests how herbal medicine can be integrated into mainstream orthodox medical practice.

Fontaine, Karen Lee. *Healing Practices: Alternative Therapies for Nursing.* Upper Saddle River, NJ: Prentice-Hall, 1999. 452pp. $35.30. paper.

Although primarily written from a nursing perspective—"I believe that we need a merger of alternative approaches with our Western-based nursing practices," Fontaine provides a highly detailed summary of the background claims of alternative medicine, preparation of practitioners, concepts, diagnostic methods, treatments, and evidence of research studies. Separate chapters deal with traditional Chinese medicine, Ayurvedic medicine, naturopathy, homeopathy, pressure point therapies, and so on. Each chapter details background, concepts, view of health and illness, diagnostic methods, and treatment. Of particular value are the up-to-date references at the end of each chapter together with relevant Web sites. Frequent reference is made in the text to both professional and popular books. Excellent, well-written digests of alternative healing practices that offer a gateway to both the professional and popular literature on a wide range of therapies.

Hess, David J. *Evaluating Alternative Cancer Therapies: A Guide to the Science and Politics of an Emerging Medical Field.* New Brunswick, NJ: Rutgers University Press, 1999. 260pp. $35.

A largely successful attempt by a cultural/medical anthropologist to bring together the voices of the leaders of the alternative and complementary cancer therapy community with the objective of identifying theories, experience, and points of agreement and disagreement. Those interviewed include key leaders, advocates of alternative therapies, and leading clinicians and researchers. Eighteen in-depth summaries and interviews shed light on the evaluation of therapies, what the patient needs, and organizations that can help. This is an excellent book on the social and political context of complementary and alternative medicine. A short interview with former congressman Berkley Bedell, who helped establish the Office of Alternative Medicine at NIH, sheds light on the initial CAM beachhead achieved within the federal establishment.

Holistic Health Promotion and Complementary Therapies: A Resource for Integrated Practice, Loose leaf binder. Gaithersburg, MD: Aspen, Last updated, October 1999. $145.

This is a loose leaf product "designed as a practical aid for all settings and individual practitioners wishing to integrate the best of holistic health promotion and 'alternative' modalities with conventional practice." The content includes both practitioner guidelines and reproducible patient handouts. Section One gives a concise overview of essential concepts and terminology; Section Two, Modalities, presents the rationale for a variety of complementary therapies citing relevant research studies; Section Three, Applications, explores options and presents tools for implementing the integrative approach according to specific conditions, patient groups, and types of care settings; while Section Four, Integrated Practice Development, offers invaluable insights and protocols for program planning and design. This is a comprehensive workbook with informative definitions, descriptions, and implementation suggestions.

Integrative Medicine Access: Professional Reference to Conditions, Herbs & Supplements. Loose-leaf binder. Newton, MA: Integrative Medicine Communications, 2000. No pagination. $299.

This is a massive and comprehensive database that is "a combination, a system, of information products designed for use by health professionals seeking clinically valuable information on prevalent medical conditions, dietary supplements, herbs and other complementary adjuncts to a total treatment plan." The total information system is comprised of integrated components to provide quick answers to diverse questions. The components include professional conditions, monographs, professional herb monographs, professional supplement monographs, patient education condition monographs, patient education herb monographs, patient education supplement monographs, and a cross reference guide. The monographs allow the health professional to review a standard medical model of diagnosis and treatment protocols of a known or suspected condition and to select alternative and complementary modalities. The herb and supplement monographs detail medicinal uses, indications, pharmacology, dosages, warnings/precautions, and so on. The corresponding patient education monographs, intended as handouts, clearly summarize basic facts on, for example, Fever of Unknown Origin in terms of signs/symptoms, causes, what to expect at the provider's office, complementary and alternative therapies, and special considerations. An extensive Cross-Reference Guide permits a quick search of 30 category lists (Herbs by Uses and Indications, Supplements by Side Effects, Conditions by Signs and Symptoms, and so on). This loose leaf guide provides the basis for a number of spinoff information products of the same publisher: *Quick Access: Professional Guide to Conditions, Herbs and Supplements; Quick Access Patient Information on Conditions, Herbs & Supplements;* and *Quick Access Consumer Guide to Conditions, Herbs & Supplements.*

*Milton, Doris, and Samuel Benjamin. *Complementary & Alternative Therapies: An Implementation Guide to Integrative Health Care.* Chicago: Health Forum/American Hospital Association, 1998. 172pp. $299.

A text that focuses on when, and when not, to use alternative therapies and how to integrate them into conventional medical practice. The authors state that ""integrative health care is much more than merely adding in some 'new' technologies, such as herbal preparations or acupuncture. Integration embraces patient self-empowerment and acknowledges the critical importance of leaving decision-making authority and many of the tools of healing within the patient's domain." The contents of the book address the challenges of the new paradigm. Chapter One provides an overview of environmental factors influencing the development of integrative health care; Chapter Two describes a wide variety of the most commonly used CAM therapies; Chapter Three outlines strategy for forming a planning group, design goals and objectives, and incorporating CAM into existing systems; Chapter Four deals with implementation and project development; Chapter Five lists the main tasks necessary to evaluate the outcomes of an integrative health care project; Chapter Six discusses business issues; while Chapter Seven focuses on legal and regulatory issues. Appendices list resources (books, journals, organizations, and Web sites), and examples of integrative health care projects.

*Novey, Donald W. *Clinician's Complete Reference to Complementary & Alternative Medicine.* St. Louis, MO: Mosby, 2000. 855pp. $49. paper.

The cover of this text shows a bridge and is intended to "symbolize a means to go from one way of thinking to another, traversing a gulf of changing perspective." The contents are presented in such a manner as to allow the reader to "lift off into new ways of approaching illness and treatment." In all, 64 CAM therapies are described by more than 90 contributors, each an expert in his field of practice. Section One of the book concisely summarizes the philosophy and basic concepts of complementary medicine. Section Two, the bulk of the book, reviews therapies utilizing a standard layout to facilitate appropriate application. The template used involves origins and history, supposed mechanism of action, indications and reasons for referral, practical applications, the research base (evidence-based, risk and safety, efficacy, function, research opportunities), credentialing and training, relevant organizations, and suggested readings. Section Three presents an array of diagnoses with a prioritized list of therapies applicable to each diagnosis, ranked according to their applicability and effectiveness. The composite ratings of the contributors reflect five levels, ranging from Level 1 (therapy ideally suited for this condition) to Level 5 (equal among many adjunctive therapies). Rankings are given for 24 therapies. This is an excellent book that assists conventional practitioners in understanding complementary therapies, answering patients' questions, and making judicious referrals.

Quick Access Professional Guide to Conditions, Herbs & Supplements. Newton, MA: Integrative Medical Communications, 2000. 472pp. $49.

This is a bound version of *Integrative Medicine Access: Professional Reference to Conditions, Herbs & Supplements* (Integrative Medical Communications, 2000). More than 100 conditions monographs provide a standard medical model of diagnosis and treatment. Each monograph provides a definition, etiology, signs and symptoms, differential diagnosis, treatment options including drug therapy and complementary and alternative therapies—nutrition, herbs, homeopathy, complications/sequelae, and prognoses together with references. Herb monographs profile herbs in terms of constituents, commercial preparations, medicinal uses/applications, pharmacology, dosages, side effects/toxicology, warnings, and contraindications. Supplement monographs provide substantive and well-referenced information on the use

of dietary supplements. A Cross-Reference Guide offers multidimensional access by medical category, signs and symptoms, uses/indications, side effects, interactions with other drugs, herbs and supplements, and so on. In depth, authoritative information organized for multi-purpose lookup. An excellent reference guide.

Tiran, Denise, and Sue Mack (editors). *Complementary Therapies for Pregnancy and Childbirth,* 2nd edition. London, UK: Baillière Tindall/Harcourt, 2000. 319pp. $34.95. paper.

Two British midwifery educators have assembled a series of contributed articles that describes how complementary therapies can be incorporated into maternity care through the use of homeopathy, osteopathy, chiropractic, acupuncture, herbal medicine, massage, reflexology, shiatsu, hypnosis, and hydrotherapy. One chapter describes how CAM can be employed for the relief of physical and emotional stress. Although oriented primarily to the British scene, this is a valuable professional text of interest to all women contemplating the use of alternative medicine in pregnancy. The text is remarkably lucid and within the comprehension of most consumers.

Other Relevant Titles

Cross, John R. *Acupressure: Clinical Applications in Musculo-Skeletal Conditions.* Butterworth-Heinemann, 2000. $55.

Deng, Tietao. *Practical Diagnosis in Traditional Chinese Medicine.* Churchill Livingstone, 1999. $99.

Charman, Robert A. (editor). *Complementary Therapies for Physical Therapists.* Butterworth-Heinemann, 2000. $52.50.

Fiatarone-Singh, Maria A. *Exercise, Nutrition, and the Older Woman: Wellness for Women Over Fifty.* CAC Press, 2000. $79.95

Fields, Tiffany. *Touch Therapy.* Churchill Livingstone, 2000. $29.95.

Finando, Donna, and Steven Finando. *Informed Touch: A Clinician's Guide to the Evaluation of Myofascial Disorders.* Healing Arts Press, 1999. $30.

Fugh-Berman, Adriane. *Alternative Medicine: What Works: A Comprehensive, Easy-to-Read Review of the Scientific Evidence, Pro and Con.* Lippincott, Williams & Wilkins, 1997. $14.95.

Li, Thomas S.C. *Medicinal Plants: Culture, Utilization and Phytopharmacology*. Technomic Publishing Company, 2000. $134.95.

Maffetone, Philip. *Complementary Sports Medicine*. Human Kinetics, 1999. $55.

Micozzi, Marc S. (editor). *Fundamentals of Complementary and Alternative Medicine*. 2nd ed. Churchill Livingstone, 2000. $39.

Marquardt, Hanne. *Reflexology of the Feet*. Thieme, 2000. 210pp. $35.

Mayer, E.A., and C.B. Saper. *The Biological Basis for Mind Body Interactions*. Elsevier, 2000. $223.

Nurse's Guide to Alternative Medicine. American Health Consultants, 1999. $199.

Nurse's Handbook of Complementary Therapies. Springhouse, 1999. $29.95.

Olshansky, Ellen. *Integrated Women's Health: Holistic Approaches for Comprehensive Care*. Aspen, 2000. $39.

Oschman, James L. *Energy Medicine: The Scientific Basis*. Churchill Livingstone, 2000. $35.

Physician's Guide to Alternative Medicine. American Health Consultants, 1999. $199.

Price, Shirley, and Len Price. *Aromatherapy for Health Professionals*. 2nd ed. Churchill Livingstone, 1999. $35.

Redwood, Daniel. *Contemporary Chiropractic*. Churchill Livingstone, 1997. $45.

Salvo, Susan. *Massage Therapy: Principles & Practice*. Saunders, 1999. $50.

Sharma, Hari. *Contemporary Ayurveda: Medicine and Research in Maharishi Ayurveda*. Churchill Livingstone, 1998. $31.

Standish, Leanna, Nary Lou Galantino, and Carlo Calabrese. *AIDS and Complementary and Alternative Medicine*. Saunders, 1999. $45.

Stux, Gabriel. *Basics of Acupuncture*. 4th ed. Springer-Verlag, 1998. $27.

Swayne, Jeremy. *Homeopathic Method: Implications for Clinical Practice and Medical Science*. Churchill Livingstone, 1998. $37.50.

PROFESSIONAL JOURNALS

Advances In Mind-Body Medicine
Fetzer Institute
Journals Marketing Department
Harcourt Publishers
P/O/ Box 156
Avenel, NJ 07001
$105, quarterly

*Alternative and Complementary Therapies: A Bimonthly Publication for Healthcare Professionals
Mary Ann Liebert Publishers
2 Madison Avenue
Larchmont, NY 10538
$69, bimonthly

Alternative Health Practitioner: The Journal of Complementary and Natural Care
Springer Publishing
536 Broadway
New York, NY 10012
$68, quarterly

Alternative Medicine Review
P.O. Box 25
Dover, ID 83825
$95, bimonthly

*Alternative Therapies in Health and Medicine
InnoVision Communications
101 Columbia
Aliso Viejo, CA 92656
$59, bimonthly

American Herbal Pharmacopeia and Therapeutic Compendium
American Herbal Pharmacopeia
P.O. Box 5159
Anta Cruz, CA 95063
$19.95 for each issue; 6 issues a year

American Journal of Acupuncture
221840 41st Avenue #102
Capitola, CA 95010
$45, quarterly

American Journal of Chinese Medicine
Institute for Advanced Research in Asian Science and Medicine
P.O. Box 555
Garden City, NY 11530
$110, 3 times/yr

American Journal of Clinical Hypnosis
American Society of Clinical Hypnosis
33 West Grand Avenue #402
Chicago, IL 60610
$55, quarterly

Chinese Medical Journal
42 Dongsi Xidajie
Beijing 100710
P.R. China
$40, monthly

Chiropractic Technique
National College of Chiropractic
200 East Roosevelt Road
Lombard, IL 60148
Quarterly; available online at http://
   www.national.chiropractic.edu

Complementary Health Practice Review
[formerly *Alternative Health Practitioner: The Journal of
   Complementary Medicine*]
Springer Publishing Company
536 Broadway
New York, NY 10012
$42, three times a year

*Complementary Therapies in Medicine
Journals Marketing Department
Harcourt Publishers
P/O/ Box 156
Avenel, NJ 07001
$93, quarterly

*FACT: Focus on Alternative and Complementary
Therapies*
Department of Complementary Medicine
University of Exeter
Pharmaceutical Press
P.O. Box 151
Wallingford, Oxfordshire, U.K.
$89, quarterly

*Integrative Medicine: Integrating Conventional and
Alternative Medicine*
Elsevier
655 Avenue of the Americas
New York City, NY 10010-5107
$109, quarterly

International Journal of Aromatherapy
Journals Marketing Department

Harcourt Publishers
P/O/ Box 156
Avenel, NJ 07001
$46, quarterly

International Journal of Integrative Medicine
Impakt Communications
P.O. Box 12496
Green Bay, WI 54307-2496
$73, bimonthly

**Journal of Alternative and Complementary Medicine:
Research on Paradigm, Practice, and Policy*
Mary Ann Liebert Publishers
2 Madison Avenue
Larchmont, NY 10538
$93, bimonthly

Journal of the American Chiropractic Association
American Chiropractic Association
1701 Clarendon Boulevard
Arlington, VA 22209
$90, monthly

Journal of the American Institute of Homeopathy
American Institute of Homeopathy
23200 Edmonds Way
Edmonds, WA 98026
$45, quarterly

*Journal of Cannabis Therapeutics: Studies in Endogenous,
Herbal, and Synthetic Cannabinoids*
Haworth Herbal Press
10 Alice Street
Binghamton, NY 13904-1580
$6, quarterly

Journal of Chinese Medicine
Eastland Press
1240 Activity Drive, Ste D
Vista, CA 92083
$45, Quarterly

Journal of Chiropractic Humanities
National College of Chiropractic
200 East Roosevelt Road
Lombard, IL 60148
Free, quarterly; available online at http://
   www.national.chiropractic.edu

*Journal of Herbal Pharmacotherapy: Innovations in
Clinical & Applied Evidence-Based Herbal Medicinals*
Haworth Herbal Press

10 Alice Street
Binghamton, NY 13904-1580.
$40, quarterly

Journal of Holistic Nursing
Sage Publications
2455 Teller Road
Thousand Oaks, CA 91320
$58, quarterly

Journal of Hypnotherapy
American Board of Hypnotherapy
16842 Von Karman Avenue #475
Irvine, CA 92714
Included in membership, quarterly

Journal of Manipulative and Physiological Therapeutics
Mosby
6277 Sea Harbor Drive
Orlando, FL 32887
$99, nine issues per year

Journal of Orthomolecular Medicine
16 Florence Avenue
Toronto, ON M2N 1E9
Canada.
$55 (U.S.), quarterly

Journal of Traditional Chinese Medicine.
(Co-sponsored by the China Association of
    Traditional Chinese Medicine and Pharmacy and
    the China Academy of Traditional Chinese
    Medicine)
3121 Park Avenue, Ste. J
Soquel, CA 95073
$90.56, quarterly

Massage Therapy Journal
American Massage Therapy Association
820 Davis Street, Ste 100
Evanston, IL 60201-4444
$25, quarterly

*Medical Herbalism: A Journal for the Clinical
Practitioner*
Bergner Communications
P.O. Box 20512
Boulder, CO 80308
$36, quarterly

Natural Pharmacy
Mary Ann Liebert Publishers.
2 Madison Avenue
Larchmont, NY 10538
$7, monthly

Natural Products Letters
Harwood Academic Publishers
Gordon and Breach Publishing Group
2 Gateway Center
Newark, NJ 07102
$83, bimonthly

Nutrition Science News
New Hope Natural Media
P.O. Box 195
Buffalo, NY 14205-9805
$79, monthly

Phytotherapy Research
John Wiley
P.O. Box 18667
Newark, NJ 07191-8667
$895, eight issues per year

Review of Aromatic and Medicinal Plants
Harwood Academic Publishers
2 Gateway Center
Newark, NJ 07102
$45, monthly

Scentsitivity
National Association for Holistic Aromatherapy
836 Hanley Industrial Court
St. Louis, MO 63144
Included in membership, quarterly

Scientific Review of Alternative Medicine
Prometheus Books
59 John Glenn Drive
Amherst, NY 14228-2197
$50, semi-annually

Yearbook of Chiropractic
Mosby
6277 Sea Harbor Drive
Orlando, FL 32887
$83

PROFESSIONAL NEWSLETTERS

Alternative Medicine Alert
American Health Consultants
3525 Piedmont Road
Building 6, Ste. 400
Atlanta, GA 30305
$19, monthly

Alternative Therapies in Women's Health
American Health Consultants
3525 Piedmont Road
Building 6, Ste. 400
Atlanta, GA 30305
$199, monthly

Complementary & Alternative Medicine at the NIH
National Center for Complementary and Alternative
   Medicine Clearinghouse
P.O. Box 8218
Bethesda, MD 20907-8218
Free, quarterly

Complementary & Alternative Medicine Select
Oakstone Medical Publishing
6801 Cahaba Valley Road
Birmingham, AL 35242
$199, monthly

Complementary Medicine for the Physician
W. B. Saunders Co.
6277 Sea Harbor Drive
Orlando, FL 32821-9816
$87, 10 issues per year

Herb & Dietary Supplement Report
Integrative Medicine Communications
1029 Chestnut Street
Newton, MA 02464
Free, weekly; available online at http://
   www.onemedicine.com

Homeopathy Today
National Center for Homeopathy
801 North Fairfax Street #306
Alexandria, VA 22314
$40, included in membership, monthly

The Integrative Medicine Consult
Integrative Medicine Communications
1029 Chestnut Street
Newton, MA 02464
$189, monthly

OneMedicineALERT
Integrative Medicine Communications
1029 Chestnut Street
Newton, MA 02464
Free, weekly; available online at http://
   www.onemedicine.com

Practical Reviews in Complementary and Alternative Medicine
Jointly sponsored by the Albert Einstein College of
   Medicine, Montefiore Medical Center, and the
   American Holistic Medical Association
Educational Reviews
6801 Cahaba Valley Road
Birmingham, AL 35242
Audiocassettes.
$99, quarterly

SECTION 7

CD-ROM Information Products

*Recommended products are denoted with an asterisk.

Alt-HealthWatch
Softline Information
20 Summer Street
Stamford, CT 06901
$1,495
$1,795 with quarterly updates
Also available online from Ebsco

> This database was sold in April 2000 to ccplanet.com (3600 Interlocken Boulevard, Broomfield, CO 80021), which will make Alt-HealthWatch available on CD-ROM and online to the library market through the EBSCOhost service. *Alt-HealthWatch* is a full-text and image database of some 50,000 articles from international peer-reviewed professional journals, magazines, proceedings, association publications, and consumer newsletters, together with special reports and book extracts. Each article is indexed according to 225 subject categories, 11 article types, and 17 publication types. The 225 therapies, modalities, and perspectives include chiropractic, naturopathy, homeopathy, energy medicine, and aromatherapy.

Alternative Remedies
Harcourt/Mosby Health Sciences
11830 Westline Industrial Drive
St. Louis, MO 63146
1998
$51.95

> This database covers over 5,700 treatable medical conditions, more than 1,200 supplements, 6,600 herb names, and 15,000 chemical and organic constituents. The spectrum of natural remedies includes Chinese herbs, Ayurvedic herbs, homeopathic remedies, vitamins, minerals, and aromatherapy oils. Searching can be accomplished by action, constituent name, or by medical condition. Footnotes are referenced from more than 200 books, journals, and other publications. Several hundred color photographs are used to illustrate the textual material.

Clinical Pearls Database
ITServices
3301 Alta Arden. Suite 2
Sacramento, CA 95825
$160. Annual updates $75.
Not available for MacIntosh.

> This is a database ("for the progressive lay person or hasty professional") on nutrition and complementary therapies, containing 18,000 fully referenced article summaries, 265 interviews of top researchers ("The Experts Speak"), and disease protocols. Between 1,500 and 2,800 summarized articles are added annually. The disk also contains the text of the *Clinical Pearls News*, a monthly newsletter that features summaries and commentary on published articles together with a monthly disease protocol.

The Complete German Commission E Monographs:
Therapeutic Guide to Herbal Medicine
American Botanical Council/Integrative Medical
　Communications
1029 Chestnut Street
Newton, MA 02464
1999
$99

This CD-ROM version of *The Complete German Commission E Monographs: Therapeutic Guide to Herbal Medicines* (American Botanical Council, 1998), provides access to 380 monographs of herbs and fixed combinations proven to be of value for therapeutic value together with indications for use. Searches can be made by indications of usage of approved herbs, and by contraindications, side effects, pharmacologic action, and interactions of herbs with conventional drugs.

Guide to Alternative Medicine
ISIS Interactive Inc
7910 Woodmont Avenue. Suite 327
Bethesda, MD 20814-3015
$29.95

Guide to Alternative Medicine features extensive coverage of alternative systems of medical practice, diet and nutrition, botanical medicines, manual healing, mind-body interventions, pharmacological and biological treatments, and bioelectromagnetic applications. A link on the disk can be used to transfer the user to the IBIS Web site to receive updated information.

Guide to Vitamins, Minerals, and Supplements
ISIS Interactive Inc
7910 Woodmont Avenue. Suite 327
Bethesda, MD 20814-3015
$17.95

This CD contains information on over 100 vitamins, minerals, amino acids, and supplements outlining natural sources, reasons for use, speculated benefits, interactions with other drugs, dosage and usage information, warnings and precautions, overdose information, adverse reactions, and side effects.

Heilpflanzen-Herbal Remedies. 3rd edition
PhytoPharm US Inc
Institute for Phytopharmaceuticals
292 Fernwood Avenue
Edison, NJ 08837
1999
$129

Over 700 plants are described in this product, with respect to names, scientific synonyms, history, etymology, and botanical detail. More than 800 drugs are included with information on pharmacology and effect, application and dosage, drug specification (source plant, purity, forms of drug), toxicology with contraindications and interactions, and component substances, including amounts and indications in accordance with the Commission E monographs. Drug descriptions contain lists of references to the specialist literature.

Herbal Guide
Arc Media
5330 Main Street #210
Buffalo, NY 14221-5360
1998
$12.95

Offers basic guidelines on use, dosage, and safety for more than 100 popular herbs for the treatment of 250 common ailments. An inexpensive and quick access to basic information with full-color photographs of herbs.

Herbal Medicine: Expanded Commission E Monographs.
American Botanical Council/Integrative Medical
　Communications
1029 Chestnut Street
Newton, MA 02464
1999
$49.95

This is a CD-ROM version of *Herbal Medicine: Expanded German Commission E Monographs: Therapeutic Guide to Herbal Medicine* (American Botanical Council, 2000). In this expanded database, intended to supplement *The Complete German Commission E Monographs: Therapeutic Guide to Herbal Medicine* (American Botanical Council, 1999), attention is focused on the 100 herbs most commonly used in the United States with data on common names, pharmacopeial names, chemistry, pharmacology, and the uses approved by Commission E.

*IBIS Integrated BodyMind Information System
IBISmedical.com
Integrated Medical Arts
4790 S.W. Watson Avenue
Beaverton, OR 97005
1998
$895

This is a computerized encyclopedia and treatment formulary of natural medicine. The product references 282 common medical conditions and identifies relevant treatments from more than 12 systems of integrative medicine and alternative therapies. For each condition, there is a discussion of the etiology, signs and symptoms, differential diagnosis, course, and prognosis. Treatment modalities are described for each condition. Modalities discussed include those of western botanical medicine, Chinese medicine, homeopathy, mind/body, and so on. There is good coverage of theoretical considerations, practical uses, indications and contraindications, precautions, and toxicity. A major reference source for natural medicine.

Interactions: The IBIS Guide to Drug-Herb and Drug-Nutrient Interactions
IBISmedical.com
Integrated Medical Arts
4790 S.W. Watson Avenue
Beaverton, OR 97005
$99.95. Single user.

This is a CD-ROM and online reference guide to the interactions between prescription and over-the-counter medications, herbs, and nutritional supplements. The purpose of the database is to make information available to physicians and other health care professionals so that they can avoid prescribing a medication that will have undesired interactions with herbs or other natural products that the patient is already taking. Typical questions answered are: can St. John's wort and Prozac be taken at the same time; are calcium supplements a risk when taking digoxin; and are herbs safe before surgery. Drugs are listed by brand name, generic name, or drug class. Information on interactions can be obtained by clicking on the "interactions" option for each drug, herb, or nutrient combination. Each herb entry includes a "linical section" describing the properties, therapeutic uses, and typical dosages for that herb. The data are based on the scientific literature from reputable sources.

The Natural Pharmacy: The Complete Home Reference to Natural Medicine
Healthnotes Inc.
1505 SE Gideon, Suite 200
Portland, OR 97202
1999
$24.95

A CD-ROM version of Skye Linninger's *The Natural Pharmacy* (Prima, 1999), which is a documented digest of the therapeutic use of nutritional supplements, herbs, and homeopathic remedies. The usefulness of a wide range of products is specified for almost 200 common medical problems.

*Natural Products Explorer
Facts and Comparisons
111 West Port Plaza. Suite 300
St. Louis, MO 63146-9976
$199, annual

This database combines *The Review of Natural Products* and *The Complete German Commission E Monographs: Therapeutic Guide to Herbal Medicines*. The disk contains nearly 700 monographs from both of these print publications. Searching is possible by variables such as trade, scientific, or common names; uses; side effects; or interactions. The in-depth monographs are based on scientific research about natural products, taking into account biology, history, chemistry, pharmacology, medicinal uses, toxicology, and patient information. A Web link is supplied to PubMed.

The Review of Natural Products
111 West Port Plaza. Suite 300
St. Louis, MO 63146-9976
$139

The database is similar in content to the *Natural Products Explorer* but without the *Complete German Commission E Monographs*.

SECTION 8

Complementary and Alternative Medicine Sources on the Internet

by Tom Flemming, MA, MLS, AHIP

INTRODUCTION

The U.S. National Center for Complementary and Alternative Medicine (NCCAM) defines the scope of its mandate as follows:

Complementary and alternative medicine (CAM) covers a broad range of healing philosophies, approaches, and therapies. Generally, it is defined as those treatments and healthcare practices not taught widely in medical schools, not generally used in hospitals, and not usually reimbursed by medical insurance companies.[1]

As a definition, this statement leaves much to be desired in that it lacks precision and works mainly by exclusion rather than by explanation or enumeration. In fairness, the NCCAM clarifies its scope of interest by offering an explanation of the five Domains of Complementary and Alternative Medicine, together with examples:

1) **alternative medical systems,** such as traditional oriental medicine, ayurveda, and other indigenous, traditional medical systems from the Americas, Africa, and Tibet, for example, as well as homeopathy and naturopathy

2) **mind-body interventions,** such as meditation and hypnosis; dance, music, and art therapies; prayer and mental healing

3) **biologically based therapies,** including herbal, special dietary, orthomolecular and biological

therapies (such as laetrile and shark cartilage to treat cancer and bee pollen to treat autoimmune and inflammatory diseases)

4) **manipulative and body-based methods,** such as those used by chiropractors, osteopaths and massage therapists

5) **energy therapies** which use biofields — such as Qi gong, Reiki, and Therapeutic Touch — or electromagnetic fields to treat asthma or cancer or to manage pain. [2]

Whatever one's understanding of the term: *complementary and alternative medicine* (CAM), it is likely to be broad and somewhat amorphous, rather more like a laundry list than a precisely articulated exposition. This breadth and variety of topics, approaches, and options is apparent to the Internet seeker of information on alternative medicine even after only the most cursory of searches.

A quick glance at Yahoo's Health section (http://www.yahoo.com/Health) reveals a selection of more sites on alternative medicine than anyone can reasonably browse. 562 alternative medicine sites were listed on 21 April 2000. It should be noted that no search engine in the world lists all the sites on any topic. Depending on the coverage of the engine used, and the way in which it classifies sites, searches on specific CAM topics yield many more than 500 sites, even with respect to quite specific and relatively minor topics. Who would have thought that there are 2,380 documents on Reiki on the Web? Yet that was the result of searching the Dogpile Web Catalog (http://www.dogpile.com/). On the same day, Yahoo listed 562 CAM sites. The quantity of CAM material on the Internet is constantly increasing and the breadth and variety of its sources, creators, and producers partially explains the burgeoning availability of what was, in generations past, almost secret information in the form of "folk remedies" passed on by practitioners to their followers, often by word of mouth.

Who Provides CAM Information?

Among the producers of CAM information on the Internet—some of which will be cited later in this chapter—are the United States (and other) government; major medical associations and health care organizations; the traditional print and broadcast media (newspapers and television, as well as radio stations and services); voluntary organizations and associations; businesses and commercial interests; pharmaceutical and medical device manufacturers; HMOs and insurers; community groups; and individuals. Some of these entities wish to promote certain practices; others work to denounce the same (and other) practices; yet others take a disinterested approach to the CAM topic they present with a focus on the public good. Some have an evident commercial purpose. There are also sites that sponsor and promote research into CAM; sites that expound the virtues (or failings) of certain practices, theories, therapies, and modalities; and yet others that proselytize for (or against) their specialty with all the fervor of "old time religion." Caution should be exercised to avoid being overwhelmed by enthusiasm and candor and not to mistake energetic argument for "righteousness."

The whole gamut of promoters — from practitioners with years of training and experience and scientific evidence to offer to the newly arrived promoter of a trendy therapy — can mount Web sites these days and publish just about anything, and sometimes, it seems they do. At times, the presentation is so slick that it is difficult to detect the flaws. It is often difficult to distinguish the good from the bad or questionable from the reliable information. While recognizing value in much of the health information available on the Internet, John S. Gould, MD, suggests that

> Along with the good comes a host of potential problems, including useful devices and medications with specific indications that the lay person often cannot discriminate from inappropriate or unapproved uses. ...

There was a time when educated people could easily recognize "snake oil salesmen." They drove horse-drawn wagons, wore funny hats, had similar sales pitches suggesting a cure for everything, and sold magnets, radium tonics, cocaine, and all manners of foul-tasting "herbals." Today, the wagon is in cyberspace; the message is the same but more neatly packaged, and the contents may be less dangerous in and of themselves, but still represent a delay of good treatment and a waste of money. With a simple "click", the patient spends hundreds of dollars on useless remedies, and goes on to complain about the cost of legitimate modalities and extols all of this to us.[3]

Yet, contrary to the widespread belief, promoted in part by the medical profession of which Dr. Gould is a member, that a medical school education is required to sort it all out, there are steps that an increasingly educated public, aided by good information services and appropriately trained librarians, can take to recognize today's "snake oil salesmen" and to use the wealth of CAM information on the Internet intelligently.

Usage of CAM Information

In the early 1990s, studies were showing the growing popularity of CAM in the United States. The authors of a study published by the highly regarded *New England Journal of Medicine* estimated that one-third of the population in the United States used some type of CAM, and that of those who used CAM, many did not see a CAM provider, but opted for self-treatment. This study also found that many of the people using CAM therapy were middle class adults; 44 percent were college educated. Surprisingly, the study revealed that: "About 425 million visits were made to CAM providers, exceeding by about 47 million the number of visits made to all primary care physicians combined."[4] A second, follow-up study was done and results were published in 1998; this second study confirmed a "dramatic" increase in the use of, and expenditures related to, CAM in the United States between 1990 and 1997.[5]

In Canada, the Nonprescription Drug Manufacturers' Association reports, in its fact sheet on *Canadian Consumers and Alternative Medicine*, that "In 1997, more than four out of 10 Canadians (42%) reported using alternative medicines and practices."[6] The Canadian Institute for Health Information (CIHI) recently published a report, drawing on figures from the 1998-1999 National Population Health Survey, which indicates that 2.5 million Canadians visited a chiropractor and that nearly 2 million used the services of other complementary and alternative practitioners in 1998-1999.[7] Furthermore, among those who treated their own colds and flu symptoms, 38 percent used herbal or vitamin supplements and another 26 percent used home remedies. Where do people get the information on which they make these treatment decisions? The Internet is certainly one of the sources of such information because it has so much health-related content and is both accessible and relatively inexpensive.

Every day we read that more and more people are using the Internet to find health information. In April 1999, *The Ferguson Report* carried news of a Harris Poll which concluded that:

> 60 million adults — 68 percent of those who use the Internet — have used the World Wide Web to find health information. 91 percent of these online health seekers said that the last time they went online, they were able to find the health information they wanted....The US online population has increased from 9 percent in 1995 to 44 percent in 1999, a 489 percent increase.... Not only are more people going on line but they are doing so much more often.[8]

Many of those online users are well-educated people who can be expected to read carefully and to understand what they read. In any search for health information, they do not wish to limit themselves to sites offering strictly conventional medicine and therapeutics. Although many will not know how to differentiate among "alternative," "complementary," or conventional medicine, they can be helped to recognize the snake oil salesmen. Questions related to the quality of the health information people read on the Internet will arise, whether they are dealing with CAM or with other health care topics, and it is both possible and desirable to educate users to be critical consumers of such information.

Educating Users of CAM Information

As information brokers, librarians have a responsibility to participate in the process of educating themselves and their users to discriminate between information that is credible and likely to be helpful, and that which is not. This does not imply that librarians can or should eventually replace doctors as arbiters of the good and the bad, or what is relevant health information for specific individuals. Health information retrieved from the Internet is just that — information — even when it is correct and timely. *Information* is different from *advice*; only a seasoned practitioner whose education and knowledge of an individual's health history and circumstances

are focused together on a health problem can turn health information into health advice that is worthy of action. The presentation of CAM (and other health) information on the Internet often takes undue abuse from those who do not appreciate this distinction between *information* and *advice*, or from those who have seen the results of such a confusion. Librarians and information scientists have a role to play in making these distinctions and in educating the public with respect to the quality of the health care information people encounter on the Internet and elsewhere.

Recently, there have been efforts from both the government and the private sector to deal with the quality of health care information on the Internet. Everyone is concerned with providing the tools that will enable the layperson to make some sense out of the health claims we encounter daily on the Internet and in print. These efforts concentrate on establishing the criteria by which it is possible to recognize worthy health care information.

Quality of Health Information on the Internet

Between November 1996 and May 1998, Mitretek Systems and its Health Information Technology Institute, with support from the Agency for Health Care Policy and Research (AHCPR), convened three Health Summit Working Group (HSWG) meetings to develop criteria for use in assessing the quality of health information on the Internet. The working groups included representation from many interested disciplines: library and information science, medicine, health care consumers, the technology industry, and government. One result of this work is a "White Paper" and a policy paper, both of which are intended to evolve over time through trial and error, comment and revision.[9] These documents offer insight into the identification and evolution of a set of seven criteria devised by the HSWG by means of which an assessment of health information on the Internet can be made. In summary, the criteria are

- **Credibility:** includes the source, currency, relevance/utility, and editorial review process for the information.
- **Content:** must be accurate and complete, and an appropriate disclaimer provided.
- **Disclosure:** includes informing the user of the purpose of the site, as well as any profiling or collection of information associated with using the site.

- **Links:** evaluated according to selection, architecture, content, and back linkages.
- **Design:** encompasses accessibility, logical organization (navigability), and internal search capability.
- **Interactivity:** includes feedback mechanisms and means for exchange of information among users.
- **Caveats:** clarification of whether site function is to market products and services or is a primary information content provider.[10]

Other efforts to make health information on the Internet more trustworthy are also underway. Concerned about what it calls "interactive health communication" ("the interaction of an individual—consumer, patient, caregiver, or professional—with or through an electronic device or communication technology to access or transmit health information, or to receive or provide guidance and support on a health-related issue"),[11] the Office of Disease Prevention and Health Promotion of the U.S. Department of Health and Human Services convened a panel of experts in many aspects of health and technology, which ultimately produced its report in April 1999. Among its conclusions was the belief that interactive health communication (IHC) has the potential to change the way consumers and health care providers communicate with each other. The panel identified four groups of stakeholders (consumers, health care professionals, IHC developers, and policy-makers) and expressed the belief that an evidence-based approach to development and diffusion of IHC makes most sense to all the stakeholders. The panel did not focus on devising criteria against which sites could be measured, but concluded that evaluation must involve all the stakeholders at an early stage in the development of any IHC application and that several different sorts of evaluation can each contribute to the improvement of health-related outcomes of IHC.

Two more efforts in the field of quality control of health information on the Internet deserve attention: these are the HON Code, and the relatively new guidelines from the American Medical Association for its own sites. The Health On the Net Foundation (http://www.hon.ch/home.html) has, since 1996, promoted what is widely known as the HON Code, a set of eight principles which promote basic ethical standards among presenters of health information on the Internet and require the disclosure of the sources and purpose of the

information consumers read on a health care Web site.[12] The eight principles deal with the following areas of concern: 1) authority (advice will be given only by qualified practitioners, or will be identified as coming from a non-qualified source), 2) complementarity (information given should support relationship between patient and professional), 3) confidentiality (privacy of medical/health information given is paramount), 4) attribution (clear references to source data, and dates indicating currency), 5) justifiability (claims should be supported by evidence), 6) transparency of authorship (identification and contact addresses for authors or the Web master), 7) transparency of sponsorship (identification of sources of support) and, 8) honesty in advertising and editorial policy. The code is a completely voluntary one. Webmasters can display the HON Code symbol on their sites claiming to follow its principles even when it is clear that they do not adhere to them.

The American Medical Association has long been in the forefront of efforts to ensure valid and useful health information to the many who access its Web site.[13] From 1995 to the present, various versions of guidelines, first for advertising on its sites and, more recently, guidelines covering a broader range of electronic information issues, have been released. In March 2000, the association published its most comprehensive code for information on Web sites under its jurisdiction, fully cognizant of the fact that these guidelines will be noticed, and perhaps followed, by other producers of health information for the public who look to the AMA for leadership.[14] Although more detailed and with greater depth of explanation, they are not significantly different from the others mentioned above in relation to content. However, they go well beyond other efforts in the areas of advertising, privacy and e-commerce. There are four main areas in which the AMA guidelines elucidate standards: 1) principles for content, 2) principles for advertising and sponsorship, 3) principles for privacy and confidentiality, and, 4) principles for e-commerce. They specify, among other things, that advertising on any Web site related to health cannot influence content and for that reason advertising may not appear adjacent to an article on the same subject. Similarly, the AMA guidelines are explicit about the use of *cookies* (files stored on the user's computer or server which are used in navigation and tracking that can collect data about the user's interests), because such technology may imperil privacy and confidentiality. The e-commerce principles also deal with the security of Internet business/financial transactions and privacy.

The preceding are areas in which all of these codes seem to address common issues: 1) validity, accuracy, currency and relevance of health information content, 2) clarity of authorship, attribution of authority and indication of sponsorship (if any), 3) recognition of the importance of support for the patient-provider relationship, 4) maintenance of consumer expectations of privacy and 5) honesty and integrity in the presentation of information, claims for benefit and advertising, and a general insistence on ethical conduct in the design and exchange of information.

While it may be difficult for consumers to evaluate the content of disciplines they have not studied, it is certainly possible for anyone with intelligence and a will to learn to acquire the knowledge needed to deal with many health care topics. People can be taught to mistrust or to avoid information that is unattributed, and claims that are made with no validation or authority indicated. Most people have a sense of what is unethical or undesirable in business practices and have a healthy concern for safeguarding their privacy. If consumers are helped to be sensitive to these issues in dealing with health care information in general, they will then be able to apply the same principles to dealing with information about complementary and alternative medicine. We all need to be prepared to make judgments about the usefulness and reliability of the health information we encounter, whether it is in print or in electronic format. As Barbara F. Schloman points out in a very useful article, a set of common evaluative criteria is beginning to emerge from both the health care and the library communities.[15] Users can learn to ask the right questions and should be taught not to rely entirely on their own abilities to discern the validity of health site claims, but also to involve health care providers in the evaluation of what they read and want to use as the basis for making health care decisions.

Evidence of Efficacy

The shift toward evidence-based clinical practice is one of the most significant trends in contemporary health care education and clinical practice. Practitioners of all disciplines are learning to evaluate the efficacy of what they do, or to adopt practices for which validity can be demonstrated. Consumers are, in this manner, not alone in their concern for validity in the information they encounter about health care claims. Many who seek a practitioner's advice will encounter someone who is equally concerned about the efficacy of a proposed therapy, and equally unsure how to determine where the balance of evidence offered falls. There is much that is done in health care without evaluated scientific proof of efficacy because it seems to have worked for most people over a period of time. Often, if a practice does no harm, and a patient's condition improves, the unscientific conclusion reached is that the practice has worked without investigation of how the therapy produced the improvement (or even if it did). CAM is becoming much more widely known than in the past at a time when evidence-based medicine is clamoring for demonstration of the value of health care practices. As we are learning to become more critical of everything we read on the Internet, CAM is being charged with the responsibility to demonstrate not only that it does no harm, but that it is actually beneficial in a manner that much of conventional medicine has, until now, avoided. As we all become more demanding consumers, health care of all kinds will have to demonstrate its claims or lose its followers. The critical attitude indicates personal adoption of responsibility for our own health and a turning away from the old paradigm of medicine in which you blindly followed what the doctor told you to do because he knew and you did not.

In the new paradigm, each individual becomes responsible for his or her own health, and health care professionals become partners in the effort to maintain or regain it. Many who focus on the preventive health maintenance aspects of CAM view it as an investment against the potentially disastrous consequences (financial as well as physical) of ill health. Others — particularly in the United States — who have little or no health insurance, consider doing their own information research as a practical necessity. Thus, many are learning to do the research that will lead to information on which good health decisions can be made after consultation with an expert. As the twentieth century gives way to the twenty-first and the Internet gains importance as a "free" source of information on almost every topic, and as the number of connections to the Internet burgeons annually, people look — naturally enough — to databases and other collections on the Internet for health information. MEDLINE is a name almost every seeker of health information knows, or quickly learns, and PubMed is becoming more heavily used as a source of

MEDLINE data. This suite of databases, offering the scientific literature of health and health care from 1966 to the present, is now practically barrier-free, thanks to legislation making it available to the public and to software which makes it possible for even the first-time searcher to obtain useful information on almost any health care topic that you can type into the search form on a PubMed screen.

MEDLINE for CAM Research

Is MEDLINE a useful database to search for CAM information? The MEDLINE database indexes over 3,000 periodicals in the various disciplines of the health sciences annually. You can retrieve information on practically any health care concept but that does not make it an excellent source of information on every health care topic, and coverage of alternative medicine is not currently one of its strengths. MEDLINE does cover approximately a dozen journals devoted to CAM (*Alternative Therapies in Health and Medicine, Journal of Manipulative and Physiological Therapeutics*, the *Journal of Natural Products*, and the *Journal of Traditional Chinese Medicine*, to name a few), but there are many more which MEDLINE does not index. MEDLINE covers only 3 of the 16 journals available on chiropractic, for example.[16] Many articles relevant to CAM issues do appear in journals that are indexed in MEDLINE, and it is always worth searching MEDLINE if you want to retrieve articles on CAM topics from "mainstream" or "conventional" medical journals. Because of cooperative efforts between NCCAM and NLM (the producer of MEDLINE), the *Medical Subject Headings* (MeSH) vocabulary used to search MEDLINE is getting better at providing appropriate language for searching alternative medicine concepts. Furthermore, the staff of the NCCAM have extracted about 180,000 citations on CAM topics from MEDLINE from 1966 to 1999 and created the *Complementary and Alternative Medicine Citation Index* (http://nccam.nih.gov/nccam/resources/cam-ci/), which can be searched free of charge via the NCCAM Web site. Since all the appropriate major journals are not indexed, alternative and complementary medicine is not well-covered in the MEDLINE database.

The NCCAM site (http://nccam.nih.gov/nccam/databases.html) suggests an array of databases in addition to MEDLINE, which can usefully be searched by those seeking citations to the literature of CAM. One

of the real disappointments of seeking literature in this field, however, is that if you do not find it in MEDLINE, the literature that is retrieved elsewhere is often not rigorously scientific. The journals selected for coverage in MEDLINE are commonly of high scientific quality; conversely, health journals that are excluded from MEDLINE are, often, less demonstrably rigorous. If you are looking for information on CAM, it would be a mistake not to search MEDLINE, but searching MEDLINE is not enough in itself.

Other Bibliographic Database Choices for CAM

Other bibliographic databases that purport to offer access to CAM topics are commonly much smaller than MEDLINE, covering far fewer periodical titles and far less time. An example is *Allied and Complementary Medicine* (A-MED), a database created by the British Library, available through both DIALOG and DATASTAR. A-MED covers about 400 biomedical and other journals, and offers citations from 1985 to the present. *Manual, Alternative and Natural Therapy* (known as MANTIS), also available through both DIALOG and DATASTAR, claims to cover health care disciplines not well-represented in "major medical databases." It has references from over 1,000 journals, many of which are peer-reviewed. It concentrates on indexing the literature of manual, chiropractic, and osteopathic medicine; some unknown quantity of retrospective indexing has obviously been done to enhance this database since, according to its DIALOG bluesheet, it covers a period of literature ranging back to 1880. It is created by Action Potential, a company with headquarters in Denton, TX.

The massive European biomedical database created by Elsevier — *Embase* — is the only other database of size and scope equal to (or greater than) MEDLINE which covers CAM on a regular basis. *Embase* covers approximately 3,300 journals in health care from about 70 countries annually and because, like MEDLINE, it covers the disciplines of health care so broadly and comprehensively, it cannot fail to include literature on CAM topics as a matter of course. It also reflects a European approach to medicine, in the same way that MEDLINE reflects a North American viewpoint. Each covers a core of the same major titles and augments that core with lesser-known journals selected mainly from its respective "sphere of influence." Thus, while MEDLINE covers U.S. regional medical journals of good quality, *Embase* tends to pick up European journals of lesser stature but significant import. European medicine has long been more interested in certain physical therapies and herbal products than is common in North America, and searches in *Embase* bear out this observation. Unfortunately, *Embase* is not always searched in North American health sciences libraries because of its great expense online. When MEDLINE is free, widely available and demonstrably comprehensive for most areas of medicine and health care, few are willing to go to the expense of searching another database that is likely to result in much overlap along with a few unique citations.

Other products are entering the database market now that the field of CAM is becoming popular. There are both CD-ROM databases and tools on the World Wide Web, which will appeal to particular segments of the researching public. One of the biggest factors for the inexperienced in doing literature searches is the time it takes to do the search, scan and evaluate the citations, and then locate the journals or other publications in which the desired article or articles appear. CD-ROM or Web services which allow instant linking to the full text source after identification in a search are inevitably popular with researchers. This makes services like Gale's *Health Reference Center* (HRC) and the newly created Gale *Health & Wellness Resource Center* very highly regarded. Although at present there is no extensive coverage of CAM overall, this will be offered in the near future in the form of an Alternative Medicine add-on module to their *Health & Wellness Resource Center*. In other health care databases, CAM topics will doubtless appear because more mainstream journals are publishing articles on alternative therapies.

The *Cochrane Library* is another source of information, particularly about the efficacy of CAM practices, that may be of great use to consumers.[17] The Cochrane Collaboration "is an international organization that aims to help people make well informed decisions about health care by preparing, maintaining and ensuring the accessibility of systematic reviews of the effects of health care interventions."[18] Its *Library* — perhaps its best-known product — is an electronic collection (both in CD-ROM format and on the WWW) of the full text of its own reviews and protocols in a suite of databases, which are available by subscription. It is not a bibliographic database, and does not index journals at all. Instead, it offers the full text of reviews of the literature on the efficacy of particular health care practices, which have been compiled by various Cochrane centers around the world. The reviews are highly authoritative and very comprehensive and are updated from time to time as new evidence warrants changes. The work of the Cochrane Collaboration is the underpinning and foundation of the evidence-based clinical practice movement, which is currently sweeping through health care education and practice.

A quick search of the CDSR (Cochrane Database of Systematic Reviews), which is the major database in the *Cochrane Library*, yields reviews on a small number of CAM topics. There are currently studies of the efficacy of a Tibetan herbal preparation for intermittent claudication, mind-body therapy for fibromyalgia, massage therapy for various conditions, homeopathy for acne, garlic for arterial occlusive disease, acupuncture for osteoarthritis and for asthma, and research on the efficacy of chiropractic and other manual therapies, osteopathy, together with other CAM practices. As of May 2000, abstracts of the systematic reviews in the CDSR appear in MEDLINE, so that searches on any CAM topic in the MEDLINE database will retrieve citations to Cochrane reviews if they exist on that topic. While there may not yet be enough material in the Cochrane Library on alternative medicine to make it worth paying for access to the work of the Cochrane Collaboration for CAM information, it is nevertheless one of the main credible sources of information on the efficacy of all health care practices, both conventional and alternative.

Many of the databases mentioned above can be accessed through public libraries and commercial services. MEDLINE is the only one which is likely to be available directly to the public without charge as it is heavily subsidized by the U.S. government. All of the others are commercial products which require subscriptions or payment of some sort to make them available for searching. Libraries do subscribe to these services, however, making the information accessible among their own clientele.

Research into CAM on the Internet

In addition to the bibliographic database sources of information about CAM previously discussed, there are untold thousands of sites on the Internet which can be mined for other information about unconventional health care practices. One of the newest and largest of these Internet sources is called ClinicalTrials.gov (http://clinicaltrials.gov/). Like MEDLINE, it is created by the National Library of Medicine. ClinicalTrials.gov provides patients, family members, health care professionals, and members of the public easy access to information on clinical trials for a wide range of diseases and conditions. Various CAM practices are among the therapies and interventions being tried. The database first became available early in the year 2000; it is intended to become a central listing of clinical studies sponsored by the NIH, other federal agencies, the pharmaceutical industry, and nonprofit organizations.

By typing into the search box at ClinicalTrials.gov concepts or terms representing CAM practices, the user can identify trials—both completed and those that are still recruiting—which involve the condition or practice searched. The entries for trials retrieved reveal what the trial is intended to accomplish, the inclusion (eligibility) criteria, contact information, and other useful details. Sometimes publications leading up to the trial are cited; for completed trials, publications resulting from the study are often cited. While CAM modalities are not involved as yet in a high percentage of the trials listed, this is likely to change with time and the nonbibliographic database is likely to become ever more valuable to those looking for information about the efficacy of CAM therapies.

It is one of the aims of this chapter to list and describe more than 60 of the best and most useful CAM sites on the Internet. Everyone who has ever searched for such information has favorites and knows some of the "tricks" involved in finding what they consider to be useful. Some go directly to their favorite CAM links when seeking information on a new topic because these sources have proven useful in the past. Others head, instead, for search engines and Internet catalogs, which list large numbers of hits on any topic, preferring to explore new territory with each new topic. Search engines such as: Alta Vista (http://www.altavista.com/), Google! (http://www.google.com/), FAST (http://www.ussc. alltheWeb.com/) and Dogpile (http://www.dogpile.com/), and Web catalogs like Yahoo (http://www.yahoo.com/), Excite (http://www.excite.com) and Hotbot (http://www.hotbot.com) offer to the searcher the advantage of turning up large quantities of information on most CAM topics. Yet the large quantity of information retrieved on many of these topics is at the same time a major disadvantage of these very efficient search engine/catalogs. Many retrieve sites that merely incidentally mention a desired topic along with sites that cover it in depth. While it is now common for search engines to show a "relevance" indicator, or to rank sites retrieved in a way that indicates their likely utility to your query, it is

frustrating that there are frequently far more sites collected in response to a query than one has time to examine. What is additionally annoying is the fact that not only do you have to determine the relevance of what is retrieved but also it is necessary to assess its validity, level of confidence, and its appropriateness. Considerations such as these send the smart and regular consumer of health care information on the Internet back, time and time again, to a few well-chosen and trustworthy sites which offer sufficient scope and reliability to be helpful in future searching.

Search engines and catalogs, in general, are good and valid beginning points when you have the time and skills needed to evaluate information widely and quickly, or when you fail to find anything on your topic elsewhere. They serve the neophyte searcher for CAM less well because they often overwhelm with apparently relevant material and leave one swamped when it becomes obvious that the skills required to sort through the competing claims of the many sites retrieved are lacking. The skill required to evaluate Web sites quickly can be acquired but it takes practice and a sharp and critical eye. It is often helpful to identify several comprehensive, reliable sources of information within the scope of your topic and to return to them repeatedly. If your trusted sites are gateways—offering links to other sources of information—and are frequently updated, you will find them invaluable as time savers and pointers to useful information. You should be able to identify sites of high quality among those listed at the end of this chapter. It is possible that even sites of very good quality will not always answer all your CAM questions, but if your favorites can be relied upon for only 50 to 75 percent of your queries, this is a profitable strategy.

A Critical Approach to CAM Information

Although it is time consuming, it is important to evaluate the health care sites you choose to rely on for information. A personal approach that will work for informal, "on the fly" decisions can be extracted from the collected wisdom of the HSWG, the HON Code and the work of the AMA previously described. The crucial question: "Can I trust this information?" or "How far can I trust this information?" is not one with which any of us is totally unfamiliar. We all buy books and other sources of information, or have done so in the past, and have made these decisions without a great deal of anxiety. Evaluating a health care Web site involves many similar considerations.

One of the first, simple things to ask of any Web site is: "Who is responsible for this information?" This is akin to asking for the name of the author of a book in that if you know the author's reputation (or that of the publisher), you have a sense of how trustworthy the information contained in the book will be. If the Web site is created by a reputable organization or individual, it is reasonable to expect the information offered there to be credible. Look for information about the author or sponsoring organization on the Web site; there will often be a section called: "About Us." Read such information for what it has to offer about sources from which the content is derived. If there is no attribution of responsibility for information presented anywhere on the site, move on to another site fairly quickly. Anonymous information is not highly trustworthy. When information about the creators of the site is available, determine whether the credentials of the creators are relevant and whether they seem to have expertise and experience with the topic. The level of confidence you have with the content of any Web site is completely a matter of your comfort level; when in doubt, look further for corroboration or refutation of what you read.

The purpose of the site can also be extremely important. Sites created by commercial organizations are, naturally enough, often concerned with selling you something. If you are looking for straight information on a topic with which you are unfamiliar, avoid commercial sites until you have enough apparently unbiased information to be able to distinguish a "sales pitch" from the "straight goods." All information carries the stamp of its creator/compiler, but familiarity with a topic permits the extraction of the commonly accepted truth from the tainted presentation. Endeavor to inform yourself widely before turning to obviously biased sources of information. Look at the audience for whom the site is intended in that this may tell you something about the approach and level of pitch. Just because a site is sponsored by a pharmaceutical company does not mean that it should be avoided. Pharmaceutical manufacturers can be just as altruistic as other organizations. Be aware when using information from such a source, however, that what you encounter is not likely to be at odds with the manufacturer's financial interests, and deal with it accordingly.

Better quality CAM sites will be well-designed. They will allow interactivity between users and creators; at the very least, they will allow you to contact the Webmaster with a query. Information on the site will be documented and sources of authority will be quoted. Research will be evident. Opinions will be clearly stated, and any advice given will be "owned" by someone whose credentials you can determine and judge for yourself. If the advice is given by a patient, for instance, you can decide whether it is reliable. Many patient-created sites on the Internet are extremely highly regarded sources of information on very rare conditions, but you can find just as many (if not more) that are soapboxes for cranks, and it is necessary to distinguish the one from the other. The date of compilation (and the dates on references quoted) is another clue to the trustworthiness of information. Not all the information in health care needs to be "up-to-the-minute," but you must be able to tell whether it is likely the information being offered is outdated. Other design issues, such as navigability and logical and consistent arrangement of the site, are important quality considerations. If the links offered are not working, and the last indication of update is many months ago, your confidence in the quality of the information may well falter. Simple things like the attention paid to spelling, grammar, and layout are other valid indicators of the quality of a site. Basic questions such as: "Can I access the site reliably, every time I want to use it?" are also important quality indicators. If you cannot access it, or if sections are missing, or "under construction" on a regular basis, suspend judgment, and move on until its creators can make the site stable and robust enough to warrant your consideration.

Be extremely cautious of CAM and other health care sites with lots of advertising which ask you to sign in, or require personal information from you prior to use. Privacy issues are matters of great concern with respect to health care. Most of us want our health and medical records treated with great circumspection and only made available to others who need to know, and only with our consent. There are many warnings about Web sites that collect information about their visitors and then sell it, or make it available to interests that want to sell products to a targeted market. An article appearing in the Health & Wellbeing section of Toronto's *The Globe and Mail* recently warned cancer patients against commercial and "for profit" Web sites, which offer highly sophisticated services to this particular group:

> Their pitch to consumers is that their for-profit sites can offer far more sophisticated services than the non-profits can afford. But to offer them for free, they must run ads and enter partnerships with sponsors.

More important, in exchange for access to sophisticated medical data and expert advice, the companies are asking patients to give personal data that, in turn, will be sold to advertisers and business partners, and used by the Web sites to create products to sell back to patients. Medical privacy, already a hot-button issue on the Internet, is especially relevant for cancer patients, who may face discrimination in everything from employment and insurance to social situations.

[Some companies] see opportunities for e-commerce targeting cancer patients, including syringes and colostomy bags, home health-care and private-duty nursing services, and even flower delivery.

As on any medical Web site, patients should read the conditions, disclaimer and privacy statements. All typically promise to treat health-related information confidentially, but say anything patients transmit or post to the sites can be used for any purpose.... The cancer sites make clear they will share demographic data with pharmaceutical companies, and use information about member patients for market research.[19]

It is one thing to give personal information freely after reading warnings such as those that appear on the cancer sites described above. It is quite another to have information collected from you involuntarily via the *cookies* used in navigating many Web sites. These little programs have great potential to gather and store data about the interests of Web consumers and their responses to seemingly innocuous questions. This potential has been recognized by the AMA and addressed in its recently published guidelines (cited in endnote 14), but not all Web creators will follow the AMA guidelines. Consumers of CAM information on the Internet need to be as aware of the potential threat to their privacy posed by *cookies* as do those who visit any other sites that ask for responses to questions. If you do not wish to become the target of some marketer, do not offer any more information about yourself and your habits or interests than you have to on the Internet. This can also be regarded as a Web site quality issue and health care sites that collect information about you either with advance warning or surreptitiously are sites that should be avoided, if at all possible. They represent a threat to your privacy.

These are the "rule of thumb" criteria for evaluating the quality of Web sites on CAM topics. With practice, one learns to apply them broadly and to make gross judgments about what to accept and what to avoid relatively quickly. It is important to develop a critical, or skeptical, approach to information. Even when you are comfortable with the information, you must remember (unless you happen to be an expert in the field) that the information retrieved is not guaranteed to be useful to any particular individual's health care. It is only information, not advice. Information you find on the Internet should always be presented to your health care practitioner—the trusted professional who knows you and your health history, and who has relevant experience and expertise—who can help you determine its value as advice.

The Future of CAM on the Internet

Dr. Tom Ferguson is Adjunct Associate Professor of Health Informatics at the University of Texas Health Science Center and a senior associate at Boston's Center for Clinical Computing, a medical computing think tank at the Harvard School of Medicine. He has been studying people he calls "net savvy consumers" for some time and although he shuns the epithet of "futurist," his work reveals a lot about the direction health information on the Internet is likely to take. The "empowered medical consumers" whom he has been studying are self-carers or self-helpers who fit the new paradigm of health care for the twenty-first century. They accept responsibility for maintaining their health and consult expert health care professionals when they are ill. They seek information about maintaining and enhancing their health and furthermore, when ill, want to participate in decisions about treatment of their illnesses. They use the Internet heavily as a source of general information and second opinions.

In a presentation to the Year 2000 meeting of the Medical Library Association, Dr. Ferguson described some of the most active of these self-helper groups as "disease tribes."[20] These "tribes" collaborate, sharing their information and experience of a disease or condition, and sometimes putting their work out for review by experts. They often produce medical information of very high quality on topics about which the professionals treating them know relatively little. Furthermore, he says, when it comes to producing quality medical information resources on the Internet, there is no guarantee that the professionally produced information coming from medically qualified sources is the best that there is. Patient sites often excel because, although their creators

certainly don't know everything a physician might know, ... they don't need to. Good clinicians must have an in-depth working knowledge of the ills they see frequently and must know at least a little about hundreds of conditions they rarely or never see. Online self-helpers, on the other hand will typically know only about their own disease, but some will have an impressive and up-to-date knowledge of the best sources, centers, treatments, research, and specialists for this condition. A smart, motivated, and experienced self-helper with hemophilia, narcolepsy, hemochromatosis or any number of rare genetic conditions may well know more about current research and treatments for their disease than their own primary practitioner. And when it comes to aspects [of] illness that some clinicians may consider secondary—e.g., practical coping tips and the psychological and social aspects of living with the condition—some experienced self-helpers can provide other patients with particularly helpful advice. The things clinicians know and the things self-helpers know can complement each other in some interesting and useful ways.[21]

Although not all of these self-helpers are producing CAM information on the Internet, most do not choose to restrict their quest for relief to conventional medicine. They try things out, and then let the world know whether what they tried works. Among those seeking enhancement of their health, rather than cures for their illness, there are many who turn to preventive practices, systems and ways of living that fall well within the boundaries of CAM. Vegetarianism and other diet-based approaches to wellness, meditation and massage to reduce stress and maintain equilibrium, manual therapies to help the body align and balance properly, and various spiritual approaches to health and wellness are all promoted by self-helpers and self-carers as means of staying well and out of the hands of the illness industries. All of these ideas and many more related ones can be found on the Internet.

Do-it-yourself care is bound to become more common as good sources of information become available and health care costs rise. In the U.S., large numbers of people are without insurance and thus have added incentive to provide their own health care. In countries such as Canada and the United Kingdom where universal health insurance covers everyone, self-care will also thrive wherever people reject medicalization and choose to retain a measure of autonomy over their return to health from illness. With pharmaceutical companies marketing their wares directly to the public, shortages of healthcare practitioners (especially in rural or remote areas), information about health and disease freely available to anybody with computer access, and governments waking up to the fact that more and more people want money spent validating some of the relatively

noninvasive therapies folk-medicine has passed down from one generation to the next, the future of complementary and alternative medical information sources on the Internet is fairly assured. What is not so certain is whether we will be adequately prepared to use this rich resource wisely. The reviews that follow are an attempt to make a step in the right direction.

EVALUATIONS OF CAM WEB SITES

The ranking system employs a graduated scale of four stars (****) at the top, through one star (*) at the lower end to indicate the relative value of these useful and noteworthy sites. The reviews are organized as follows:

A. Comprehensive Sites
B. Sites for Specific CAM Therapies/Topics
  a. Acupuncture, Oriental/Chinese Medicine
  b. Aromatherapy
  c. Ayurvedic Medicine
  d. Cancer, Alternative Therapies
  e. Chiropractic
  f. Diet (Vegetarian, Macrobiotic) Supplements
  g. Herbs and Herbal Remedies
  h. Homeopathy, Naturopathy, Osteopathy
  i. Reflexology
  j. Reiki
  k. Spirituality and Meditation
  l. Therapeutic Touch
  m. Skepticism/Fraud

A. Comprehensive Sites

About.com: Alternative Medicine
http://altmedicine.about.com/health/altmedicine/
Accessed on: 22 May 2000   *Ranking*: ****

Sponsor: *About.com* is a unique Internet resource with a network of over 700 highly targeted environments, each overseen by a subject specialist guide. The guides collect and present link directories, original content, special features, and e-shopping on each topic. The *Alternative Medicine* guide at *About.com* is Terri Ramacus, a professional Reiki Master/Teacher. There are a number of other *About.com* sites, such as Chiropractic and Herbal Medicine, that fall within the subject scope of CAM.

Description: The *About.com* sites are all visually busy, with boxes and columns offering access to a variety of related topics, features, shopping opportunities, links, and search engines. Take your time; get used to it; there is lots to be explored on these sites. On the *Alternative Medicine* site, there are separate *Chat* and *Discussion* opportunities; there is *News*, a guide to the whole spectrum of CAM disciplines and a library of articles on many alternative medicine topics. You can, of course, search the site for information not immediately apparent on the top page, or you can explore CAM via a list of topics down the left-hand column: *Ayurveda Medicine, Botanical Medicine, Energy Medicine, Oriental Medicine, Scientific Studies*. There is a similarly comprehensive list of specific therapies. If you cannot find adequate information related to your topic on the general *Alternative Medicine* site, you can always move to one of the CAM-related *About.com* pages (with a different subject specialist guide) for related topics, such as *Chiropractic, Vegetarian Cuisine,* or *Exercise*. The guides personalize the approach to any topic by organizing the resources according to their own understanding of how the material could, or should, be used and they often provide their own original content. Through a partnership with another Internet information provider *OnHealth.com, About.com* is now providing access to even more topical information about alternative and complementary medicine through links to *OnHealth* articles.

Alternative Medicine

http://alternativemedicine.com/

Accessed on: 19 June 2000   *Ranking*: *

Sponsor: Burton Goldberg, the founder and publisher of **AlternativeMedicine.com**, is a businessman with an avid interest in CAM. He lays it on the line at the outset:

> Two systems of health care are available in this country today: conventional Western medicine and alternative medicine. Conventional practitioners are medical doctors who practice by the book, and commonly align themselves with the multibillion dollar pharmaceutical industry.... These doctors practice medicine that is superb when it comes to surgery, emergency and trauma.

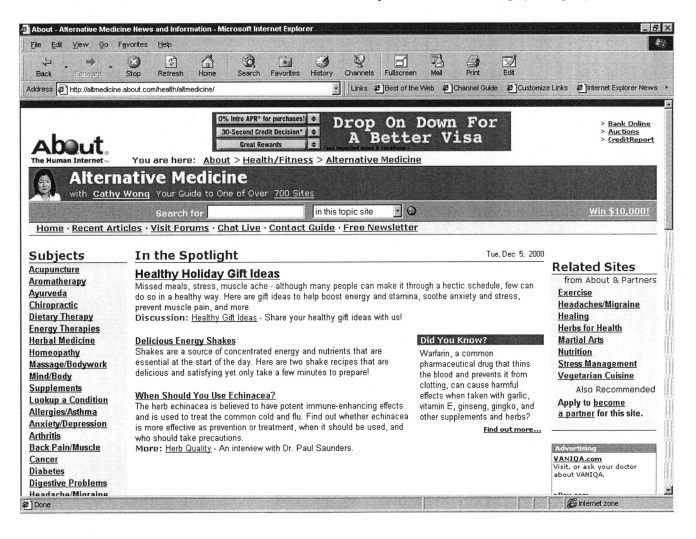

But there's no question that alternative medicine works better for just about everything else, especially for chronic degenerative diseases like cancer, heart disease, rheumatoid arthritis, and for more common aliments.

Description: With the *credo* above ringing in your ears, you won't be surprised that Burton Goldberg's Web site offers *Provocative Essays* (by Mr. Goldberg himself), and *Political Issues*, as well as a *Message/Discussion Board* to engage you on its homepage. Mr. Goldberg is as unabashedly a promoter of CAM as others (notably Dr. Stephen Barrett, of **Quackwatch**) are opposed to it. The site advertises *Alternative Medicine* magazine, available by paid subscription, and a free weekly e-mail newsletter. Once registered with the site, you qualify for discounts when buying books and magazines, and products from the NutriClub (coming soon). No privacy statement can be found anywhere on the site indicating how information collected from registrants will be handled. The site offers access to an amazingly small collection of clinics and educational organizations (or their Web sites) for such an enthusiastic supporter of CAM. No information about how these sites were selected appears, but we recall that Mr. Goldberg is a self-proclaimed businessman, so it is possible that a fee is collected prior to the appearance of any recommendation on the site. It is somewhat disturbing that Mr. Goldberg does not seem to offer any scientific evidence for his recommendations. An article on Tahitian Noni juice, posted on 19 June 2000, makes quite fantastic claims and mentions a clinical trial, but does not provide any citation to published evidence that can be independently examined. The site is highly commercial and offers no indication that anyone with any scientific qualifications is behind the promotion of products and therapies freely recommended here. Mr. Goldberg's Web site seems to want you to believe that the choice between CAM and conventional medicine is a political one, not one based on independent, objective evidence of what works, even if it cannot yet be explained. The site is attractive and easily navigated and does a lot to promote CAM, but I am not sure that this kind of business promotion is what will win the hearts and minds of intelligent people.

Alternative Medicine Homepage

http://www.pitt.edu/~cbw/altm.html

Accessed on: 22 May 2000   *Ranking*: **

Sponsor: Charles B. Wessel, compiler of the *Alternative Medicine Homepage*, is Coordinator of Affiliated Hospital Services at the Falk Library of the Health Sciences, University of Pittsburgh, in Pittsburgh, PA.

Description: The *Alternative Medicine Homepage* is a Web site with a simple, well-designed and attractive presentation that offers a rich resource of briefly annotated pointers and links to a wide variety of information sources. The compiler uses a classification developed in 1992 by a conference of the Office of Alternative Medicine of the NIH and provides access to resources under headings such as: *Alternative systems of medical practice, Bioelectromagnetic applications, Diet, nutrition and lifestyle changes, Herbal medicine, Manual healing*, and *Mind/body control*. There is a list of resources for alternative therapies of specific conditions and the AIDS and Cancer lists are particularly noteworthy. The site also offers information about mailing lists and newsgroups in relevant areas, directories of practitioners of CAM therapies, and government resources with respect to CAM (mainly U.S. government, but with a few Canadian references, as well). There is also a list of Pennsylvania resources, providing highlighted access to resources specifically of interest in the community where the site originates. The collection is not an exhaustive one but it presents specific information sources that its compiler believes to be of value and thus has a very personal appeal. It is not frequently updated, but has existed for slightly over six years and is well-regarded. Finally, it is worth noting that a page offering "studies" of CAM therapies is available. While not exhaustive by any means, the studies offer useful information.

Ask Dr. Weil

http://www.pathfinder.com/drweil/

Accessed on: 22 May 2000   *Ranking*: ****

Sponsor: Dr. Andrew Weil is a leader in the integration of Western medicine and the exploding field of alternative medicine. A graduate of Harvard Medical School, he teaches at the University of Arizona in Tucson, specializing in alternative medicine, mind/body interactions and medical botany. He is also the author of eight books on CAM topics.

Description: Dr. Weil's site is very different than many of those reviewed. At the center of his home page every day is a new question related to health or illness, which he answers in a way that brings various CAM issues to the fore. Dr. Weils' answers are well-researched and complete with references and links to other Web sites that are helpful in making his point. In this way, the

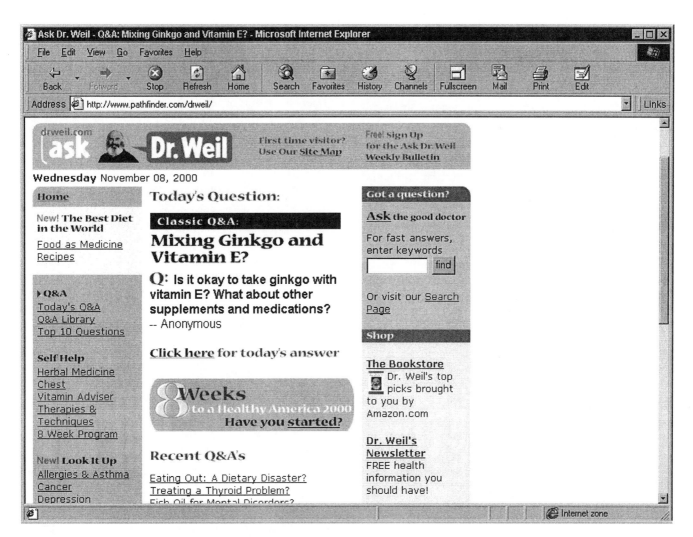

interactivity of this site is highlighted and nothing is static. The questions and answers Dr. Weil gives are all archived and can be retrieved by date, or by topic, using an onsite search engine. Other features on the site include various self-help resources such as *The Herbal Medicine Chest*, which is reconstituted for each season and stocked with herbs to combat the ills or threats of that time of year; *The Vitamin Advisor*, which has the reader answer a series of questions before responding with a generalized prescription for dietary supplements intended to promote health and energy; and the *Find A Doctor* section which allows searching for doctors, managed care plans and other health care providers in the United States. You can undertake to follow the principles in his famous book, **8 Weeks to Optimum Health** by interacting with the *8 Weeks to a Healthy America* section of the site. There are recipes from Chef Alice Waters of *Chez Panisse* Restaurant, who espouses the "fresh, local, seasonal" principle for culinary success.

Be warned that advertising and shopping (for books and vitamins, in particular) are prominent here. There is much that is unique and helpful in spite of the commercialism that probably makes it all possible. You will receive an extremely helpful and friendly introduction to herbalism and dietary preventive medicine from Dr. Weil.

Ask NOAH about: Alternative (Complementary) Medicine

http://www.noah.cuny.edu/alternative/alternative.html

Accessed on: 22 May 2000   *Ranking*: **

Sponsor: New York Online Access to Health (NOAH) is a project that brings together the unique assets and experience of four New York partners who have worked together on a variety of projects for 26 years: The City University of New York, The Metropolitan New York Library Council, The New York Academy of Medicine and The New York Public Library. The contributing editor for the *Alternative Medicine* section of NOAH is Robert Lasner, a Health Sciences Librarian at the New York Academy of Medicine Library.

Description: The resources offered by NOAH go far beyond those being considered in this review. *Alternative Medicine* is only one of the many topics or collections of resources put together by the partners in this highly valuable and trustworthy information project. NOAH's Webmasters and editors select the best explanations and chunks of text from various Web sites and pull it all together with an outline that promotes a consistent and rational presentation of information. They use FAQ's (*Frequently Asked Question* documents), bibliographies, and statistical presentations from many sources in a massive effort to catalog the Web on each health care topic they select. They list local and worldwide resources, not in an attempt to include Web sites comprehensively or exhaustively, but in order to be logical and informative about CAM. Everything is listed in simple menus which you can follow sequentially, or select from, at random. Unfortunately, not all of the links are checked often enough and several were dead at the time of this review. While there is often information in Spanish to complement the English information, this is not the case with the *Alternative Medicine* topic.

HealingPeople.com
http://www.healingpeople.com/ht/index.tmpl

Accessed on: 4 June 2000   *Ranking:* ***

Sponsor: **HealingPeople.com** uses the slogan: "Your Source for Complementary and Alternative Medicine" and has a very large advisory board of practitioners in a great many health care disciplines, both conventional and alternative.

Description: The topics dealt with on the **HealingPeople.com** Web site cover a wide range of CAM: Chinese/Oriental Medicine, Homeopathy, Aromatherapy, Bodywork, Ayurveda, and Western Herbalism, Nutrition & Lifestyle, and Cancer Risk Reduction. There is even a section on Pet Health where you will find articles on homeopathic remedies and chiropractic care for your pets, as well as acupuncture for animals, flower remedies and holistic veterinary care. Clicking on any of the topic headings takes you into an encyclopedia and offers a selection of articles related to the topic. The site offers both a general and a professional encyclopedia, although the latter is so brief that one is led to believe that it was not finished at the time of

review. The *Practitioner Listings* support searching for practitioners by discipline, specific qualifications, name, geographic location and languages spoken; practitioners using the site can register for listing in the database. There are a number of useful and simple FAQs on CAM topics and visitors to the site can register for chat and discussion groups which offer free e-mail and a newsletter, as well as fast check-out when shopping on the site for the herbs or other health care products (homeopathics, aromatherapy products, vitamins & dietary supplements, books, etc.) available for sale. There is a search engine and a map which makes navigating this large site somewhat easier. The graphic design is sophisticated and attractive; the privacy statement is prominent and claims to allow for the blocking of cookies in the near future. Secure shopping is available online, but the site allows for telephone sales if you do not want to send your credit card information over the Internet.

The Healing Spectrum
http://www.inforamp.net/~marcotte/index.htm

Accessed on: 22 May 2000   *Ranking:* ***

Sponsor: Diane Marcotte was a banker for 38 years before leaving that profession to concentrate on her mail-order book business and her work as a healer.

Description: **The Healing Spectrum** draws on both alternative and allopathic (conventional) medicine for its exposition of nondrug, nonsurgical methods of preventing and treating illness, and healing. This is another site that acts as an annotated bibliography of electronic information resources, offering an enormous number of links to resources the compiler judges to be of value. There are directories of practitioners, associations, journals, magazines and newsletters, holistic centers, schools and research sites and even a section on holistic health for animals. You can locate resources, both alternative and allopathic, related to specific diseases and much information on "related topics" such as caregiving, environmental issues, channeling, dowsing, electromagnetic fields, *feng shui*, religion, vegetarianism, labyrinths, and more. There is a whole section on the Chakra System and auras, while another offers a large variety of inspirational quotations. You can buy books on this site from the compiler's business, as well as from Amazon.com, and the Canadian roots of the site are evident throughout. There is a search engine which helps retrieve details from this massive site.

Health Care Information Resources — Alternative Medicine

http://www-hsl.mcmaster.ca/tomflem/altmed.html

Accessed on: 22 May 2000   *Ranking*: **

Sponsor: Tom Flemming is Head of Public Services in the McMaster University Health Sciences Library in Hamilton, ON, and the author of this chapter.

Description: Not one to be accused of false modesty, this author has included his own Web site in this list of valuable resources because, in terms of Internet collections in the field of CAM, it has a venerable pedigree. It was created on 1 July 1995 and has been updated frequently ever since. The *Alternative Medicine* page currently has nearly 250 links to CAM sites ranging broadly through all the disciplines and modalities in the field. The *Alternative Medicine* page is part of a larger collection of Health Care Information Resources (HCIR), which are updated daily. The site offers annotated links to CAM topics ranging from *Acupuncture, Oriental/Chinese Medicine and Shiatsu* through *Zero Balancing*, and touching upon such little known practices as *Cheirology, Rolfing,* and *Urine Therapy,* as well as the more standard practices of *Apitherapy, Chiropractic, Herbs and Herbal Remedies,* and *Reiki.* While merely a collection of large static lists of links without any search engine to aid those lost in the hinterlands, the site has its own logical organization and is designed for browsing the vast array of available information. Links to commercial sites are generally excluded, unless no noncommercial site on the topic is available. To be included all sites must offer valuable and freely accessible useful information. Canadian sites are of particular interest in this resource and French language sites are offered whenever these can be found. There are links throughout the *Alternative Medicine* page to related resources in other sections of HCIR, such as those to the *Fraud* page, the *Consumer Advocates* page, and many links to relevant sections of the *Health Care Disciplines & Education* page, for CAM education.

Healthfinder

http://www.healthfinder.gov/default.htm

Accessed on: 6 June 2000   *Ranking*: **

Sponsor: healthfinder® is a gateway to reliable consumer health and human services information developed by the U.S. Department of Health and Human Services.

Description: There are two sections of healthfinder® that may interest people who want to know more about CAM. There is a menu choice for *Alternative Medicine* under *Hot Topics* and one for *Fraud and Complaints* under *Smart Choices.* This Web site works through menus so that anyone who can read and click a mouse can use it. Under the *Alternative Medicine* menu choice, one finds four more lists from which to select items of interest. *Is it for me?* offers selections which link to definitions, doctors, journals and research, as does *Alternative Therapies* and the other topics found here. The healthfinder® Web site is a directory service that points the information seeker to other Web sources of information. The selection of CAM sites available here is not overly large, but the sites are well-chosen. The *Fraud and Complaints* section of healthfinder® is also reliable and easy-to-use. Its presentation of resources from various U.S. government and other agencies is done so as to help the user "Learn how to avoid health scams and the potential harm that may result from inappropriate care and misleading or false claims. Know who to call to research or complain about such claims." It has three sections: 1) how to recognize a quack or scam, 2) reporting product complaints and, 3) reporting provider complaints. Each of the sections offers a simple, clickable list of links to articles available, usually on the Web sites of agencies such as the FTC and the FDA. There are also links to organizations—like the National Consumers League, the Health Care Financing Administration—that can be expected to have regulations or to provide assistance that will be relevant in cases of health care fraud. The lists of links under *Product Complaints* and *Provider Complaints* similarly identify regulatory organizations or offer information and assistance in pursuing complaints about products or providers.

HealthWorld Online

http://www.healthy.net/

Accessed on: 6 June 2000   *Ranking*: ***

Sponsor: **HealthWorld Online** tries to provide a tool that will allow individuals to take full responsibility for their own health care. Its vision is to support what it calls "self-managed care", both when ill and in wellness. **HealthWorld Online** is committed to fulfill the public and professional demand for reliable, integrative health, wellness and medical information, products, and services.

Description: **HealthWorld Online** "offers a series of information centers and discussion forums where consumers, health professionals and the media can explore information and share views on the growing, integrated connection between conventional medicine and the various forms of natural health and medicine—what the mainstream calls 'alternative and complementary' medicine." There are a Natural Health Clinic, a Nutrition Center, a Fitness Center, a Natural Health Library, and so on. CAM modalities and topics appear everywhere. Some of the best information that the site has to offer appears in several lengthy essays in the *Alternative Medicine Center*. Here you will find a *Guide to Understanding Alternative Medicine* (http://www.healthy.net/CLINIC/therapy/guide.asp) in three parts, by Mary and Michael Morton. The essays are lengthy, but very readable, and in explaining the differences between conventional medicine and CAM they make CAM more easily understood. The same *Alternative Medicine Center* (http://www.healthy.net/clinic/therapy/) has extensive resources to offer on each of nearly two dozen CAM modalities, under the headings *Systems of Traditional Medicine* (e.g., acupuncture, chiropractic, osteopathy) and *Alternative and Complementary Therapies* (e.g., aromatherapy, chelation therapy, fasting, flower remedies). A major complaint about this site is that it works through menus that seem interminable and load very slowly. It is a very text-oriented site and requires some concentration in order to be appreciated fully.

National Center for Complementary and Alternative Medicine

http://nccam.nih.gov/nccam/

Accessed on: 18 June 2000   *Ranking*: ***

Sponsor: The **National Center for Complementary and Alternative Medicine** (NCCAM) is a part of the U.S. National Institutes of Health (NIH) with a mandate from Congress to "facilitate the evaluation of alternative medical treatment modalities" to determine their effectiveness. Its primary purpose, therefore, is to conduct and to support basic and applied research and training on complementary and alternative medicine. The NCCAM began life in 1992 as the Office of Alternative Medicine (OAM), within the Office of the Director, National Institutes of Health. It was elevated to the Status of Center within NIH in 1999 and thereby acquired greater ability to initiate and to fund research.

Description: The Web site of the NCCAM is a great, sprawling collection of important information about complementary and alternative medicine in the United States. It has sections for "consumers and practitioners" and for "investigators" because these groups are the major stakeholders in its territory. For consumers and practitioners, the NCCAM offers a brief FAQ of eight questions, which focus on helping practitioners and the public understand its role. There is an explanation of its own classification of complementary and alternative medicine, which has recently contracted from seven to five categories. There are also small collections of NCCAM fact sheets and consensus reports (likely to grow as the research of the Center comes to fruition). The NCCAM offers access to a group of federally produced databases (MEDLINE, MEDLINE*plus*, CAM Citation Index, CRISP, Clinicaltrials.gov) from which CAM information in the scientific literature of health care can be identified. Each of these databases can be searched for free, at the click of your mouse. There is information about the NCCAM Clearinghouse, whose role is to disseminate information to the public, media, and health care professionals to promote CAM research, awareness, and education. Further, the site offers information about clinical trials opportunities, research funded by the NCCAM and other federal government resources of potential interest to site visitors. There is an equally important collection of introductory and explanatory information for investigators about research policies, applications and guidelines, funding opportunities and other relevant items. You can also find on the site a list of the nine research centers around the U.S. which are funded by the NCCAM to evaluate alternative treatments for chronic health conditions such as addictions, aging, arthritis, cardiovascular disease, cardiovascular disease and aging in African Americans, chiropractic, craniofacial disorders, neurological disorders, and pediatrics (http://nccam.nih.gov/nccam/research/centers.html). The NCCAM site is valuable in that it provides a framework for the vast array of CAM topics and offers an introduction, as well as access, to some further information via the Clearinghouse, which responds to written questions from the public. It is disappointing in that it does not offer a public collection of information on each of the modalities it classifies, nor does it summarize what is known, or even what is being investigated with respect to each of them. That is probably demanding a lot at this point in the development of seriously organized and funded research into CAM, but one hopes that such an approach will soon be possible. There are two final sections on this site which offer detailed information about the NCCAM, its history and organization, and news and events about research into CAM disciplines. The site is well-organized, carefully worded, attractive and easy-to-navigate. There is a site-specific search engine, which can help you locate something that you have seen before on this site (but cannot recall where), an index (which lays out the topics on various pages) and a list of "What's New" so that you can approach information topics chronologically by the date on which they were added to the site. Much has changed on this site even during the writing of this chapter; keep your eyes on it as it develops! This is one site that is bound to become more valuable as research proceeds in CAM.

OneBody.com

http://www.onebody.com/index.jhtml

Accessed on: 26 June 2000   *Ranking*: ****

Sponsor: OneBody.com had its beginnings three years ago as an independent medical company developing and managing programs that brought conventional and alternative medical practitioners together for health plans in seven U.S. states. By going on the Web, the company is offering its expertise directly to the individual consumer and health care practitioner. They offer information, connections with practitioners and a variety of services for consumers and practitioners.

Description: OneBody.com claims devotion, both on- and offline, to bringing alternative, complementary, and traditional medicine into harmony. The medical advisory board comprises people with M.D., D.O. and D.C. qualifications; the Web "content team" also appears to have very diverse and appropriate qualifications. Information that will help the public make decisions about treatment modalities is the major product of this

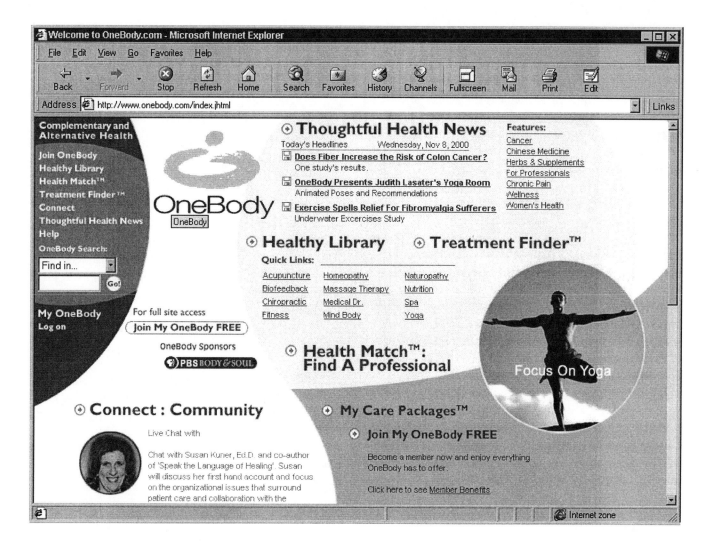

site. In addition to the *Thoughtful Health News* and its *Archives* of topical articles which explain health news to a lay audience, there is the *Healthy Library*, which offers credible, thoroughly referenced information to help consumers make informed treatment decisions and to help practitioners understand evidence-based applications of CAM. *Quick Links* to topics such as *Acupuncture*, *Chiropractic* and *Nutrition* are prominently displayed, but *Chronic Pain*, *Stress* and *Women's Health* also appear among the extensive list of other topics also accessible on this site. Each topic has a basic introduction, which is signed by someone whose credentials are identified, and there are citations to articles on which the introduction is based. There is depth in the article reviews accessible on each topic. The **OneBody** reviewers evaluate writing on the topic under discussion using a standard format which allows easy consultation and quick evaluation by the reader. The aim of each of the articles on a topic is to present the existing evidence for it, and to leave readers in no doubt as to whether the therapy is recommended. You can use the *Treatment Finder* to identify various approaches to dealing with, for example, *Allergic Rhinitis*, *Back Pain*, *Heart Attack* and *Menopause*, while the *Health Match* can identify a practitioner in the geographic area of your choice. There is a valuable and extensive glossary of terms used in the CAM discussions. Each of the articles can be e-mailed or printed, using little icons prominently placed at the top of the article that make the task easier. There is also a list of conferences arranged by discipline and, within each discipline, by date; entries are hyperlinked to Web sites, when known, and contacts are always given so as to make possible communication with the organizers. All of the above features are freely accessible without any registration. If you are willing to register, even more is offered. By registering for free membership on the site, you can collect or create "packages" of information from the site to mail to family and friends who might benefit from such concern, consult profiles of health professionals available on the site during a search for a practitioner, and use a tool called *Word of Mouth* to obtain references about your choices, and communicate with other members, experts, authors and researchers in a discussion forum. Similar benefits are available to practitioners who register; they can list themselves and their services via a free Web page service offered by the company, and participate in discussion with other practitioners registered on the site. The *Privacy Policy* is lengthy and full of legalese, but read carefully; it does say that **OneBody** will not release personal or contact information without your consent. Information collected via your use of the site and through "cookies" can be used by the company and by other companies which offer their services on the **OneBody** site. The site is attractive, easy-to-navigate and almost always rewarding. If you want fast results, you can always use the on-site search engine.

OneMedicine.com
http://onemedicine.com/

Accessed on: 18 June 2000   *Ranking:* *

Sponsor: **OneMedicine.com** is IntegrativMedicine's online service, designed to facilitate Web-based access to a suite of breaking news, advisory, reference and training services. Integrative Medicine Communications, the parent body, is a Newton, MA, based information services company combining the best of alternative medical practices with conventional medicine for optimal health care. The company was founded in 1998, and is a private, venture capital–backed organization.

Description: The **OneMedicine.com** Web site makes a lot of claims for which I can find no evidence. It states that it is the world's most complete integrative medicine information resource, but unless you are willing to register as a "member" and provide your name, e-mail address and zip/postal code (at the minimum) together with occupation and postal addresses as well, you are denied the opportunity to see the material on which they base this claim. Furthermore, they say that all products are *peer reviewed by a 50-member board of expert health care professionals.* Unlike other sites reviewed for this chapter which list their "experts" with credentials when making such a claim, there is no such list on this site. I looked carefully for a detailed privacy statement before I filled in the minimal information required but I did not find any. After logging in with as little information about myself as I could provide and still get in, a two- or three-line privacy statement was displayed; it said that any information a "member" provides would only be used internally. This is hardly reassuring. I was asked whether I would like to receive mailings from selected advertisers and declined; I was also asked if I wanted to receive "alerts", and if I am currently a paid subscriber to another service offered by IntegrativMedicine. Then, when I tried to access the "member" choices on the site, I was denied access. The *News & Articles* section of the site, available to all without membership, does not bear out the claim to be, "The world's most complete integrative medicine information resource." There were fewer than a half-dozen "news" items on the page, none bearing any obvious date of posting on the initial screen, although when you access the titles, you discover the date on which the article excerpted in the headline is published. In the *Focus* section, I found articles about the "pioneers" of integrative medicine—clinicians who are currently treating patients with both conventional and alternative therapies—and selections from the *OneMedicine Archives*. These selections looked to be interesting and informative, but offer very spotty coverage of CAM on a site that claims to be complete. The *Resources* section offered a calendar of upcoming conferences of potential interest to practitioners (in the main), and a *CAM Primer* with an article "adapted" from its original appearance in the *Annals of Internal Medicine*. The *CAM Primer* also contains links to a series of other brief articles on major CAM modalities, but it would be hard to describe any of those examined as comprehensive. Now, it may be that—for members—there is more expansive detail, but that wasn't hinted at anywhere. What is suggested, though, by the offer: *Learn how to get more from* **OneMedicine.com** *with a free, 30-day trial membership*, is that after your trial membership is over, there is a charge for continued use of the site. Nothing I saw here suggested to me that I should pay money to get at the rest of the site. Certainly, a second review of information in the *About Us* portion of the site indicates that the public may not be the primary target audience for this site; it claims to be: *an online subscription service designed for medical professionals interested in integrating conventional and alternative medicine into their practices*, and offers arrangements for licensing other organizations to use its content on their Web sites. It may be that this is a unique service and that there are Webmasters crying out for content they can't create for themselves who welcome this kind of offer. I am not persuaded, however, that the content on this site is of sufficiently high interest or quality that any member of the public with access to the many other sites reviewed here would want to pay to use this service.

WholeHealthMD.com

http://www.WholeHealthMD.com

Accessed on: 22 May 2000   **Ranking**: ****

Sponsor: *WholeHealthMD.com* is a partnership between several companies in the health-care field: American WholeHealth and Rebus. Their Web site offers consumers the added convenience of being able to purchase health-related products through an e-commerce partner, WholeFoods Market.

Description: *American WholeHealth Inc.* is a provider of integrative medicine services at centers located in Chicago, Washington, DC, Denver, and Boston. Each center has conventionally trained doctors and alternative medicine specialists on staff. *Rebus Inc.* is a consumer health and wellness publisher based in New York; Rebus publishes the *University of California, Berkeley Wellness Letter, The Johns Hopkins Medical Letter*, and the *WholeHealthMD Advisor*. Their joint venture Web site is slick, attractive, user-friendly and current. It offers *Healing Centers* which combine conventional and alternative therapies to help manage illnesses from A to Z. Each condition is presented by a specialist whose qualifications and biography are offered, and each follows a standard presentation: introduction, summary of the condition (cause, symptoms, treatment, self-care, etc.), list of supplements which may help, useful vitamins and sometimes several articles for further reading on the topic. The *Healing Kitchen* section of the site extols the virtues of healthy eating and cooking via guest chefs and "food remedies" that target specific conditions. The section also offers reasons why, for example, eating foods rich in calcium, manganese, bromelain, vitamin D and ginger may be helpful to those who suffer back pain. You can ask questions on the site and have them answered by integrative medicine experts and you can access the archive of previously answered questions. A "reference library" groups articles into categories such as therapies, foods, supplements, drugs, and fundamentals. A useful feature of the reference articles is the ability to send the article to a friend by e-mail, or to access a "printer-friendly" version of the text. There is an ever-changing selection of news related to CAM interests, and as is more and more common all the time, a section called WholePeople, where you can shop, presumably, for things that will make you "whole" (food, travel, the natural home, etc.). The site is pleasing, informative and authoritative. Overall, the service offered here is valuable and the sales pitch is not intrusive.

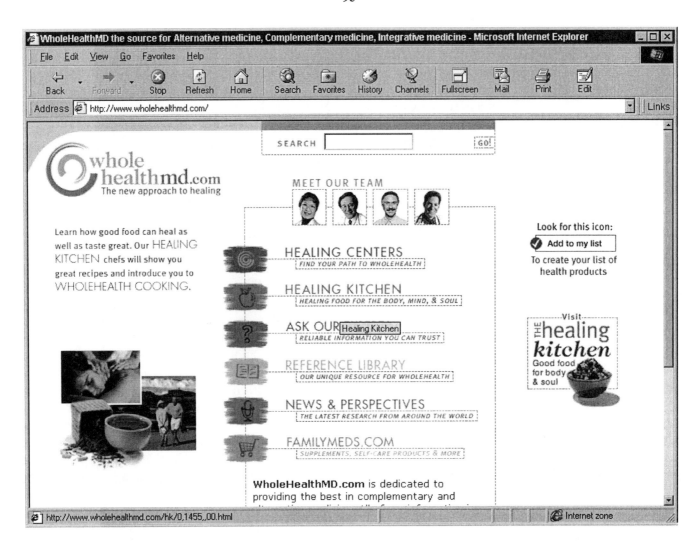

B. Sites for Specific CAM Therapies/Topics

a. Acupuncture, Oriental/Chinese Medicine

American Academy of Medical Acupuncture
http://www.medicalacupuncture.org/

Accessed on: 25 May 2000   *Ranking*: ***

Sponsor: The AAMA is the sole physician-only professional acupuncture society in North America, accepting members from a diversity of training backgrounds. Physician members represent all of the disciplines of medical acupuncture currently practiced in the United States and Canada.

Description: The site of the AAMA is also home to the Medical Acupuncture Research Foundation (MARF), a charitable, nonprofit organization which serves as the research arm of the AAMA. The site has sections for members which are strictly "off-limits" to the public. The AAMA promotes "medical acupuncture" an integrative medicine practice described as: "acupuncture performed by a doctor trained and licensed in Western medicine who has also had thorough training in acupuncture as a specialty practice. Such a doctor can use one or the other approach, or a combination of both as the need arises, to treat an illness." Presumably, "traditional acupuncture" would be performed by a specialist in Traditional Chinese Medicine whose supplementary armamentarium would be Chinese herbal medicine. Under the heading of *Public Information*, there is a lot more material (articles on how acupuncture works; treating cancer with acupuncture; a FAQ; information from the NCCAM on acupuncture; a searchable bibliographic database) that is well–laid out and easy to use. You can search for a medical acupuncturist in the United States, find out which AAMA members have hospital privileges and check out the status of regulations for acupuncturists in each state. The journal of the association (*Medical Acupuncture*) is available in full text on the site from early 1998 and selected full text articles from earlier issues are also accessible on the site. There is also a searchable collection of research articles compiled by MARF. Some screens can be visually cluttered and, at times, text has to be centered to fit the screen, but it is generally graphically clear and eye-friendly.

American Association of Oriental Medicine
http://www.aaom.org/

Accessed on: 24 May 2000   *Ranking*: **

Sponsor: The American Association of Acupuncture and Oriental Medicine (AAAOM), was formed to be the unifying force for American acupuncturists who are committed to high ethical and educational standards and a well regulated profession to ensure the safety of the public. Originally involved in regulation and education of acupuncturists alone, it recently changed its name to reflect the fact that acupuncture is just one part of the entire scope of oriental medicine.

Description: The AAAOM Web site focuses on offering information about the profession and how to find a school in the United States for the potential student of oriental medicine. There are lists of educational institutions and opportunities, and an essay on comparing them to facilitate a choice about where to study. There are proposed statutes, under the heading *Legislation*, along with information showing states that regulate acupuncture and oriental medicine practitioners. There is also a list of state associations. The public may find the list of books and publications available for sale to be of interest, but it is disappointing to discover that the access to *Articles* is by password and they are not available to the casual user of the site. Overall, the site is text-heavy and graphically simplistic; it is not hard to navigate, but it is necessary to get used to the irritating Java Script boxes which keep popping up with messages when you change pages.

British Acupuncture Council
http://www.acupuncture.org.uk/

Accessed on: 25 May 2000   *Ranking*: **

Sponsor: The British Acupuncture Council (BAcC) represents 1,800 acupuncturists who have extensive training in acupuncture and the Western medical sciences appropriate to the practice of acupuncture.

Description: Members of the BAcC are the acupuncturists in Britain who are not physicians. They practice the full range of traditional acupuncture but without a Western medical diagnosis as a point of beginning. Their site explains carefully the difference between what they do and the more limited acupuncture practice of "medical acupuncturists." Under the heading *Acupuncture Treatment*, they offer a good explanation of what you should expect if you consult a traditional acupuncturist. Many of the links to sections of the site were not working when reviewed. It was not possible to access their directory, information about training, or information under the headings *Health & Safety*, and *Research*. Their journal (*European Journal of Oriental Medicine*) is accessible on the Web site, but only articles in the current issue are available in full text. However, abstracts of articles in earlier issues can be viewed. The site is graphically clean and simple to use, when it works, but is either "under construction" (without warning) or simply promises more than it can currently deliver.

British Medical Acupuncture Society
http://www.medical-acupuncture.co.uk/

Accessed on: 24 May 2000   *Ranking*: ***

Sponsor: The British Medical Acupuncture Society (BMAS) was formed in 1980 as an association of medical practitioners interested in acupuncture. There are now 1700 members who use acupuncture in hospital or general practice and there are also sections for dentists and veterinarians. The BMAS opposes unfounded therapeutic claims and recommends the practice of acupuncture by health care professionals.

Description: The BMAS site falls into the category of "integrative" medicine rather than "alternative" medicine. Certainly, acupuncture is a CAM modality, but the members of the BMAS are doctors, dentists or veterinarians, not "alternative" practitioners. The site offers content both for members and for the public, but—to its credit—relatively little of the content is actually restricted to members. Members will find the information about scientific meetings, courses, regional groups and society news of interest and can access the contents of the *Journal of the British Medical Acupuncture Society* (with selections available in full text), and the full text newsletter *The Point*. Although intended for members, access for others is not restricted. Software reviews and videos are also listed. For the public, there are articles in a section entitled *Hot Topics*. There is also general information for patients about acupuncture and how to locate medical acupuncture practitioners in the United Kingdom. The society has an axe to grind in that acupuncturists are not regulated in Britain and the BMAS argues that the public's only guarantee of quality acupuncture treatment is to choose to be treated by a member of the BMAS, who is also a medical doctor. This stance is not belabored or intrusive. A section of the site is set aside for feedback and for sending questions. The site is graphically simple, well–laid out, and logically organized.

Chinese Medicine and Acupuncture in Canada
http://www.medicinechinese.com/

Accessed on: 25 May 2000   *Ranking*: *

Sponsor: unknown

Description: This site commits one of the worst errors possible in terms of health information on the Internet in that nothing is said about the sponsor of the site or who takes responsibility for it, nor is there any statement of purpose. It is not possible to determine, from anything I can find on the site itself, what its aims or affiliations are. Yet the site is remarkably well-organized, simple to use, helpful and well-used. There is a lengthy explanatory or introductory essay (with a menu and individual links to all of its sections) on the history of Traditional Chinese Medicine (TCM), including the principles and the treatments used in the discipline. While some of the parts of this essay seem to be dealt with rather briefly — with only about ten lines on the 10,000-year history of TCM—there are good links to offsite sources of further information so that the reader can skim quickly through the presentation all at once, or linger over sections, following up the offsite links as desired. There is a collection of linked articles on how TCM is used to treat various disorders, diseases and conditions such as depression, irritable bowel syndrome and cancer. Unfortunately, many of these links are offsite and were not working when accessed. An additional problem is that credentials for the authors of these articles are not evident. Similarly, articles in the "library" have been mounted onsite and the links are under better control than those in the previously-mentioned section, but again the credentials for many of the authors are not apparent. The authority behind such material is not indicated. A really useful feature of this site is the information it offers about regulation of TCM practitioners in various Canadian jurisdictions. As health care is a matter of provincial jurisdiction in Canada,

health care practitioners are regulated at the provincial level. CAM practitioners have not, until recently, been regulated in Canada, so the section on government regulations is very useful. There are also lists of schools and associations of TCM in Canada, and a list of schools in China where practitioners can study. In addition, there are testimonials from patients, a brief FAQ, a useful (but unannotated) list of links to other TCM sites on the Internet, and an invitation to search the bibliographic database of **Acupuncture Progress,** which is said to contain 30,000+ citations of articles in acupuncture science published in 1,500+ journals in China and abroad since the year 1950. This was not working when accessed. Finally, some other useful features on this site are chat, a message board (or forum) and "interest groups" which help those who use this site (and a brief look at messages in the forum indicates that people from all over the world have used it) connect with each other. There is a lot of potential here but the site needs a lot of work in order to realize its potential.

National Certification Commission for Acupuncture and Oriental Medicine
http://WWW.NCCAOM.ORG/

Accessed on: 24 May 2000   *Ranking*: *

Sponsor: The National Certification Commission for Acupuncture and Oriental Medicine (NCCAOM) is a U.S. organization that promotes nationally recognized standards of competency and safety in acupuncture, Chinese herbology, and Oriental bodywork therapy for the purpose of protecting the public. It is accredited by the National Commission for Certifying Agencies.

Description: The NCCAOM site gets full marks for being useful to practitioners and to the public wanting to locate practitioners. It is easy to use, if somewhat plain and dull in appearance, but it does not offer information about the discipline to the uninitiated or to the consumer wanting to find a general presentation on acupuncture or oriental medicine. It is really intended for the practitioner. The site offers information about the NCCAOM certification programs, examinations, fees, forms, and eligibility criteria for certification. There is a searchable directory of its over 9,000 diplomates. It will be of interest to any member of the public wanting to know what conditions practitioners have to meet before certification or wishing to explore the history of the regulation of acupuncture in the U.S. While one would like more introductory information about the disciplines being certified, this site offers a small collection of links and leaves it at that. It is hard to fault such a site for not doing something they probably do not feel is necessary because others are doing it, and it is for that reason the site gets only one star.

SinoMD.com

http://www.sinomd.com/putong/etcm/index.htm

Accessed on: 26 June 2000　　*Ranking:* **

Sponsor: **SinoMD.com** is a company of doctors, researchers, writers, technicians, designers and marketers all working to provide the best and the most complete information on TCM available on the Internet. The site is a business venture between three partners: China Academy of Traditional Chinese Medicine, Hong Kong SinoMD (China) and the China National Corporation of Traditional and Herbal Medicine; it was launched on 22 April 2000 and has offices in Hong Kong and Beijing.

Description: SinoMD.com offers *Health News* at the top of its home page and, surprisingly, it is almost always recent. Who would have thought there was something newsworthy every day about such an ancient tradition of health care? Clearly the people behind this excellent site have a Western sense of how to catch your attention. There is no fractured English here and there are no misspellings of common English terms. There is an amusing chronicle—regularly updated and complete with cartoons—of "Joe" who is undergoing acupuncture treatment to aid his attempts to quit smoking. The dialogue often tries too hard to be ironic (and achieves sarcasm, instead), but reveals a Chinese sense of how Westerners like to be "jollied along" on being introduced to a strange new topic. Beneath the somewhat strained attempt at humor, though, we learn a lot about acupuncture. There is a section with information on Chinese herbs although, as yet, not nearly enough. One hopes that the collection of information on Chinese herbs will grow as the site matures. Other sections of the page, such as *Health Food*, present information on diet therapies for specific common ailments (hypertension, hiccups, toothache, vomiting, etc.), and foods that nourish your *Qi*, *Yang* and *Yin*. While the ingredients used may not all be common in Western grocery stores, it is probable that they can be located in the Chinese groceries ubiquitous in larger North American cities. Under the heading *Common Ailments*, there is a presentation of how TCM deals with chronic conditions from *arthritis* to *obesity*. A section on the Culture of Traditional Chinese Medicine delves into the background of notions that are commonplace in Chinese health care, offering essays on history, diagnosis, diet, and the use of herbs in TCM. The site also offers a brief introduction to Tibetan Medicine. There are glitches in the writing of HTML code for this site—images that do not load properly or characters out of place and links that lead to unfinished pages—that show up on the screen, which clearly ought not to be there. It is a very new site that tries to create an electronic bridge from the ancient Orient to the modern West. Already its achievement indicates that it is worth watching. As China and the Chinese develop more expertise in Western ways, we can expect this site to grow in sophistication and content, and to become more valuable in translating the Chinese experience of health care into terms we can understand and embrace.

b. Aromatherapy

AromaWeb

http://www.aromaWeb.com/

Accessed on: 27 May 2000　　*Ranking*: ***

Sponsor: **AromaWeb** is owned by Wendy Robbins. A resident of Michigan, Ms. Robbins has a B.A. degree with a concentration in marketing from the University of Michigan School of Business Administration. She is primarily self-taught in aromatherapy and is a current student in a yearlong aromatherapy course from the Australasian College of Herbal Studies, a state licensed school located in Oregon.

Description: **AromaWeb**, as one might expect from the academic qualifications of its creator, is intensely commercial. There are multiple ads and sales pitches but you can ignore them if you wish and simply concentrate on the significant information the site has to offer. In spite of the aura of commercialism there is nothing to buy on this site except advertising space. Ms Robbins is not selling oils directly. Despite its commercialism, this is the best site on aromatherapy. It has the following features: an archive of articles, oil profiles, a bookshelf, a business plaza, a newsroom, lots of links to other aromatherapy resources, and information about how to advertise on the site. In the article archive, in addition to the usual essays on what aromatherapy is all about, and the history of aromatherapy (which are worth reading), there are articles on the ingredients in aromatherapy oils, tips for buying quality essential oils, information on proper storage of essential oils, blending , substituting, using in massage, and so on. The profiles of more than 70 different essential oils are impressively complete and include references to other sources of information on the oil discussed. The business plaza provides listings not only of vendors of oils and aromatherapy necessaries, but of schools where the practice can be learned, and of practitioners. The bookshelf has the usual link to Amazon.com, so that you can actually buy the books described here. A feature known as the "recipe box" provides instructions for mixing your own oils for particular purposes (such as stress relief, arthritic joints, stuffy noses). There is a search engine to search the site. The site also offers news, polls and upcoming events of interest to aromatherapists and people who are interested in aromatherapy. The graphic presentation is attractive and uncluttered, in spite of the banner ads. Tracking where you are on the Web site is made easy by means of a small menu on the left-hand side of the screen. **AromaWeb** offers visitors a pleasant and surprisingly educational experience despite its business orientation.

Guide to Aromatherapy
http://www.fragrant.demon.co.uk/

Accessed on: 27 May 2000   *Ranking:* **

Sponsor: This site is the work of Graham Sorenson, in Wales. Little information is given about Sorenson or his credentials but there are contact telephone and fax numbers and an e-mail address at the bottom of the first page of the site. You can also view a photo of Mr. Sorenson in an article (dated 18 April 2000) about his work in aromatherapy from a Welsh newspaper, the *Western Mail*, available on the site.

Description: The **Guide to Aromatherapy** is a British commercial Web site. However, there is minimal advertising, and lists of suppliers of essential oils. Aromatherapy seems to be the avocation of the site creator rather than his profession. After retiring from the RAF (Royal Air Force), he took up Web design and aromatherapy, both of which are offered on his site. Sorenson offers information on the use of essential oils (extracted from flowers, herbs, spices, woods and fibers, usually by distillation, expression and solvent extraction) in aromatherapy—for massage, baths, compresses, inhalations, vaporizations, and in perfumes. There is a

lengthy alphabetic list of oils (sources, traditional uses, safety information) and a section on "carrier" oils, which are mixed with essential oils to dilute and extend them. A useful glossary of terms used in aromatherapy is also found on the site. Although there are more than 200 books on aromatherapy offered on this site, most of the titles are listed only with an author's name with no date of publication or publisher shown. Books in French, German, and Dutch, however, have much more information with ISBNs and prices given for some of these. There is also a lengthy list of suppliers of oils and practitioners of aromatherapy in the U.K. This site is somewhat eclectic, but useful, informative and low-key relative to other aromatherapy sites.

International Federation of Aromatherapists
http://www.int-fed-aromatherapy.co.uk/

Accessed on: 27 May 2000   *Ranking:* **

Sponsor: The **International Federation of Aromatherapists** (IFA), a registered charity in the United Kingdom, is the longest-established international aromatherapy organization. The Federation has been at the forefront of developments within the aromatherapy profession since its foundation in 1985 and has pioneered the use of aromatherapy in hospitals, hospices, special care units and general practice.

Description: The IFA Web site takes a very serious approach to the business of introducing the public to aromatherapy. There is no hint of "commercialism." The introductory essay on aromatherapy indicates that the twentieth century business of aromatherapy can be traced back to the work of a French chemist who used lavender essential oil serendipitously to soothe a burn and was so amazed at the results that he subsequently began a lifetime study of the therapeutic effects of essential oils. The essay continues by explaining the way in which aromatherapy works, and what to expect from aromatherapy treatments. The searchable directory of practitioners does not appear to be of much use to North Americans, as searches for practitioners in Canada and the United States result in almost no hits. There is a list of educational institutions in the U.K. where aromatherapy can be learned, but no information about the educational standards by which members are prepared. The site is easy to navigate and pleasing to view.

National Association for Holistic Aromatherapy
http://www.naha.org/index.html

Accessed on: 27 May 2000   *Ranking*: ***

Sponsor: The **National Association for Holistic Aromatherapy** (NAHA) is an educational, nonprofit organization in the United States dedicated to enhancing public awareness of the benefits of true aromatherapy. NAHA is actively involved with promoting and elevating academic standards in aromatherapy education and practice for the profession.

Description: The **National Association for Holistic Aromatherapy** Web site offers a wide variety of resources to the visitor. The mission of the association is to disseminate educational material about the medicinal use of aromatic plants and essential oils. In this endeavor, it addresses itself to the public, to trade and professional associations and to business owners and practitioners. The site offers information about the association itself and about aromatherapy: "The practice of true aromatherapy centers on the inhalation and application of 'essential oils' --- volatile essences of plants obtained primarily through steam distillation from various parts of certain plants." The holistic aromatherapist uses both the essential oils and the "hydrosols" or "watery" parts of the distillation process. In its educational role, the site disseminates information about a dozen schools which are "in compliance" with the NAHA guidelines. The *Standards of Training* are also available. The site offers access to the NAHA journal, called **Aromatherapy Journal**. At the moment (as of May 2000), only two articles from the journal are accessible, but the promise is that "An electronic version of the journal (in pdf format) will be available in the next few weeks." Although shopping is advertised, it was likewise not available at the time of review but is also promised within "the next few weeks." Finally, the site offers a toll-free telephone number for contacting the association to obtain further information, as well as an e-mail address.

c. Ayurvedic Medicine

Ayurvedic Institute

http://www.ayurveda.com/

Accessed on: 27 May 2000   *Ranking*: **

Sponsor: The **Ayurvedic Institute** is a nonprofit, private, post-secondary educational institution established in the state of New Mexico in 1984 to teach and provide the traditional therapy of East Indian Ayurveda including herbs, nutrition, panchakarma detox, acupressure massage, yoga, Sanskrit, and Jyotish (Vedic astrology).

It is headed by Dr. Vasant Lad, a world renowned Ayurvedic physician from India.

Description: The Web site of the **Ayurvedic Institute** is really an information brochure for an educational institution, with a description of services available for purchase. High on the site menu is information about the academic calendar, student services, and courses. Services features available include an offering of the *Panchakarma Department*—a sort of Ayurvedic spa—offering traditional Ayurvedic procedures for purification and rejuvenation that include oil massage, herbal steam treatment, *shirodhara*, cleansing diet, herbal therapy and so on. These services are available, by appointment, for stated prices. There is also an *Herb Store*, with a catalog of Ayurvedic products that can be downloaded in a variety of MSWord formats, or in RTF; online ordering was not available at the time of review, but was promised. Since Yoga is often linked with Ayurveda ("Yoga helps with enlightenment and Ayurveda helps with perfect health"), it is no surprise to find a section of the site devoted to that science. The real value of this site to those interested in CAM lies in the information it offers about the principles and practices of Ayurveda and Yoga. Although it is not possible to compare what you see here with what can be read in a textbook, what is found here will intrigue and may lead to further study. There is a plan to offer online ordering of books from the Ayurvedic Press in the near future. The graphics and design of the site are rudimentary, but do not detract from the experience.

Center for Natural Medicine and Prevention of the College of Maharishi Vedic Medicine

http://mum.edu/CNMP/

Accessed on: 28 May 2000   *Ranking*: **

Sponsor: The **Center for Natural Medicine and Prevention** (CNMP) is the research division of the College of Maharishi Vedic Medicine in Fairfield, IA. Late in 1999, the NIH, through its National Center for Complementary and Alternative Medicine, awarded the CNMP nearly $8,000,000.00 to establish the first research center specializing in natural preventive medicine for minorities in the United States. It is one of nine NIH-supported centers in the United States for studying natural medicine, and the only one with a specialization in minority health. The Center will study the effectiveness of Maharishi Vedic Medicine approaches for the treatment and prevention of cardiovascular disease in high-risk aging populations.

Description: The Web site of the CNMP is a rudimentary construction, at best, and relies heavily on the Web site of the College of Maharishi Vedic Medicine (http://mum.edu/CMVM/mvm.html) for content. There is a mission statement for the center, a press release announcing the recent grant of money from the NIH, an "overview" of the research to be done, a list of faculty and staff at the Center and a list of publications hyperlinked to abstracts. On the college Web site, you can read about the holistic approach of Maharishi Vedic Medicine and can consult scientific studies of its benefits. The Maharishi is often quoted, saying things that sound quite mystical and belief-oriented. Transcendental Meditation is among the tools used in the Maharishi's brand of Vedic medicine, and is one of the modalities for which scientific documentation is offered. The site emphasizes the preventive and natural approach of the Maharishi's system of care and there is much talk of the noninvasive and nondangerous nature of natural medicine in contradistinction to iatrogenic illnesses and the many hazards of "modern medicine." There is a great deal more promotion of the system than revelation of the principles behind it. The program of instruction includes pulse diagnosis, vedic architecture (building construction for optimal health), the vedic system of predicting the future, and transcendental meditation, which includes Yogic Flying.

National Institute of Ayurvedic Medicine

http://niam.com/corp-Web/index.htm

Accessed on: 27 May 2000   *Ranking*: ***

Sponsor: The **National Institute of Ayurvedic Medicine** (NIAM) was established in Brewster, NY, in 1982 by Scott Gerson, M.D., who is the only medical doctor in the United States to hold degrees in both Ayurveda and conventional allopathic medicine. Dr. Gerson's medical practice has combined Ayurveda and conventional medicine for more than fifteen years.

Description: The **National Institute of Ayurvedic Medicine** Web site focuses on Dr. Gerson and his work, which integrates ancient Indian medicine with conventional Western medicine. Dr. Gerson has impressive credentials and links with Indian schools and teachers. He continues, after years of study and practice, to work on the academic and research frontiers to promote the understanding and practice of Ayurveda, a holistic system of healing which evolved among the Brahmin sages of ancient India some 3,000-5,000 years

ago. His site centers around an explanation of the *Basic Principles of Ayurveda*, and a list of medicinal plants which require some understanding of the principles of Ayurvedic pharmacology. There is information on Dr. Gerson's current research in conjunction with the National Cancer Institute and the Richard and Hinda Rosenthal Center for Alternative and Complementary Medicine at Columbia University. The latter project involves the collection of data on Ayurvedic herbal medicines useful in the treatment of various women's diseases and conditions. There is also further information on research projects, which the NIAM is conducting on its own. Several sections of the Web site offer information on educational projects of the NIAM. A school of Ayurvedic medicine is being established and a correspondence course is available. Ayurvedic herbs, jams, teas, massage oils and essential oils are available for sale on the site but there is no sense of commercialism. The site is attractive and easy to navigate and very helpful to the beginner or to those who simply want to know more about what is often regarded as an "arcane" topic.

d. Cancer, Alternative Therapies

Annie Appleseed Project

http://www.annieappleseedproject.org/

Accessed on: 28 May 2000   *Ranking*: ***

Sponsor: The **Annie Appleseed Project** Web site is created by Ann Fonfa, a woman from New York City who was diagnosed with breast cancer in January 1993. She has survived by informing herself about her options and pursuing those which seemed to her most likely to be of benefit. She has become an advocate and an activist, while urging others to do the same.

Description: While the cancer that Ann Fonfa experienced was breast cancer, her Web site does not concentrate on breast cancer alone. Breast cancer in men is discussed, other female cancers are a part of the focus (ovarian, in particular), and cancers of all types are included. The message of this site seems to be that you can help yourself tremendously by becoming involved in your fight against any kind of cancer. Even though your prognosis may not be good, your job is to stay alive, any way you can, until a cure is found. Fonfa collects information personally and through assistance from collaborators and offers it to the public, sowing the "seed" of information about alternative therapies for cancer much like Johnny Appleseed spread apples across America in the folk legend. This site is a treasure-trove of "leads" and of good solid information on a bewilderingly large collection of alternative cancer therapies. The headings used in the list of links on the left-hand side of the screen do not always reveal fully what you are going to find if you explore. Under the heading: *Treatment: Consumers' View of Alternative Medicine* is a series of about 26 information items on *The Revici Method, Hydrazine Sulfate, Detoxification Techniques, Mushrooms, MGN-3, IP6*, and much more that was not hinted at in the heading. Similarly, the heading *Relevant Studies* is the caption for more than 20 articles on topics such as curcumin/genistein, green tea, fish consumption and the like, each of which, when accessed, may reveal further articles cascading away from that page. Exploring this site at length is important if you want to exploit it fully. There is information about treatment at the Gerson Clinic in Mexico, about African-American breast cancer issues, ovarian cancer, multicultural issues, and environmental issues in cancer of all sorts. Fonfa addresses health care professionals directly in a special section of the page. She asks them to use her site to inform themselves about what their patients are doing to supplement the treatment received from doctors, and to learn something about alternative therapies that they may not have known about previously. She fully supports the proper evaluation of alternative therapies, noting that the promises of conventional therapy have not always been kept. On the downside, there is no information about the evaluation of these therapies on the site at all and everything is offered as though it could be of potential value to someone. The onsite search engine is powerful and very useful in such a large collection. The site is well-designed and very simple to use, as well as being attractive. All of the main links are always visible on the left-hand side of the screen, although you may have to use the bar at the bottom of your screen to move the text space into view to read the information on each page.

Unconventional Cancer Therapies

http://www.bccancer.bc.ca/uct/

Accessed on: 4 July 2000   *Ranking***

Sponsor: The British Columbia Cancer Agency (BCCA) operates a comprehensive program of cancer control for the people of British Columbia, in collaboration with many partners. It provides these services through a program including prevention, early detection, diagnosis and treatment, community programs, rehabilitation, supportive care, research and education. The service is run through provincial programs and regional cancer centres throughout the province. **Unconventional Cancer Therapies** is the work of librarians at the agency under the direction of David Noble.

Description: The Library/Cancer Information Centre of the BC Cancer Agency offers the third edition of its **Unconventional Cancer Therapies** free of charge on the BCCA Web site; a printed version is also available for sale in three-ring binder format. The information is formatted into a list of 46 monographs on substances or therapies—those about which the library is most frequently asked—which have been used outside the practice of conventional cancer therapy to "cure" or relieve the distress of cancer. The monographs have all been revised or updated in the year 2000. Some of the suggested substances are specific—such as Essiac, and Ginseng—others are broader, or more inclusive of varying substances—like Livingston therapy, or vitamins—and yet others—like psychic surgery, and holistic medicine—are not substances at all. Each monograph begins with a standard acknowledgement, stating that patients often supplement oncologist-approved regimens of treatment with "alternative" therapies of some sort. Each monograph provides a summary of what is known about the substance or therapy, and a history, through extensive quotation from sources that are cited at the end of the monograph. The claims made for the substance or therapy are clearly stated, and an account of any known evaluation, toxicity and costs follow. The presentation is careful, matter of fact and easy to use, but the constant quotation from sources tends to distance the agency (and the reader) from the information offered. Feedback is welcomed and a form is provided for that purpose. The cumulative effect of reading this information is the realization that there is very little scientific publication about some of the unconventional therapies described; use (of all therapies that I read) is discouraged and the overall approach to complementary therapy in this source is extremely conservative. Visit this site if you really want to know why current science says you ought not to use CAM therapies for cancer, but don't expect to find much that is positive or supportive about complementary and alternative cancer therapies here. The **Unconventional**

Cancer Therapies is only part of the BCCA site, though, and there is also a lot of non-CAM information about conventional cancer drugs available on this site under the heading: *Patients and Public Information* (http://www.bccancer.bc.ca/).

University of Texas Center for Alternative Medicine Research

http://www.sph.uth.tmc.edu/utcam/

Accessed on: 28 May 2000   *Ranking*: ***

Sponsor: The **University of Texas-Center for Alternative Medicine Research** (UT-CAM) is one of the centers established by the National Center for Complementary and Alternative Medicine at the National Institutes of Health to evaluate alternative therapies. UT-CAM is the only CAM center focused solely on alternative and complementary cancer therapies and co-funded by the National Cancer Institute.

Description: Given the uniqueness and importance of the mission of the UT-CAM, it is a real disappointment to discover a message on their Web site that the center is no longer operational. While no explanation is given on the site, there is a note indicating that the Web site will remain available at least until December 2000. The main content of this site consists of a list of about 30 therapies reviewed by the center. Much like the British Columbia Cancer Agency (see listing under Unconventional Cancer Therapies above) in its conception, it is quite unlike the BC site in results and general tenor. The reviews here focus on providing details about the scientific studies that have evaluated the therapies discussed. The reference lists are exhaustive and annotated. Since there is so much detail in terms of the science involved for each substance reviewed, there is little of the negative tenor found in the BC site. It is important to note that the conclusions about many of the therapies may not be different than those in the BC materials (where the same substances/therapies are reviewed), but the approach is more detailed. Some may find this plethora of detail hard to use, but it does reflect the fact that the ultimate verdict is not yet in on many therapies and that research will continue for some time before a final answer to the question "Does it help?" can be given. A note on the home page indicates that the reviews on this site were last updated in 1998 and, presumably, since the center

is no longer operational, no further updates of these reviews will be available. A FAQ list offers brief answers to questions about the work of the UT-CAM, how to find the scientific reviews on therapies covered, and what you should ask a CAM practitioner before beginning treatment. The list of *Resources & Links* is extensive and helpful. It will be a significant loss if this site disappears as planned.

e. Chiropractic

American Chiropractic Association Online

http://www.ACAToday.com/

Accessed on: 28 May 2000   *Ranking*: ****

Sponsor: This site is the official Web site of the American Chiropractic Association.

Description: The **American Chiropractic Association Online** Web site offers information about the association and the profession. There are sections for the public and for members. The section for the public called *About chiropractic*, has information about the benefits of chiropractic treatment, FAQs to answer common questions, tips for consumers, and data on education for the profession. There is a chiropractic doctor locator that allows a search for members of the association in any area of the United States the searcher chooses to specify. One of the main sections of the home page quickly identifies what the association calls *Hot Topics* and a scan of this section will alert the visitor to things that affect the practice of chiropractic in the United States today. The publications section offers abstracts of articles in the last three issues of the *Journal of the American Chiropractic Association*, and the suggestion that full text is available to members in the members' section of the site. Another official publication of the association, the *Journal of the Neuromusculoskeletal System,* is linked to the site but only for subscription information. Neither abstracts nor full text are available free. A government affairs section indicates the issues on which the profession is currently lobbying governments in the United States, and legislative updates and issue briefs are accessible on the site. Two more sections— *Chiropractic Information and Reference* and *Public Relations and Chiropractic in the Media*—offer a wealth of information on practically any chiropractic subject you can imagine. The site is really a marvelous source of reference on chiropractic in the United States.

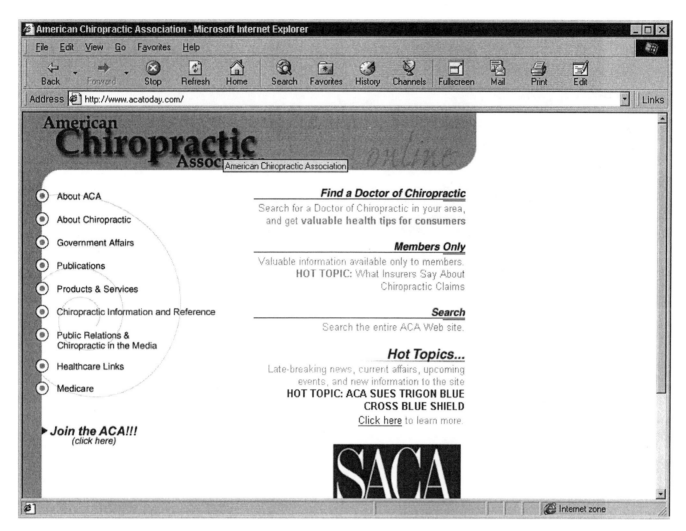

Chiropractic in Canada

http://www.ccachiro.org/

Accessed on: 28 May 2000   *Ranking*: ****

Sponsor: **Chiropractic in Canada** is the official Web site of the Canadian Chiropractic Association.

Description: The **Chiropractic in Canada** Web site is available in both English and French. Topics are chosen with a view toward promoting the profession and making it more familiar to the public. There are articles that define what chiropractic does, and that discuss the philosophy behind the discipline. Yet other articles explain how chiropractors are licensed in Canada, and how chiropractic care is paid for. For those thinking of becoming a chiropractor there is a whole section with information about the post-secondary schooling requirements, what is involved in the course of study, and choosing a school in Canada or the United States. The site offers yet other sections such as history, research, a large collection of links to sites of interest to chiropractors, and—in an attempt to involve the public—sections for feedback, public surveys, and a collection of FAQs that answer basic questions about chiropractic treatment. You can also locate a chiropractor near you by entering the first half of your postal code. Easy-to-navigate, attractive and informative; the site is not without advertising.

The Chiropractic Page

http://www.mbnet.mb.ca/~jwiens/chiro.html

Accessed on: 28 May 2000   *Ranking*: **

Sponsor: **The Chiropractic Page** is maintained by John Wiens, D.C., who practices in Winnipeg, MB. Dr. Wiens graduated from the Canadian Memorial Chiropractic College in 1980 and has been in his current practice for 20 years.

Description: The first thing to be noted about **The Chiropractic Page** is that it is divided into separate parts

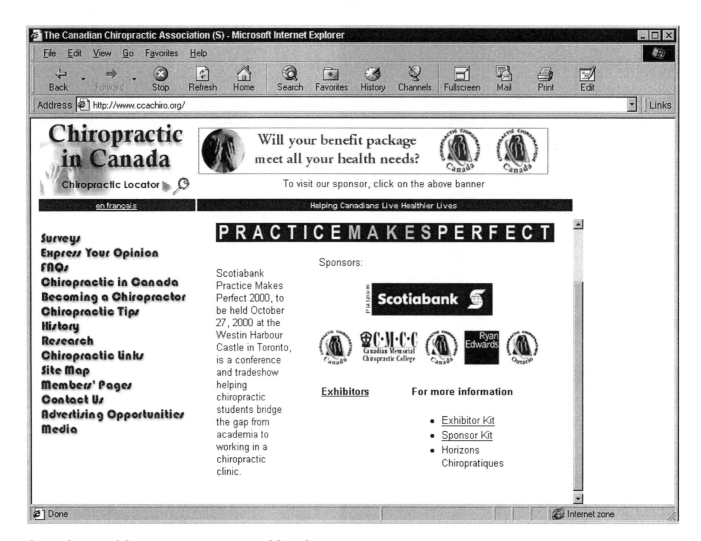

for students and for prospective patients, although it is possible to view the whole site via a third section called *The Full Chiropractic Page*. A fourth point of access is for those who want to know about *Chiropractic in Manitoba*. Each of these parts consists of a selection of links to material about chiropractic on other Web sites. Basically, Dr. Wiens has created a guide to chiropractic information on the Internet and separated it into that which will primarily interest students, and that which will primarily interest patients, prospective patients, and the curious. The patient resources chosen are practical; you can search for a chiropractor near you in the U.S. on the *healthgrades.com* site, and in Canada on the *Chiropractic in Canada* site. Links for students are equally carefully chosen—you can go to the U.S. Bureau of Labor Statistics Web site and read the entry for "Chiropractors" in the *Occupational Outlook Handbook*. There are also links to the Association of Chiropractic Colleges and the American Chiropractic Association site and to all

of the chiropractic colleges in North America which have Web sites. Dr. Wiens also offers links to products and services for chiropractors, software, research (organizations, databases, journals), mailing lists of interest to chiropractors and their patients, and to Internet resources. The site does nothing startling in terms of providing resources, but it keeps its links up-to-date and offers one chiropractor's view of his profession and how others may want to approach it.

f. Diet (Vegetarian, Macrobiotic) Supplements

About.com: Vegetarian Cuisine
http://vegetarian.about.com/food/vegetarian/

Accessed on: 28 May 2000   *Ranking*: ***

Sponsor: Your guide for the *About.com* **Vegetarian Cuisine** pages is Tiffany Refio, who has been a vegetarian for 10 years.

Description: Like the other *About.com* sites, **Vegetarian Cuisine** is visually busy and replete with subject collections of articles on practically any related topic imaginable. A sample of topics from the basic collection includes *Why Vegetarian?* through: *Macrobiotic, Fruitarian, Organic, Weight Loss, Cooking Classes.* Practically anything you might want to know about vegetarianism is discussed here. It is possible to shop for books and videos on vegetarian topics and find related *About.com* pages (*Animal Rights, Ecotourism, Herbs for Health,* etc.). As is necessary with such an abundance of material in cascading arrangements off the main page, there is a good search engine which allows you to locate material that is hidden under headings that do not mean much. I searched for "tofu", for instance, and found 428 hits on this site (mostly recipes and tips for handling) which are displayed in chunks of ten at a time. If you are ever at a loss for a recipe at dinnertime, my advice is simply to visit the *About.com* site for the cuisine you would most like to eat that evening and you will be overwhelmed with recipes you can try! There is advertising on this site, as there is on all *About.com* sites, but considering the value received from the information made available by these sponsors this is tolerable. A greatly appreciated feature of the *About.com* sites is that there is almost always a box at the bottom of the page where you can enter the e-mail address of a friend and send the text conveniently without cutting, pasting, and re-formatting.

ConsumerLab.com

http://www.ConsumerLab.com/

Accessed on: 19 June 2000   *Ranking*: **

Sponsor: **ConsumerLab.com, LLC,** is a privately held company based in White Plains, NY, which provides independent test results and information to help consumers and health care professionals evaluate health, wellness, and nutrition products. The results of these tests are excerpted on its Web site.

Description: The **ConsumerLab.com** (CL) Web site provides the public with an important service in testing products such as herbals, vitamins, minerals and other supplements, sport and energy, and personal care products to determine if the products live up to the labeling claims made by manufacturers. Additionally, **ConsumerLab.com** examines the actual comparability of apparently similar products and investigates and identifies their potency, purity, bioavailability, and

consistency. The results of testing appear in *Product Reviews* which are sold by CL and excerpted on their Web site. They also license their content for use on other Web sites, thus generating revenue which makes them more independent. Two other programs—the *Guaranteed Testing Program* and the *Ad Hoc Testing Program*—are available to manufacturers who want to be able to use CL's seal of approval. A section called *CL HealthSearch* allows you to enter a term (disease, therapy or topic) and to retrieve information which CL has collected from a great variety of sources (bibliographic databases, journals, organizations and Web sites). I entered *Valerian*, and was overwhelmed with the quantity of possibly useful information retrieved, but was impressed with the ease of linking to a wide variety of information and sources. The CL site is very new (the first *Product Review* was posted to the Web on 16 November 1999) and has, therefore, only a small collection of *Product Reviews* to offer at this point. It has, however, wisely conducted reviews of well-known supplements to begin. You can already read about the test results on the content of Ginko Biloba, Saw Palmetto, Glucosamine and Chondroitin products, SAM-e, and Vitamin C. More product reviews and comparisons are promised in the near future. This is a site for the avid consumer of dietary supplements to get excited about and to visit frequently. Anticipating much interest, CL has created a mailing list to alert interested consumers to the appearance of new *Product Reviews* and updates. The site is straightforward and quite plain and is easy to use. Everything about its minimalist design supports its claims to probity, independence, and trustworthiness. Bookmark this site!

International Vegetarian Union

http://www.ivu.org/

Accessed on: 28 May 2000   *Ranking*: ****

Sponsor: The **International Vegetarian Union** (IVU) is a nonprofit-making organization with membership open to any nonprofit organization that advocates vegetarianism and is governed exclusively by vegetarians. The IVU has existed since 1908 when it supplanted the Vegetarian Federal Union founded in 1889. For the purpose of membership in IVU, vegetarianism includes veganism and is defined as the practice of not eating meat, poultry or fish or their by-products, with or without the use of dairy products or eggs.

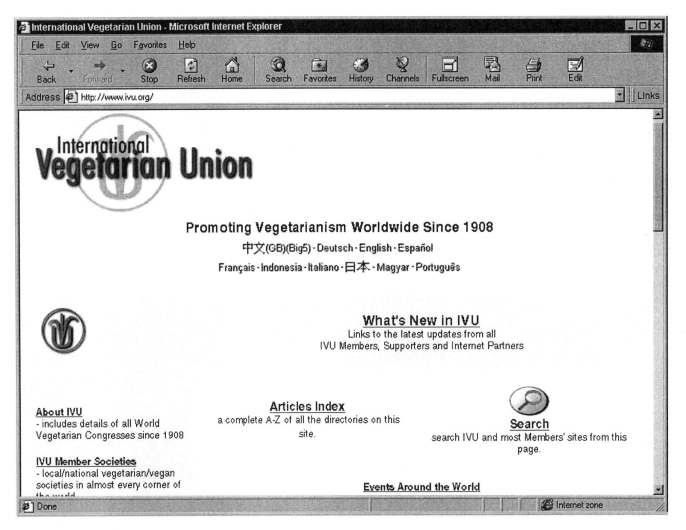

Description: There are many good vegetarian Web sites. This one is noteworthy in that it offers its resources in nine world languages (Japanese, German, English, Spanish, French, Indonesian, Italian, Chinese and Hungarian). Since the IVU is an international organization, one of the features on their Web site is a list of links to vegetarian societies with Web sites around the world. This list is supplemented with e-mail discussion lists on vegetarian topics in many world languages. The site is full of other interesting information: *Religion and Vegetarianism* deals with the major world religions (Buddhism, Christianity, Hindu/Hare Krishna/Sikh/Jain, Islam, Judaism) and offers vegetarian articles related to each. There is a list of famous vegetarians and, for those who travel to foreign countries, a list of vegetarian phrases in world languages (so that you can ask for vegetarian food when in Timbuktu). Moreover, there is a discussion list for science relative to vegetarianism and lists of published articles on vegetarian science topics (probably for copyright reasons most of the articles appear to be derived from publications connected with the organization). The *Books* section offers access to no less than three national versions of Amazon.com (U.S., Britain, and Germany) to cater to as many buyers as possible. There are message boards, forums, chat, and FAQs and, of course, there are recipes—in English, German, Spanish, Italian, Swedish and Dutch. You can search the recipe database, submit recipes, and join an e-mail list which will send recipes flooding into your mailbox. This is a very international site and one that is easy to use. There are ads, but the site is not highly commercial.

Macrobiotics Online

http://www.macrobiotics.org/

Accessed on: 28 May 2000   *Ranking:* **

Sponsor: The **Macrobiotics Online** Web site is a creation of the Kushi Institute, in Becket, MA. The Kushi Institute, a division of the Kushi Foundation Inc., is the leading macrobiotic educational center in the world. Students from around the globe attend residential-style programs on the macrobiotic approach to health and healing.

Description: "Macrobiotics is the art and science of health and longevity through the study and understanding of the relation and interactions between ourselves, the foods we eat, the lifestyles we choose to lead, and the environments in which we live," according to the Kushi Institute. "As what we choose to eat and drink and how we live our lives are primary environmental factors that influence our health and create who we are, the macrobiotic approach emphasizes the importance of proper dietary and lifestyle habits." The site offers a library of articles about diet and lifestyle, and educational material about macrobiotics. There is a strong emphasis on whole-grain cereals and vegetables, but fish and seafoods, fruits and nuts are occasionally permitted. The site highlights information about programs offered at the Kushi Institute, including health recovery and career training. There is an online store but online secure ordering is not available, and orders have to be placed by telephone, fax, mail or e-mail. There is nothing exciting about the layout or design of this site. This reviewer found that most of the links on the home page did not work so that it was necessary to type the URLs into the location line and hit the enter key in order to access related pages off the main page. There is a lot of useful information here, but the Kushi Institute's Webmaster really needs to take a look at how that information is presented and ensure, minimally, that all the links work to ensure that the whole site is easy to use.

Office of Dietary Supplements
http://odp.od.nih.gov/ods/

Accessed on: 19 June 2000   *Ranking:* **

Sponsor: The **Office of Dietary Supplements** (ODS), formally established in 1995, is a congressionally mandated office in the Office of the Director, National Institutes of Health (NIH). The ODS supports research and disseminates research results in the area of dietary supplements. Among its main objectives are the following: to explore the role of dietary supplements to improve health care; and to promote scientific study of dietary supplements in maintaining health and preventing chronic disease.

Description: Dietary supplements are not generally well-understood at this point, so one of the first important contributions made by the Web site of the ODS is to offer a complete and careful definition of *dietary supplements* which goes far beyond the common notion of vitamins, minerals, other nutrients and botanical (or herbal) preparations taken to add something to one's regular diet that is perceived to be missing or of particular benefit. Part of the reason for a painstaking definition is that in order for government to deal appropriately with such products, precise legal terms had to be drawn up which would identify exactly what is to be regulated and studied. Indeed, the details actually come from the *Dietary Supplement Health and Education Act* (DSHEA, Public Law 103-417, October 25, 1994), which is an amendment to the U.S. *Federal Food, Drug and Cosmetic Act* of 1958. The ODS site provides a hyperlink that leads to a very good explanation of the DSHEA on the Web site of the U.S. Food and Drug Administration's Center for Food Safety and Applied Nutrition. One of the other main reasons to visit this Web site at the moment is the free access it offers to the *International Bibliographic Information on Dietary Supplements* (IBIDS) database. This collection of citations to published, peer-reviewed, international, scientific literature on dietary supplements draws upon medical and scientific databases already in existence. Literature in IBIDS currently comes from AGRICOLA, MEDLINE, and an agricultural database known as AGRIS International. There are plans to mine other databases for appropriate citations to add to IBIDS in the future. A second database, to be known as CARDS (*Computer Access to Research on Dietary Supplements*), will eventually offer access to federally supported research in progress on subjects of interest. A page called *Other Relevant Links* is very worthy of examination in that it brings together a great many Web sites of agencies and organizations engaged in similar or related work both in and outside the U.S. There are announcements, news releases, conference advertisements, and information about grants, awards, and partnering opportunities also available on this site. A number of federal government publications (mainly conferences and bibliographies) are available in PDF or HTML formats on the site. As interest increases and more research on dietary supplements becomes available, this will be a site to watch.

The Vegetarian Society of the United Kingdom
http://www.vegsoc.org/

Accessed on: 28 May 2000   *Ranking*: ****

Sponsor: The **Vegetarian Society of the United Kingdom** is the oldest vegetarian organization in the world and is the leading voice and authority on vegetarianism. It works to accomplish its goals by raising awareness of vegetarianism and surrounding issues through campaigning, educating, providing information, research and working with the food industry.

Description: The Web site of the Vegetarian Society offers a variety of interesting features not found elsewhere. *New Veggies* explains the choice to people who may be contemplating the meat-free alternative and it offers definitions of bewildering terms and arguments in favor of the vegetarian choice. There is a section for youth and school children with school activities for teachers, vegetarian pen pals, and a virtual classroom with resources divided into "primary" and "secondary" categories for easy use by teachers. In the *Health and Nutrition* section, there are resources to deal with questions such as whether vegetarians get enough protein and other essential nutrients. Beyond that, there is a wealth of information about vegetarianism for people at all stages of life. There is information on special diets for allergies, gluten-free diets, and how vegetarian choices can reduce your risk of a whole host of diseases that are now being discovered to be food-related. A *Leisure & Lifestyle Directory* lists hotels, guesthouses, B&B's, as well as caterers and restaurants in the United Kingdom which offer vegetarian choices. The *Cordon Vert Cookery School* occupies a part of the Web site offering recipes, articles on vegetarian food and drink, and cookery classes. The usual features—a search engine for the site, news, and shopping —round out this site.

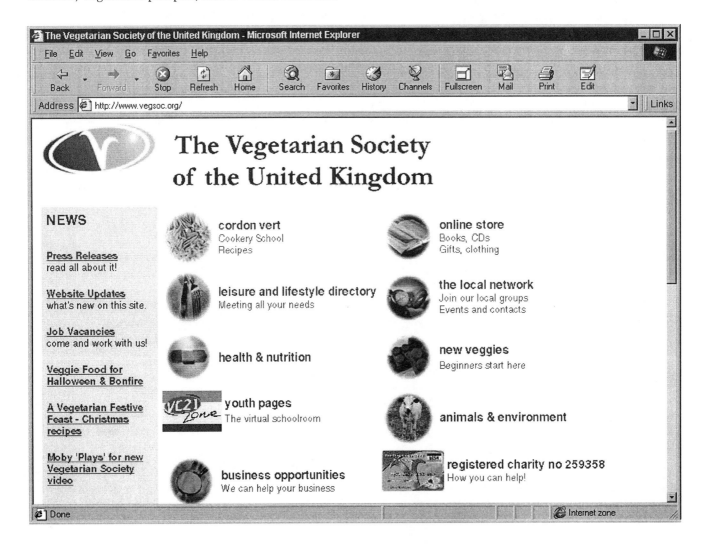

g. Herbs and Herbal Remedies

About.com: Herbs for Health

http://herbsforhealth.about.com/health/herbsforhealth/

Accessed on: 28 May 2000   *Ranking*: ***

Sponsor: Juli Kight is your *About.com* guide to herbs; she has been working with herbs for about 15 years and is a member of the Herb Research Foundation, the National Center for Homeopathy, the Flower Essence Society, the American Herbalists Guild, and is a student of the Michael Tierra's East West Planetary Herbalism.

Description: Although, strictly speaking, the business of this site is not complementary and alternative therapeutics, the question of CAM uses of herbs is bound to arise wherever herbs are discussed. The list of subjects in the left-hand column on this site includes: *Herbs and Health, American Indian Herbs, Aromatherapy, Ayurvedic Herbs, Cancer, Chinese Herbalism*, and so on. Each subject offers a series of articles on that topic which is well-written and informative. The featured articles at the time of review were about lettuce opium, images of herbs (important to identification), and catnip. In the *Essentials* section, there are articles about herbs and allergies, herbs and pregnancy, and a FAQ for beginners. There is also a discussion forum on *Herbs and Health*, and you can join a chat group if you wish to discuss any aspect of herbs or ask a question. As on all *About.com* sites, you can shop for books and videos and subscribe to a newsletter. Related *About.com* sites are listed—on Gardening, Healing, and Vegetarianism.

Algy's Herb Page

http://www.algy.com/herb/index.html

Accessed on: 28 May 2000   *Ranking*: **

Sponsor: No information that explains who manages the page, or for what purposes it appears on the Web site, but from its subtitle "A *BBS for the discussion of herbs and their uses*," one can draw certain conclusions.

Description: The lovely old-fashioned image on the home page of **Algy's Herb Page** might have come from an old seed catalog but it offers a menu of the four main parts of this site: the *apothecary* (talk about medicinal herbs and their uses), the *potting shed* (growing, harvesting and crafting with herbs), the *greenhouse* (for promoting biodiversity and exchanging seeds), and finally the *kitchen* (for culinary uses of herbs). Under each of these menu items, a bewildering array of messages can be found posted to the discussion list. The value of the message archives provided is far from clear. The best thing about this Web site is the massive collection of links to other herb sites on the Internet, arranged into two categories: medicinal herbs, and growing herbs. The database is searchable, or you can simply see lists of all the herb sites in eight different categories. When displayed in a table, there are very brief annotations and the titles are clickable (i.e., they are hyperlinked). From many of the pages, it is difficult to return to the home page since HOME has been left off the clickable menu. This site is not really intended for the browsing public looking for alternative medicine. It probably appeals only to hard-core herbalists.

Herbal Hall

http://herb.com/herbal.html

Accessed on: 28 May 2000   *Ranking*: *

Sponsor: No information on the **Herbal Hall** site could be found to indicate who is responsible for its creation nor what it is intended to accomplish.

Description: The **Herbal Hall** Web site is one of the oldest herbal sites on the Internet. This is a site where you can actually consult herbal monographs, difficult to find in print, unless you happened to be in just the right sort of library collection. Now, on once more reviewing the site after a lapse of time, I find much of the initial attraction has worn thin. Its Reference section still offers Michael Moore's *Herbal Reference Library*, a small list of schools and herbal apprenticeships, and *Dr. Duke's Phytochemical and Ethnobotanical Databases*. But the *Books* section was last updated in 1997! The *Herb Walk* still offers a variety of sources of images of herbs and the *Herb Mail* section still offers discussion lists for nutritive and medicinal herbalism, and a quick scan of postings shows that it has been recently used. The *Medicinal Herb FAQ* is so large that it is presented in seven parts, but there does not seem to be any index external to the seven parts, nor any way to search it. The list of Links offered is unannotated and the News section seems neglected. It had only one item at the time of review. The site still has valuable features but they look dated and a bit woebegone.

The Natural Pharmacist

http://www.tnp.com/home.asp

Accessed on: 29 May 2000   *Ranking*: ****

Sponsor: **The Natural Pharmacist**, or **TNP.com**, as it is known, is a division of Prima Communications, Inc. which publishes a variety of CAM books. The slogan: "*Science* *based natural health information you can trust"* appears at the top of every page on the **TNP.com** site. The list of advisors and contributors to the site is impressive—in addition to R.N.s, M.D.s and Ph.D.s there are also many other professionals appearing in the list, such as R.D. (Registered Dietitian), N.D. (Naturopathic Doctor), D.O. (Doctor of Osteopathy) and Pharm.D (Pharmacist). These qualifications are doubtless included to substantiate the credibility of the site.

Description: TNP.com is a site with a focus on natural medicine and therapeutics, which really means herbal products and supplements. The site centers around a database known as the **TNP Encyclopedia** which offers three approaches to its contents. You can search for conditions (such as acne, peptic ulcers, or rheumatoid arthritis); for herbs and supplements (such as feverfew, red clover, or vitamin E); or for herb-drug interactions (herbs which interact with acetaminophen, for instance). If you look up a condition, the article you access will indicate whether there are any herbal or natural treatments known for that condition. Searching for *Benign prostatic hypertrophy*, identifies saw palmetto, among other natural therapies. If you choose to look up an herb, such as *Nettle*, you will find that among its uses, it is also recommended for *Benign prostatic hyperplasia*. The drug interactions section of the encyclopedia will alert you to both positive interactions of herbs and supplements with drugs you may be taking, as well as to harmful or negative interactions. Much of the information in the **TNP Encyclopedia** comes from *the Natural Health Bible* by Steven Bratman, M.D., David J. Kroll, Ph.D. and Angelo DePalma, Ph.D. All of the authors are contributors on this site. The articles found at **TNP.com** are highly referenced and authoritative. Articles on vitamins, for instance, typically offer information about requirements and sources of the vitamin, therapeutic dosages and uses, the scientific

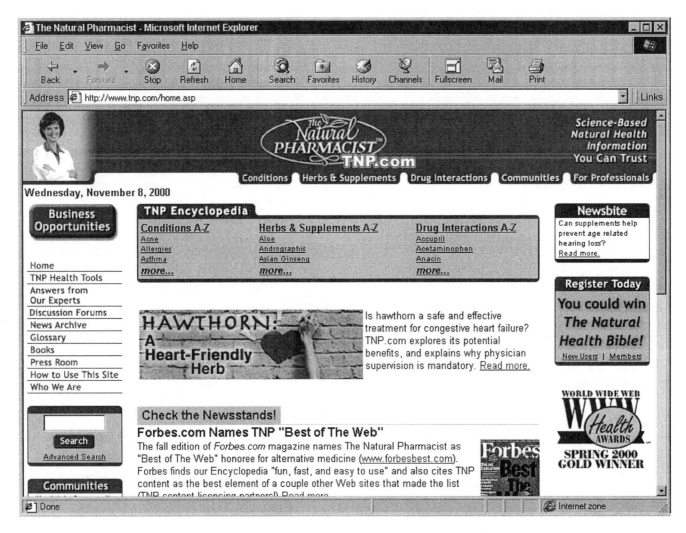

evidence for recommended use, and safety issues and interactions. The articles on various conditions in the encyclopedia are written to be skimmed quickly. In a section called *Conditions in depth,* you find more comprehensive coverage. **TNP.com** offers tools (interactive questionnaires) which help determine what supplements may be useful to you, what herbs and nutrients may alleviate common health conditions, and which herbs and nutrients may interact with any medication you may be currently taking. There are sections for people with diabetes, Alzheimer's disease, and many other common chronic conditions. There is a section for health professionals, which offers articles such as *"Brief History of Herbal Medicine," "Level of Scientific Evidence in Alternative Medicine,"* and *"Quick Guide to Clinical Evidence."* There are FAQs on a great many conditions, a news archive focusing on herbal products and treatments, a glossary of terms you may encounter in reading on the site, and a bookstore. This trustworthy site is remarkably free from sales pitches to buy vitamins, herbs and dietary supplements and commendably has no obvious commercial intent.

onhealth Alternative Herbal Index

http://onhealth.com/alternative/resource/herbs/
    index.asp

Accessed on: 29 May 2000   *Ranking*: ****

Sponsor: onhealth is a commercial venture on the Internet which has an established policy of editorial independence, a board of distinguished medical advisors, many awards, and a large presence on the Web in the area of health information.

Description: The **Alternative Herbal Index** portion of the *onhealth* site is only a small part of a larger endeavor on alternative health, which is in turn part of the overall *onhealth* Web publishing venture. The Index is noteworthy because its entries are based on the famous

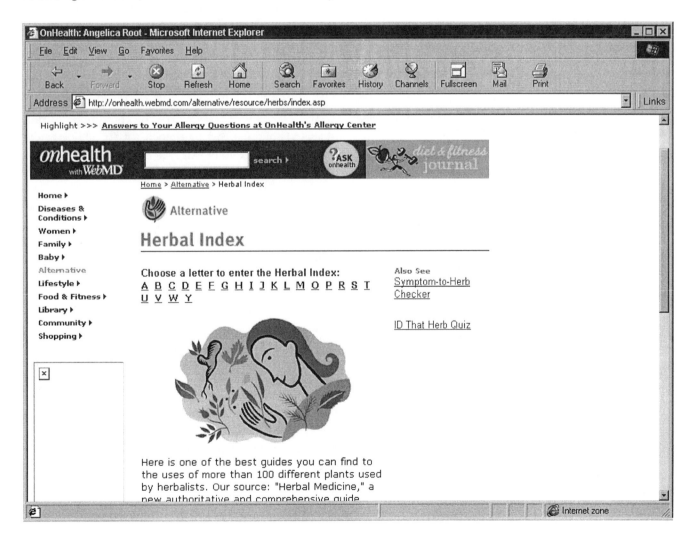

German Commission E monographs, probably the most authoritative printed source on the efficacy and uses of herbal remedies available today. There are about 100 herb entries in the *onhealth* index, each of which is lengthy and erudite but can be useful to the lay public. The entry on garlic is a case in point: after introducing the Latin and pharmacopeial names, the monograph provides a lengthy overview of uses for garlic, including a summary of the clinical trials and meta-analyses which have tested its efficacy for specific uses. There is a description of garlic, an account of its chemistry and pharmacology, uses, contraindications, side effects, interactions with drugs, dosage and administration, and a long list of references to publications cited. The entries on herbs in this list are substantial and very similar to those in any drug handbook used by prescribing physicians. Hyperlinks off to the side of the page provide access to related articles. This is a wonderful and authoritative source of information on herbs and their uses in CAM therapies.

h. Homeopathy, Naturopathy, Osteopathy

American Association of Colleges of Osteopathic Medicine

http://www.aacom.org/

Accessed on: 30 May 2000   *Ranking*: **

Sponsor: The **American Association of Colleges of Osteopathic Medicine** (AACOM) exists to serve the administration, faculty, and students of the 19-member osteopathic medical schools in the United States through its centralized application service, government relations, finance, communications, and research/ information departments.

Description: In a very real sense, osteopathy ought not to be considered a CAM discipline, since D.O.s employ modern medicine and surgery techniques, are widely accepted, and practice side by side with M.D.s in many parts of North America. Osteopaths remain somewhat "alternative" in their approach to health care, partly because osteopathy takes a holistic approach to the patient and because of the manipulative techniques osteopaths employ. The AACOM Web site is very definitely the site of an educational organization in that it addresses itself largely to the prospective student of osteopathic medicine at the same time as presenting much useful information of interest to the public. The

sections on *Osteopathic Medicine* and *Osteopathic Medical Education* offer an explanation of the philosophy of the discipline and a brief account of its origins in post–Civil War Missouri. The student can learn what to expect in an osteopathic college, or will be able to do so when the site is complete. At the time of review, chunks of material were "under construction." There is a list of the 19 colleges offering the degree of D.O., with very complete information on each, and a link to their Web sites. Several of these colleges have even more complete information on the origins and culture of the discipline and will be of some interest to those wanting to follow up and learn more about the profession.

American Association of Naturopathic Physicians

http://www.naturopathic.org/

Accessed on: 29 May 2000   *Ranking*: **

Sponsor: The **American Association of Naturopathic Physicians** (AANP), in Seattle, WA, is the professional association for licensed and licensable N.D.s (naturopathic doctors) in the United States.

Description: The AANP Web site is full of useful information if you want to know more about the practice of naturopathy in North America. Here can be found the standard features of most professional Web sites in health care: a basic explanation of what the profession does and how members are trained, a list of schools where training is offered in North America, how accreditation of these schools is managed, and a directory of members so that the public can locate practitioners. There is a "library" of articles (some of which is password-protected, for members only), and an extensive collection of links to other sites. Because naturopathy is still an "emerging" profession in health care—fighting for respect, if not for recognition—there is a section called *Politics*. This section deals with issues focusing on licensing and registration, and the legalities of practice in the various states where N.D.s are not yet licensed. *Politics* offers an interesting glimpse into a profession fighting for a place in primary care. You can buy books on this site, engage in chat, join a message board, find information about the annual convention, and so on. Unfortunately, links often open extra windows without warning and, before you know it, you have three or four of them opened simultaneously. Overall, the site has the look of one that just grew and grew through add-ons, and is now in need of some rationalization, but it is not hard to use.

Canadian Naturopathic Association
http://www.naturopathicassoc.ca/

Accessed on: 30 May 2000   *Ranking*: **

Sponsor: The **Canadian Naturopathic Association** (CNA) is a not-for-profit professional association representing the interests of naturopathic doctors and promoting naturopathic medicine throughout Canada.

Description: The following statement from the home page of the CNA Web site provides a good introduction to Naturopathy: "Naturopathic medicine integrates natural healing therapies including botanical medicine, homeopathy, clinical nutrition, hydrotherapy, naturopathic manipulation, Traditional Chinese Medicine/Acupuncture, and prevention and lifestyle counseling." Naturopathy employs a number of practices which may be thought to be specific to other CAM modalities and Doctors of Naturopathy (N.D.s) are trained to know when to refer patients who cannot be treated with the methods they employ. This site provides access to a searchable database of N.D.s practicing in Canada which can be searched by name or by province. You can also find a list of provincial associations of N.D.s and of licensing boards in the four provinces where N.D.s are licensed to practice. There is also minimal information about the four colleges in North America where N.D.s are trained with e-mail addresses and Web site links. There is a curious list of suppliers of products used by naturopaths with no street addresses or contact information (such as telephone number or postal address) shown for any of them. The *Questions & Answers* is a collection of commonly asked questions with brief answers relating to the kind of treatments N.D.s use, training, and the advantages of naturopathic care. There is a French version of the site, but it is merely a brief summary of the information available in English. The site is easy to navigate.

National Center for Homeopathy
http://www.healthy.net/nch/

Accessed on: 29 May 2000   *Ranking*: ***

Sponsor: The **National Center for Homeopathy** (NCH), in Alexandria, VA, is a membership organization with a mission: "to promote health through homeopathy." The center provides general education to the public, and specific programs for homeopaths.

Description: The *Introduction to Homeopathy* on the NCH Web site labels it as *Natural medicine for the 21ˢᵗ century*. The articles linked to this introductory page explain the discipline to the public and emphasize the gentle, safe, and effective character of this method of treatment. There is an account of how homeopathy differs from conventional medicine and a description of homeopathic medicines for those who are curious about how those minute quantities of active ingredients can be expected to effect a cure. There is an interesting account of the history of homeopathy in the United States and the legalities involved in its practice today. The site also offers access to abstracts of published research about homeopathy, lists of education and consulting services in homeopathy in all parts of the United States and Canada, and an article on training for the discipline. One of the most useful features of the site is its directory of homeopaths; since they are often difficult to identify from qualifications alone. You can search by a variety of means, but the simplest way is by geographical location. The is a serviceable and well-constructed site.

Osteopathic.com — The Osteopathic Medicine Resource
http://osteopathic.com/ocom.html

Accessed on: 30 May 2000   *Ranking*: **

Sponsor: The *StudentDoctor Network* is an independent resource that offers the **Osteopathic.com** Web site, among many other resources for student physicians. It is operated by SDN Communications, Inc., a privately held company. **Osteopathic.com** provides an international open forum for osteopathic students and serves to increase awareness of osteopathic medicine.

Description: This site offers information about osteopathic medicine and physicians, helps to locate a D.O. in the United States, and allows students and pre-meds to learn more about what lies ahead of them, educationally. There is an interesting *Osteopathic Historical Timeline*, covering 1874 to 1999, full of interesting bits of osteopathic history. *Gregory's Osteopathic Links* is a **Yahoo**-style directory of Web sites of interest to anyone interested in osteopathy. The site is small, but attractive and straightforward.

i. Reflexology

Association of Reflexologists
http://www.reflexology.org/aor/

Accessed on: 31 May 2000   *Ranking*: *

Sponsor: The **Association of Reflexologists** is a British professional organization founded in 1984 which unites practitioners concerned about training and standards in the profession.

Description: The Web site of the **Association of Reflexologists** (AoR) offers an introduction to the practice of reflexology in the United Kingdom. Under the first heading on the page *The Healing Art of Reflexology*, there is a brief introduction — for the public — of what reflexology is all about. This page has a copyright date of 1993. The next link on the homepage is to an article entitled *"Reflexology in the UK,"* which describes how reflexology came to the U.K. from the U.S. in the 1960s, gives an account of early training standards and education, the growth of organizations of practitioners, and the subsequent push for national occupational standards, and possibly, licensing, in the future. This page bears a copyright date of 1997. There is a further history of the AoR itself, and much repetition of the history of the drive toward accredited training programs and national standards. The page was last revised in 1998. The site offers access to a directory of its members in the U.K. and abroad. The directory bears a revision date of 11 May 2000. There is also information under the heading *Training as a Reflexologist*, which is directed at the prospective student/practitioner and reflects the working situation in Britain. One can also find on this site a listing of accredited courses in the U.K. and a lengthy list of books, charts, and videos on reflexology compiled by Anthony Larkin, an Irish reflexologist. This page was last updated in February 1999. There is a small collection of articles published by the association and a large list of links to other reflexology sites on the Internet, bearing no date of revision. The site is useful as an introduction to the discipline, but needs a lot of consolidation and updating. Its design is quite rudimentary.

Ontario College of Reflexology

http://www.ocr.edu/

Accessed on: 31 May 2000   *Ranking*: ***

Sponsor: The Ontario College of Reflexology (OCR) is not merely an educational institution; it is also a body of practitioners lobbying the Government of Ontario to grant them recognition as a self-governing licensing body, which would regulate the profession in Ontario.

Description: The Web site of the OCR is created by somebody who likes large buttons with words and arrows on them as navigational aids. The site advertises courses in reflexology offered by the OCR, and includes course descriptions and information about examinations, distance education courses, including correspondence courses and courses offered on the Internet. The

curriculum and credit system leading to professional qualifications is explained. Foot charts and books on reflexology are available for sale and the site supports secure online ordering. The site menu seems to meander through links to the products catalog, a bulletin board, a mechanism for feedback from the public, links to other reflexology sites, a newsletter, a directory of practitioners (certified by the OCR) throughout Canada, to the Reflexology Registration Council of Ontario, and to a list of qualified teachers of reflexology recognized by the OCR. A survey of reflexologists which is intended, when complete, to provide statistical and demographic information about the profession is being conducted via the Web site and forms can be downloaded and mailed back, or completed on the Internet and sent by e-mail. The site is busy, with boxes and arrows and navigational aids at the foot of the page, as well as along the left margin, in symbols and text. The word *overdone* comes to mind in visiting this site but there is much here. You can easily find what there is on the site.

j. Reiki

International Center for Reiki Training

http://www.reiki.org/

Accessed on: 31 May 2000   *Ranking*: ***

Sponsor: The **International Center for Reiki Training** (ICRT), in Southfield, MI, is a nonprofit organization dedicated to the re-establishment of Reiki energies in our modern world.

Description: Reiki is a technique for stress reduction and relaxation that allows everyone to tap into an unlimited supply of "life force energy" to improve health and enhance the quality of life. It is a very spiritual mode of CAM, but does not involve belief. The Web site of the ICRT is remarkable because it really helps one to understand this conundrum. It consists of a number of linked "home pages:" home page for classes, an article archive, quarterly newsletter, home page for FAQs, home page for current topics, home page for the center itself, home page for healing, home page for developing your own Reiki practice, and a home page for the global healing network. There is also a search engine for the site (because of its size) and a Reiki store that sells tapes, books, teaching materials, clothing, art prints and posters, and other paraphernalia. Although the intended audience of this site is the student or the prospective student/practitioner of Reiki, the curious public will find much to hold its attention. The FAQ section offers articles with some depth in answer to standard questions such as "What is Reiki?" and "How does it work?" The history of Reiki and its various versions or branches, named after important teachers, is fascinating and is offered here in detail. There is also a large list of Reiki Internet resources. It is necessary to do a lot of scrolling on this site since the lists offered are lengthy, and everything seems to be oriented vertically. The site is pleasantly uncluttered, though, and links on the various homepages aid in navigation.

The Reiki Page
http://Reiki.7gen.com/

Accessed on: 31 May 2000   *Ranking*: **

Sponsor: David Herron, who calls himself the "convenor" of **The Reiki Page**, is trained in Hypnotherapy, Massage Therapy, Reiki, Drisana, Cellular Electromagnetic Field Balancing (CELF), and Computer Science. By day he "heals" computer software and by night he assists people with their healing using the gifts that have come his way.

Description: **The Reiki Page** is an unassuming small Web site without much craft or design but with a lot of information about the discipline. It is divided, after a general introduction, into sections for *development* (the history and ethical principles of the discipline), *applying Reiki* (healing and practitioners), and *practitioner information* (choosing a teacher, charging for Reiki, energy healing). Much of what is conveyed here about the discipline is whispered in the reverent tone of the "convenor." Clearly, there is spirituality, or at least mysticism, at the heart of this particular branch of CAM. David Herron writes: "Reiki is very easily learned, very simple to use, and beneficial for all. It is one of many forms of healing through the use of the natural forces which were given the name Chi by ancient Chinese mystics. Some forms of healing using Chi energy forces are Chi Gong, Pranic Healing, Chelation (as taught by Barbara Brennan and Rosalyn Bruyere), and Polarity Balancing. All (apparently) use the same energies, with the difference being techniques of application and an energy quality commonly known as vibration." If you want to know more about this healing method, David Herron's site is a good place to develop a feeling for it.

k. Spirituality and Meditation

Foundation for International Spiritual Unfoldment
http://www.fisu.org/

Accessed on: 3 June 2000   *Ranking*: **

Sponsor: The **Foundation for International Spiritual Unfoldment** (FISU) is dedicated to promote and propagate the teachings of Gururaj Ananda Yogi; it is a nondenominational, nonsectarian organization located in the United Kingdom. Meditation is at the center of the practices taught by FISU and the argument that meditation is beneficial to health appears prominently on this site.

Description: The FISU Web site is graphically simple and full of clickable lists, easy enough to navigate, but not particularly conducive to a satisfying information experience. A large part of the site is devoted to a general introduction to the health benefits of meditation, but no scientific evidence or claim to this knowledge is offered. There is a lengthy and helpful FAQ, which addresses meditation and its benefits, stresses the nondenominational nature of the organization, differentiates between meditation and prayer, and gives general information about courses and their cost. The site contains separate pages of information on the original guru and his son, who continues to do his father's work, and a "satsang" (talk, or sermon) from the work of Gururaj Ananda Yogi, on *"The Purpose of Life."*

National Federation of Spiritual Healers
http://www.nfsh.org.uk/

Accessed on: 3 June 2000   *Ranking*: ****

Sponsor: The **National Federation of Spiritual Healers** (NFSH) is a registered charity in the United Kingdom which unites spiritual healers through training and support; it has a strict code of conduct, and complaints and discipline procedures. It assists those who want to find healers, both nearby, in person, and for distant healing. NFSH promotes research into healing. It is not associated with any religion.

Description: The NFSH Web site is extremely well-designed, attractive, easy to read and helpful. No page is longer than one screen, and everything on the screen is well placed to make an unhurried, restful, and very serious impression on the viewer. Links are, generally, in the center of the screen and on the left; and there is always a "back" link to the previous page. The site explains what healing is in simple terms: "Healing is the channeling of energies by the healer to re-energize the patient to deal with illness or injury," and goes on, in a brief FAQ, to explain that "faith" as normally understood (religious faith) is not necessary. The site offers information about the NFSH itself, courses, referrals (in the U.K. only), and distance healing and local centers throughout the U.K. No outrageous claims are made, rather it is discreetly pointed out that there is a very high degree of public acceptance of spiritual healing in the U.K. since 1965, when more than 1,500 hospitals gave permission for spiritual healers to attend patients upon request.

The Transcendental Meditation Program (Maharishi Mahesh Yogi)

http://www.tm.org/

Accessed on: 31 May 2000   *Ranking*: **

Sponsor: Maharishi Vedic Science is a corporation promoting health and success in life through the Maharishi Vedic Universities and Schools and Web sites such as this one.

Description: Be prepared when you access this site to be overwhelmed with text, quotations, links, and icons. The layout is frenetic. "The Transcendental Meditation® (TM®) program of Maharishi Mahesh Yogi is the single most effective technique available for gaining deep relaxation, eliminating stress, promoting health, increasing creativity and intelligence, and attaining inner happiness and fulfillment." Claims abound, and the evidence for them is collected in a bibliography of 500 scientific studies, which can be consulted on the site. Everything seems to be at a fever-pitch and may be fairly characterized as "marketing." You can learn all about Transcendental Meditation through this site, but not on it. You have to enter your telephone area code and click to be connected to the nearest Maharishi Vedic University, School or Center which, presumably, will teach you. There is no mention of fees or any of the mundane details of classes or how long it takes, just a determined sales pitch and citations to proof in superabundance that TM works.

I. Therapeutic Touch

Healing Touch International, Inc.

http://www.healingtouch.net/

Accessed on: 4 June 2000   *Ranking*: ***

Sponsor: **Healing Touch International, Inc.**, exists to meet the needs of its members (nurses, other health care professionals and lay people who provide "heart centered care"), to offer education and certification of practitioners and instructors, to set standards of practice and an international code of ethics for practitioners, and to promote "scholarly development" of healing touch care.

Description: The **Healing Touch International, Inc.** Web site is maintained at the Colorado Center for Healing Touch, in Lakewood, CO. The home page concentrates on introducing the reader to the concept of healing touch, which is "a type of alternative healing using hands-on and energy-based techniques to balance and align the human energy field." In fact, the approach used by this organization appears to be more integrative than alternative. The introduction suggests that therapeutic touch is used by nurses, doctors and other health care workers in hospitals and elsewhere to augment other therapies and to hasten healing, and is not intended to replace other modalities. In addition to its mission statement, scope of practice, code of ethics, and international standards of practice, the site offers information about courses available to those who wish to become practitioners. Healing Touch was begun by a nurse named Janet Mentgen, who had been practicing "energy-based care" in Denver, CO, since 1980. The instructional program was subsequently affiliated with, and endorsed by, the American Holistic Nurses Association (AHNA). Courses are also offered in other countries: Canada, Australia, New Zealand, and the Netherlands. The site offers access to the separate Web site of **Healing Touch Canada, Inc.** (http://www.pathcom.com/~htcanada/), and to a page on Healing Touch in the Netherlands. Other links to Australia, New Zealand and South Africa were "under construction" at the time of review. You can consult lists of practitioners throughout the United States (and beyond) on this site, and find support groups and clinics. Under the "Research" heading, there is a bibliography of more than 700 articles (updated to January 1999) in a great variety of journals (both popular and scientific) arranged in five categories for easy access: *Energy Medicine, Healing Touch, Therapeutic Touch, Holistic and Miscellaneous,* and *Spirituality.* The site offers rebuttals of articles in the recent health care press which "debunk" therapeutic touch under the heading: *White Papers,* and a full text newsletter with about nine years of backfiles supposedly available, but there was nothing accessible beyond the current issue at the time of this review. There are links to related groups, mostly affiliates in other countries, but two in particular are worth noting: the *Healing Touch Spiritual Ministry*, and *Healing Touch for Animals*. There is nothing noteworthy about the design of this site, except in a few cases where it does not work because the text overruns borders. It is generally functional, although initially slow to load.

Therapeutic Touch Network of Ontario
http://www.therapeutictouchnetwk.com/

Accessed on: 4 June 2000   *Ranking*: **

Sponsor: The **Therapeutic Touch Network of Ontario** promotes the practice and acceptance of Therapeutic Touch as developed by Dolores Krieger and Dora Kunz. It is a nonprofit organization engaged in teaching, research and patient care; it puts those in need in touch with practitioners.

Description: The **Therapeutic Touch Network of Ontario** Web site has a simple, graphically striking design and a lot of information to offer. There is a list of research papers recently collected for use in a meta-analysis by a Ph.D. nurse researcher, a list of teachers, a course list that is very vague, simply referring to the listing of teachers and suggesting a check of the course offerings at community colleges. There is also a list of practice groups where the student can learn through participation. A small list of links to related Web sites offers access to a French site in alternative medicine and several sites on energy medicine and other eclectic health care topics. Articles mounted on the site come from the network newsletter. E-mail contacts with various officers of the group are also offered.

m. Skepticism/Fraud

Alternative Health News Online
http://www.altmedicine.com/

Accessed on: 22 May 2000   *Ranking*: **

Sponsor: Frank Grazian, editor and publisher of **Alternative Health News Online**, is a Professor Emeritus of Communications at Rowan University in New Jersey and has studied many of the CAM modalities.

Description: **Alternative Health News Online** (AHNO) approaches CAM cautiously, with prominent disclaimers and warnings displayed. It promotes the philosophy that alternative medicine should be considered a supplement to traditional medicine and

not a replacement for it. Nonetheless, the site offers information on techniques and approaches that it believes are valid and worthy of consideration. There is a free weekly newsletter that you can sign up to receive, frequent health news bulletins on various CAM related topics, and the ability to search the entire site for information of interest. There are sections for diet and nutrition, mind/body control, alternative medical systems (homeopathy, naturopathy, Chinese medicine, Ayurvedic medicine, etc.), manual healing, and longevity. AHNO reads somewhat like a newspaper in that its various sections reveal the touch of an investigative journalist. The journalistic approach proves to be disappointing veneer. In the end, much of the content of the site comes from links to other sources, rather than from the compiler of the site himself. Furthermore, since each topic (e.g., phytochemicals, vegetarianism, homeopathic medicine) is afforded only one link, the apparently rich depth of the site is rather more limited than one would like, especially when the links offered are no longer active. The *Recommended Books* section seems to offer more of the journalist's touch and there is a collection of links to daily compilations of health news from major news sources, both print and electronic.

Dictionary of Alternative-Medicine Methods
http://www.acsh.org/dictionary/index.html

Accessed on: 5 June 2000   *Ranking*: **

Sponsor: Jack Raso, M.S., R.D., author of the **Dictionary of Alternative-Medicine Methods**, is director of publications at the American Council on Science and Health (ACSH), a contributing editor to *The Scientific Review of Alternative Medicine*, and the former editor of *Nutrition Forum* newsletter. Mr. Raso is also a board member of The National Council Against Health Fraud and coordinator of its Task Force on Dubious Healthcare Credentials. The ACSH "is a consumer education consortium concerned with issues related to food, nutrition, chemicals, pharmaceuticals, lifestyle, the environment and health. It was founded in 1978 by a group of scientists who had become concerned that many important public policies related to health and the environment did not have a sound scientific basis." The voice of ACSH "is a unique voice, backed by mainstream science, defending the achievements and benefits of responsible technology within America's free-enterprise system."

Description: The **Dictionary** appears on the ACSH Web site. Given the above characterization of its host (in words supplied by the ACSH itself), how could the **Dictionary** be expected to be sympathetic to CAM? It is definitely not, but on the other hand, it claims not to be antipathetic, wishing to present a non-judgmental view. The nonjudgmental approach is not maintained throughout. It must be said at the outset that the **Dictionary** does not attempt to tackle the whole of alternative medicine. Perhaps more is planned but the part presented at the moment on the Web site deals only with *Mystical, Supernaturalistic, and/or Vitalistic Methods*. It excludes, therefore, *Naturalistic (Nonsupernaturalistic and Nonmystical) Methods*, by definition. This distinction between two kinds of alternative medicine is not one to be found elsewhere. It means, among other things, that *Bach flower therapy* warrants an entry, but *chiropractic* does not. If you want an example of how "nonjudgmental" the site is, read the entry on *Bach flower therapy*. The choice of quotations and the lexicographer's habit of "supposing" what he apparently does not understand leave little doubt about the claimed impartiality. A brief glance at the list of peer reviewers and their credentials seems to confirm the notion that the deck is stacked against CAM. There are a great many M.D.s, Ph.D.s, D.D.S.s, and the like, but no peer reviewers in the list who have any obvious alternative medicine qualifications. Still, one can learn a lot about a whole variety of quite recondite topics: everything from *Abhyanga* to *Zulu Sangoma bones* is included, and there is quite a lot in between these two, the first and last entries. What it adds to the sum of our knowledge about CAM is not clear, but it certainly makes a contribution to cataloguing some of the more unusual therapeutic modalities. The site is graphically straightforward and easy-to-use, although it relies on alphabetic entry and searching of each letter of the alphabet rather than offering a site-specific search engine.

Healthwatcher: Canada's Best Consumer Health Watchdog

http://www.healthwatcher.net/

Accessed on: 6 June 2000   *Ranking*: *

Sponsor: I can find no information on the site that indicates who is responsible for **Healthwatcher**, nor any that spells out the aims and objectives of the site. There is a postal address in Waterloo, ON, but no names or identification of interests are revealed.

Description: **Healthwatcher** appears to be a journalistic effort to alert visitors to consumer concerns about health. Thus, the *Hot Topics* column on the day that the site was reviewed dealt with *Ecstasy deaths, Elk velvet antlers, Chelation racket,* and *Shark cartilage*. Many of the topics are, recognizably, within the field of CAM. In the main "news" of the day were stories about an E. coli outbreak in the water supply of a small Ontario town, and the headline: "*Quack University plans for downtown Hamilton.*" The quality of journalism on this site is not much above that in your typical grocery store tabloid newspaper. Derogatory terms are freely thrown about and sensationalism is the order of the day to grab the reader's attention. The site seems to be modeled to some extent on the **Quackwatch** site (reviewed below) and has companion chiropractic and nutrition sections, which seem designed to denigrate and belittle rather than to investigate and weigh claims. At the same time, there are collections of articles, which seem to embody serious concern about real threats to the health of children and to provide a public service. The content of the site is very mixed, expressing sympathetic concern with some health threats, a nasty sensational interest in others, and a very determined antipathy to CAM practices and practitioners. There is a lot of advertising that blinks from little boxes on every page. The effect of all this activity detracts from the value of the site. It is hard to take seriously.

National Health Care Anti-Fraud Association

http://www.nhcaa.org/

Accessed on: 6 June 2000   *Ranking*: **

Sponsor: Founded in 1985 by several private health insurers and U.S. federal/state law enforcement officials, the National Health Care Anti-Fraud Association (NHCAA) is a unique, issue-based organization comprising private- and public-sector organizations and individuals responsible for the detection, investigation, prosecution and prevention of health care fraud.

Description: The NHCAA Web site offers guidelines that define health care fraud as "an intentional deception or misrepresentation that the individual or entity makes knowing that the misrepresentation could result in some unauthorized benefit to the individual, or the entity or to some other party. The most common kind of fraud involves a false statement, misrepresentation or deliberate omission that is critical to the determination of benefits payable. Fraudulent activities are almost invariably criminal, although the specific nature or degree of the criminal acts may vary from state to state." It is as likely that cases of health care fraud will be apprehended among CAM providers as among those practicing conventional medicine. The Web site of the NHCAA makes no reference to either; it merely offers information about what constitutes fraud in health care and what kind of impact that sort of criminal behavior has on health care spending in the United States. In actual fact, since very little CAM therapy is reimbursed by health insurance in the United States, it is unlikely that the NHCAA is much concerned with fraudulent CAM practice. The site is interesting in terms of the estimated size of fraudulent activity in health care (anywhere from 3 to 10 percent of money spent on health annually in the United States, or more than $30 billion per year). The design of this site is sophisticated and attractive, although the dark backgrounds make some of the print hard to read.

Quackwatch

http://www.quackwatch.com/index.html

Accessed on: 5 June 2000   *Ranking*: **

Sponsor: Stephen Barrett, M.D., a retired psychiatrist who resides in Allentown, PA, is a nationally renowned author, editor, and consumer advocate. An expert in medical communications, he is medical editor of Prometheus Books and consulting editor of *Nutrition Forum*, a newsletter emphasizing the exposure of fads, fallacies and quackery. He is also on the list of peer reviewers for the *Dictionary of Alternative-Medicine Methods*.

Description: **Quackwatch** is "Your Guide to Health Fraud, Quackery, and Intelligent Decisions," according to the slogan used on the Web site. It is part of a "Skeptic Ring: an alliance of sites that examine claims about paranormal phenomena and fringe science from a skeptical point of view," and part of the "Consumer Action and Advice Ring: an alliance of sites that provide free consumer advice or education." Some of the site's content is translated into French, German, and Portuguese. It has three sister sites: *Chirobase*, *MLM Watch* (for multilevel marketing), and *NutriWatch*. Each of the sites consists of long lists of articles— many of them by Dr. Barrett himself, or with a co-author—on quackery; questionable products, services and theories; questionable advertisements; nonrecommended sources of health advice (not surprisingly both Deepak Chopra and Dr. Andrew Weil are "nonrecommended");

consumer protection; various consumer strategies; education for consumers and health professionals; research projects; legal and political activities; and links to like-minded sites. Many of the articles are well-researched and carefully argued and offer the considerations requisite to decision-making on alternative health care choices, but not everyone will reach and share Dr. Barrett's conclusions. There is a combative tension about the writing, which often makes it difficult to read, even when the point being made is one you are willing to concede. **Quackwatch** is a site created by a man with a mission, and that mission does not accommodate complementary and alternative medicine. Unfortunately, this pervasive negativism about CAM undercuts the impact of some of the acceptable research and common sense approaches to advertising fraud and the sales pitches of charlatans, which are also targets of Dr. Barrett's attacks. There is much good reading here and many points well-made from a particular point of view, but the site will not appeal to anyone who believes even remotely in the effectiveness of a CAM therapy. Dr. Barrett's work will appeal to skeptics and believers in the failure of CAM to offer scientific proof for anything. It will have little impact on those many who look for other types of proof or who believe in outcome rather than argument.

REFERENCES

1. National Center for Complementary and Alternative Medicine. *Frequently Asked Questions: What is Complementary and Alternative Medicine?* Retrieved from the WWW on April 21, 2000: http://nccam.nih.gov/nccam/fcp/faq/index.html#what-is.

2. Excerpted on June 19, 2000 from a document found at: National Center for Complementary and Alternative Medicine. *Major Domains of Complementary and Alternative Medicine.* Retrieved from the WWW on June 19, 2000: http://nccam.nih.gov/nccam/fcp/classify/index.html.

3. J.S. Gould. "The Menace of Cyberspace." *American Journal of Orthopedics* 28, no. 12 (December 1999): 682.

4. D.M. Eisenberg, R.C. Kessler, C. Foster, F.E. Norlock, D. Calkins, and T.L. Delbanco. "Unconventional Medicine in the United States: Prevalence, Costs, and Patterns of Use." *New England Journal of Medicine* 328, no. 4 (January 28, 1993): 246-252.

5. D.M. Eisenberg, R.B. Davis, S.L. Ettner, S. Appel, S. Wilkey, M. Van Rompay, and R.C. Kessler. "Trends in Alternative Medicine Use in the United States, 1990-1997: Results of a Follow-up National Survey." JAMA 280, no. 18 (November 11, 1998):1569-1575.

6. Nonprescription Drug Manufacturers Association of Canada. *Fact Sheet: Canadian Consumers and Alternative Medicine*. Retrieved from the WWW on May 24, 2000: http://www.ndmac.org/new/back_02_01.html.

7. *Health Care in Canada 2000: A First Annual Report*. Ottawa: Canadian Institute for Health Information, 2000. Retrieved from the WWW on May 3, 2000: http://www.cihi.ca/Roadmap/Health_Rep/healthreport2000/pdf/Healthreport2000.pdf.

8. "Data Watch: 60 Million Now Use the Web to Find Health Info." *The Ferguson Report* 2 (April 1999). Retrieved from the WWW on April 21, 2000: http://www.fergusonreport.com/articles/fr049901.htm.

9. These papers can be accessed at the Mitretek/HITI Web site; the main site address is: http://hitiWeb.mitretek.org/; and the address for the documents (in HTML and PDF formats) is: http://hitiWeb.mitretek.org/hswg/documents/default.asp.

10. Health Summit Working Group. *Criteria for Assessing the Quality of Health Information on the Internet - Policy Paper*. Retrieved from the WWW on April 22, 2000: http://hitiWeb.mitretek.org/docs/policy.html#top.

11. Science Panel on Interactive Communication and Health. *Wired for Health and Well-Being: the Emergence of Interactive Health Communication*. Washington, DC: US Department of Health and Human Services, US Government Printing Office, April 1999. Retrieved from the WWW on April 22, 2000: http://scipich.health.org/pubs/report/execsummary.htm.

12. Health on the Net Foundation. *HON Code of Conduct for Medical and Health Web sites*. Retrieved from the WWW on April 22, 2000: http://www.hon.ch/HONcode/Conduct.html.

13. W.M. Silberg, G.D. Lundberg, and R.A. Musacchio. "Assessing, Controlling and Assuring the Quality of Medical Information on the Internet: Caveat Lector et Viewor — Let the Reader and Viewer Beware." *JAMA* 277, no. 15 (April 16, 1997): 1244-1245.

14. M.A. Winker, A. Flanigan, B. Chi-Lum, J. White, K. Andrews, R.I. Kennett, C.D. DeAngelis, and R.A. Musacchio. "Guidelines for Medical and Health Information Sites on the Internet: Principles Governing AMA Web sites." *JAMA* 283, no. 12 (March 22-29, 2000): 1600-1606. Web site: http://jama.ama-assn.org/issues/v283n12/full/jsc00054.html (HTML version); http://jama.ama-assn.org/issues/v283n12/pdf/jsc00054.pdf (PDF version).

15. B.F. Schloman. "Whom Do You Trust? Evaluating Internet Health Resources." *Online Journal of Issues in Nursing*, January 28, 1999. Retrieved from the WWW on April 3, 2000: http://www.nursingworld.org/ojin/infocol/info_1.htm.

16. National Center for Complementary and Alternative Medicine. *Alternative Medicine Journals Currently in MEDLINE*, from MEDLINE and Related Databases. Retrieved from the WWW on May 1, 2000: http://nccam.nih.gov/nccam/what-is-cam/medline.html#journals.

17. J. Ezzo, B.M. Berman, A.J. Vickers, and K. Linde. "Complementary Medicine and the Cochrane Collaboration." *JAMA* 280, no. 18 (November 11, 1998):1628-1630.

18. "Mission Statement." *The Cochrane Leaflet*. Retrieved from the WWW on May 21, 2000 at: http://hiru.mcmaster.ca/cochrane/cochrane/leaflet.htm.

19. L. Landro. "Cancer Web sites Raise Privacy Issues." *The Globe and Mail*, May 2, 2000, section R, 11.

20. T. Ferguson. *Digital Doctoring: Health Online and the Empowered Medical Consumer*, the John P. McGovern Lecture, delivered at Plenary Session 1, May 7, 2000, annual meeting of the Medical Library Association, Vancouver, BC.

21. T. Ferguson. "Can Useful and Reliable Online Health Resources be Produced by 'Medically Unqualified' Persons?" *The Ferguson Report* 5 (July 1999). Retrieved from the WWW on May 21, 2000: http://www.fergusonreport.com/articles/fr079902.htm.

SECTION 9

Popular Books on Complementary and Alternative Medicine

This section contains reviews of 350 popular books relating to complementary and alternative medicine mainly published during the past three years. A few earlier, classic works are also included to provide more comprehensive coverage. The reviewed books were selected from a total of more than 500 titles examined for their intrinsic value. Criteria used for selection were based on scope, depth of coverage, balance, and the quality of the sources providing supporting evidence for the content. Preference was given to those titles that reflect an integrative approach, showing how alternative therapies can best be combined with conventional clinical practice. Books reviewed include encyclopedias, manuals, handbooks, help books, question-and-answer books, and guides.

Professional books are reviewed in Section 6.

General Works

Adams, "Patch," with Maureen Mylander. *Gesundheit: Bringing Good Health to You, the Medical System, and Society through Physician Service, Complementary Therapies, and Joy*. Rochester, VT: Healing Arts Press, 1998. 227pp. $14.95 (paper).

The author is the subject of the Robin Williams film, *Patch Adams*. Adams, the founder of the Gesundheit Institute (a home-based medical practice in West Virginia) that has treated, free of charge, more than 15,000 people, believes that humor is vital in healing the problems of individuals, communities, and societies. "It is time to join laughter with love," argues Adams, "to serve humanity through healing." Bernie Siegel comments that "behind his clownlike persona lies a great deal of wisdom, and it often falls to the court jester to speak the truth that those in power need to hear." The basic point made is that the present health care system is in trouble and that true health is based upon happiness—"from hugging and clowning around to finding joy in family and friends, satisfaction in work, and ecstasy in nature and the arts." Inspiring and uplifting.

Ardell, Donald B. *14 Days to Wellness: The Easy, Effective, and Fun Way to Optimum Health*. Revised and updated. Novato, CA: New World Library, 1999. 236pp. $14 (paper).

This is a completely rewritten edition of a book of the same title published in 1982. Once again, Ardell outlines in detail a practical wellness program, involving no more than 15 minutes each day, that includes explicit instructions with respect to a nondiet approach to weight loss, a nonmeditation approach to stress management, a nonjogging approach to physical fitness, and a nonmedical approach to super health. While offering practical detail and suggestions, the discussion is somewhat philosophical—develop a realistic perspective on the medical system, draw a picture or image of what it means to be a healthy person, begin work on your black belt in self-responsibility, consider the enormous payoffs of physical fitness and the adequacy requirements of any exercise, understand the dynamics of stress, and consider the payoffs of stress management.

Balch, James F. *10 Natural Remedies That Can Save Your Life*. New York: Doubleday, 1999. 256pp. $19.95.

The 10 natural remedies advocated include the benefits of light, water, and air; green foods (cereal grasses, barley grass, alfalfa); garlic, ginseng, and ginkgo biloba; chelation therapy; natural hormone maintenance, and vitamins C and E. Some of the therapies described are controversial—bio-oxidation therapy such as rectal insufflation (sending between 100 and 800 milliliters of an oxygen-ozone mixture into the rectum by means of an enema tube, where it is absorbed through the intestines). Balch claims that "improvements are noted for ulcerative colitis, some forms of cancer, HIV-related problems, and others." This is a rich mixture of the strange, esoteric, and the unproven. There are no references, bibliographic notes, or suggested readings.

Ballentine, Rudolph. *Radical Healing: Integrating the World's Great Therapeutic Traditions to Create a New Transformative Medicine*. New York: Harmony, 1999. 612pp. $27.50.

Ballentine (a psychiatrist, herbalist, Ayurvedic practitioner, and homeopath) believes that the field of holistic medicine has remained "as fragmented as an unassembled jigsaw puzzle." His book "aims to show how the pieces of that puzzle fit together and how the whole that results is greater than the sum of the parts." The book does a credible job of blending together proven techniques such as the use of herbal and homeopathic remedies, exercises, flower essences, Ayurveda, and traditional Chinese medicine. The major, and unique, value of the book lies in the 100-page resources section. This contains a "Self-Help Index" to what can be done for many common ailments "weighed against decades of experience and study," a simple home medicine kit, a guide to further study, (excellent analytical reviews of classic and current books on alternative medicine), a glossary, and endnotes.

Bettschart, Rol (ed.), and others. *The Complete Book of Symptoms & Treatments: Your Comprehensive Guide to the Safety and Effectiveness of Alternative and Complementary Medicine for Common Ailments*. Boston: Element Books, 1999. 953pp. $24.95 (paper).

This book is a translation of a book originally published in German in 1995. The authors' objective is to "provide a critical appraisal of individual complementary health care practices and realistically assess individual techniques used to treat the commonest ailments and symptoms." Part One of the book describes common disorders contrasting orthodox and complementary treatments. Each treatment is rated as "of little use," "maybe of some use," "not advised." The entry for sinusitis identifies 20 complementary treat-ments and rates 11 treatments as "of little use," six as "maybe of some use," and three as "not advised." The ratings were compiled by a panel of scientific experts who examined published data. Part Two is an A-to-Z review of the most popular complementary therapies available, showing the rationale of each therapy, how a therapy works, its benefits and risks, indications for use, and an assigned rating. Part Three describes the main principles of the diagnostic techniques commonly used in complementary medicine. This book succeeds in its objective of opening patients to a broader range of therapies and to make more readily available the best that mainstream and complementary medicine jointly have to offer. However, the ratings criteria are fuzzy and poorly defined.

*Bratman, Steven. *The Alternative Medicine Ratings Guide*. Rocklin, CA: Prima, 1998. 391pp. $19.95 (paper).

Trying alternative medicine can involve a great deal of confusion with trial and error. Bratman sets himself the task of evaluating alternative medicine options for some 80 common health problems in terms of the probability of success, cost-effectiveness, and ease of use. An expert panel of 18 experienced alternative practitioners was chosen not as "evangelical advocates of alternative medicine, but as dedicated and objective practitioners who have spent years discovering what methods are most useful for their patients." For each of about 80 health problems, the experts rated various possible treatments on a simple 1–3 scale, where a score of 1 indicated occasional success, and a score of 3 pointed to frequent, dramatic success. The evaluations of all the experts were then combined in order to extract a consensus opinion. Treatments were examined for conditions such as cardiomyopathy, esophageal reflux, and hypoglycemia. The result is a compilation of current practice in the form of consensus statements rather than true objective evaluations. Good.

Bratman, Steven. *The Alternative Medicine Sourcebook: A Realistic Evaluation of Alternative Healing Methods*. 2nd edition. Lincolnwood, IL: Lowell House, 1999. 275pp. $17.95 (paper).

In this second edition, Bratman states that his book "takes a hard-boiled look at alternative medicine as it is practiced in real life" by providing information and insights necessary to find a way through the maze of alternative possibilities prescribed by a licensed practitioner. Alternative medicine is defined broadly as "every available approach to healing that does not fall within the realm of conventional medicine." Most alternative practices provide treatment propelled by three ideas: the treatment must be natural, holistic, and calculated to promote wellness. A clear explanation is given with respect to naturopathic medicine, herbal medicine, homeopathy, Chinese medicine, acupuncture, chiropractic, movement therapies, and spiritual approaches. A distinction is made between the scientific approaches to healing such as naturopathy and homeopathy, and the healing arts, such as acupuncture. Specific guidance is given on how to use alternative medicine with recommended methods best suited to a number of common medical conditions. A largely successful attempt to provide a balanced approach to alternative medicine.

***Bratman, Steven, and David Kroll (series eds). *The Natural Pharmacist TNP.com.* 6 titles: Anna M. Barton and Others. *Natural Treatments for Cold and Flu.* 161pp; Dentali, Steven. *Natural Treatments to Improve Memory.* 123pp; Head, Kathi. *Natural Treatments for Diabetes.* 157pp; Hobbs, Ron, and others. *Natural Treatments for Arthritis.* 162pp; Ingels, Darin. *Natural Treatments for High Cholesterol.* 137pp; Snow, Joanne Marie. *Natural Treatments for Menopause.* 157pp. Roseville, CA: Prima/TNP.com, 1999. $9.99 each (paper).

The series editors state that their main objective is "to cut through the hype and tell you what is known and remains to be scientifically proven regarding popular natural treatments. These books are more conservative than any others available, more honest about the weaknesses of natural approaches, more fair in their comparisons of natural and conventional treatments." In this vein, the authors of each volume contrast conventional and natural treatments and review the available evidence as to efficacy and safety. The volume on arthritis, by way of example, discusses in separate chapters the scientific evidence for the use of glucosamine sulfate, chondroitin sulfate, SAM-e, herbs, and vitamins and minerals for the treatment of osteoarthritis and rheumatoid arthritis. The final chapter of each volume—"Putting It All Together"—summarizes the key information presented and identifies the major treatment choices. This is a highly informative series that represents a serious and largely successful attempt to assess the available evidence and to present an unbiased, integrative analysis. Excellent.

Bruce, Debra Fulghum with Harris H. McIlwain. *The Unofficial Guide to Alternative Medicine.* New York: Macmillan, 1998. 480pp. $15.95 (paper).

A book that intends to give "savvy consumers like you a foolproof appraisal of what works and what doesn't—the good alternative methods and the bad ones—with unbiased recommendations that are not influenced by any company, product, or organization." The authors provide a good description of alternative treatments including Chi-

nese medicine, bodywork, touch therapy, herbal medicine, mind/body medicine, and so on. Each therapy is described in terms of how it works, what it does, and the basics. Suggested therapies are also given for a wide assortment of the specific conditions contrasting conventional and alternative treatments. Two final chapters deal with legal and insurance issues and navigating through the drugstore and the health food store. While strong on description, cautions, and valuable tips, the book is weak in pinpointing "what works, and what doesn't."

***Cassileth, Barrie. *The Alternative Medicine Handbook: The Complete Reference Guide to Alternative and Complementary Therapies.* New York: Norton, 1998. 340pp. $25.

This is a serious and largely successful attempt to describe and evaluate over 50 alternative therapies such as Ayurveda, flower remedies, macrobiotics, Kirlian photography, chelation therapy, colon/ detoxification therapies, Alexander technique, rolfing, light therapy, and faith healing. Each therapy is described in a standard format—what it is, what practitioners say it does, beliefs on which it is based, research evidence to date, what it can do for you, and where to go for treatment. Where no scientific evidence exists, this is so indicated, as in the case of nine unproved biological cancer therapies described. A balanced, analytical survey of alternative medicine by a founding member of the Advisory Council to the NIH Office of Alternative Medicine. Excellent.

Castleman, Michael. *Blended Medicine: The Best Choices in Healing.* Emmaus, PA: Rodale Press, 1999. 708pp. $29.95.

Blended medicine in this instance is synonymous with complementary medicine. Castleman attempts to answer which combination of approaches works best for more than 100 diseases and health conditions. Drawing upon the expertise of a wide range of medical advisors, Castleman summarizes what can be expected from an assortment of alternative therapies such as chiropractic, homeopathy, Ayurvedic medicine, and so on. The blended approach is illustrated with reference to some 100 medical conditions such as flu, kidney stones, and osteoarthritis. In each instance, Best Choices, Other Good Choices, Medical Measures, and Red Flags are indicated. Informative, well written, and intelligently organized for easy use.

Chopra, Krishan. *Your Life Is In Your Hands: The Path to Lasting Health and Happiness.* Boston: Element, 1999. 318pp. $21.95.

Krishan Chopra is an Indian cardiologist and Chairman of the Health Care Foundation of India. His son is Deepak

Chopra, who has contributed a foreword to this book. Chopra's main point is that our thoughts and mental attitudes are the most crucial determinant of our physical state of health, our well-being, happiness, efficiency, creativity, and productivity. Mingling Indian mysticism with almost 50 years of clinical experience, Chopra deals with self-realization, self-discipline, correct diet, good sleep, regular exercise, and moderation. Emphasis is also placed on the value of meditation, practice of yoga, and the joy of service. A final chapter spells out the secrets of longevity and healthy aging. A highly readable and sensible distillation of ancient wisdom and practical guidance.

Credit, Larry P., Hartunian, Sharon G., and others. *Your Guide to Complementary Medicine.* Garden City Park, NY: Avery, 1998. 200pp. $10.95 (paper).

An introduction to a number of complementary care approaches to a wide variety of ailments. Some 37 approaches are described, including some lesser-known treatments such as lymphatic massage, polarity therapy, and Trager. Each approach is discussed in a standardized format—what it is, conditions that respond best, how it works, what to expect, costs/duration, credentials/education, how to find a practitioner, professional organizations, and recommended readings. The authors insist that "these approaches are not viewed as alternatives but as complements. In partnership with conventional western medicine, the treatments can bolster your potential for health and recovery." Interesting, informative, and easy to read.

Croft, Jack. *The Doctor's Book of Home Remedies for Men: From Heart Disease and Headaches to Flabby Abs and Road Rage, Over 2,000 Simple Solutions.* Emmaus, PA: Rodale, 1998. 674pp. $17.95.

The latest medical advice from some 400 doctors on how to deal with the aches, pains, ailments, and problems that men face each day. Amazingly, not a single one of the 2,000 tips offered requires a prescription or doctor's visit. The problems covered include bladder shyness, coughs, dry hair, fatigue, gum ailments, nosebleeds, sex addiction, swimmer's ear, and more. For each problem there is a short description, indication of the cause, solutions, alternative approaches, and preventive measures. An excellent source of browsing that reflects plain commonsense as much as medical advice.

*Dillard, James, and Terra Ziporyn. *Alternative Medicine for Dummies.* Foster City, CA: IDG Books Worldwide, 1998. 348pp. $19.99 (paper).

The authors offer a sensible, humble, balanced, and often humorous discussion of the essential features of alternative medicine. Their focus is on how to determine when alterna-

tives are worth a try, how to evaluate various alternative approaches, how to use alternatives safely, how to find a conventional doctor who is open to alternatives, and how to find an alternative practitioner. Separate chapters are devoted to Chinese medicine, Ayurveda, naturopathy, homeopathy, osteopathy, herbs and botanicals, and nutritional therapy. A yellow-page insert suggests "Best-Bet Alternatives" for specific conditions such as colds and flu, heart disease, and skin problems. Icons are used to explain the use of medical jargon, alert readers to myths and marketing hype, indicate when to see your doctor, and highlight useful tips, existence of unknowns, and warnings. A most informative and enjoyable book to read, replete with a host of clever tips, suggested sources of information, recommended Web sites, and advice on how to shop for alternative health care. Dillard is medical director for Oxford Health Plans' alternative medicine program; Ziporyn is a former associate editor of *JAMA*. Good.

The Drug & Natural Medicine Advisor: The Complete Guide to Alternative & Conventional Medications. Alexandria, VA: Time-Life Books, 1997. 880pp. $29.95 (paper).

An A-to-Z guide that combines prescription and OTC drugs, Chinese medicines, aromatherapy, homeopathic preparations, and herbal medicines. An icon identifies which type of remedy a healing substance is. Each entry provides a broad overview, availability, precautions, possible interactions, side effects, and warnings. A 16-page color guide to prescription drugs and herbs is included to facilitate easy identification of both prescription drugs and herbs (such as rosehip, ephedra, and turmeric). An alphabetical index of natural medicines is found at the end of the book listing healing substances for six natural remedies—aromatherapy, Chinese medicine, homeopathy, nutritional supplements, vitamins and minerals, and Western herbs. An excellent source, offering quick access to a wide variety of both mainstream and alternative medications.

Eden, Donna, with David Feinstein. *Energy Medicine: Balance Your Body's Energies for Optimum Health, Joy, and Vitality.* New York: Tarcher/Putnam, 1999. 378pp. $25.95.

A detailed manual that describes techniques for working with the body's energy systems to optimize physical vitality and mental acuity. Working with energy can strengthen the immune system, alleviate pain and depression, and relieve common complaints such as colds and tension headaches. The eight energy systems described are the meridians, the chakras, the aura, the Celtic weave, the basic grid, the five rhythms, the triple warmer, and the strange flows. Eden and Feinstein explain the basic tools that are needed to create an internal environment that is conducive to health and healing. An appendix lists resources designed to lead the reader to competent practitioners of energy medicine.

The Editors of Time-Life Books. *The Medical Advisor: The Complete Guide to Alternative & Conventional Treatments.* 2nd edition. Alexandria, VA: Time-Life Books, 2000. 1152pp. $39.95 (paper).

This book is a revised edition of a paperback published in 1997 at the very modest price of $19.95. The second edition has been updated and expanded. Valuable features include a Dictionary of Conventional Medicines and Alternative Therapies; General Guidelines to Health; Emergencies/First Aid; Visual Diagnostic Guide; and an Index of Conventional and Natural Medicines that lists in alphabetical order the most commonly used medicines and herbal remedies. The core of the book still consists of entries for 3000 ailments. Each entry describes symptoms, when to call the doctor, tests and diagnostic procedures, treatment (conventional and alternative options), at-home management, and prevention. This remains an ambitious and enormously successful attempt to combine in one volume the best of conventional medical practice and the benefits of alternative therapies. Extensive use is made of color illustrations, tables, and sidebars to enhance the text. First rate, despite the jump in price!

**Feinstein, Alice (editor). *Better Homes and Gardens Smart Choices in Alternative Medicine.* Des Moines, IA: Better Homes and Gardens Books, 1999. 358pp. $24.95 (paper).

A reference book that presents "the bright side of alternative medicine" stressing the wonderful healing potential of many forms of alternative medicine while admitting that quality control continues to be a major issue. Excellent summaries are provided for 26 major forms of alternative medicine such as Ayurveda, Chinese medicine, magnet therapy, and therapeutic touch. The distinguishing characteristic of the book is the highlighting of what works, common uses of each form and how it is used, possible side effects, safety and warnings, how to choose a practitioner, and resources (books, journals, organizations). In short, a highly readable and informative source of practical information that is aimed at helping transform a parallel system of alternative health care into the new paradigm of integrative medicine. Splendid!

Froemming, Paul. *The Best Guide to Alternative Medicine.* Los Angeles: Renaissance Books, 1998. 304pp. $16.95 (paper).

Froemming, in an introductory chapter, analyzes what is "alternative" about alternative medicine and summarizes the differences in philosophy between conventional and alternative medicine. "Ultimately" states Froemming, "the convergence of western and alternative medical practitioners has led to a new type of medicine, called integrative medicine that utilizes the best elements from both practices." To facilitate consumers' choice of new ways to view health problems through alternative health practices, Froemming offers "the best of alternative medicine." Part One of his book discusses the keys to vitality and balance (Ayurveda and Chinese medicine, nutrition, water, exercise, and breathing); Part Two analyzes the mind/body connection; Part Three deals with disease prevention and longevity; Part Four offers a guide to 25 leading alternative therapies; and Part Five illustrates natural remedies for some 25 common health problems. Contains a bibliography, glossary, recommended Internet sites, and a directory of alternative medicine resources.

Gallagher, Sean P., and Romana Kryzanowska. *Pilates Method of Body Conditioning: Introduction to the Core Exercises.* Philadelphia: Bainbridge Books, 1999. 208pp. $19.95 (paper).

Pilates, a German immigrant and physical fitness expert, developed an exercise method called "Contrology" that was adopted by well-known dancers such as Martha Graham and George Balanchine. The Pilates Method combines the best of Western and Eastern traditions, blending the mind and body and viewing them as a unity with one another. The Eastern approach to exercise is a path to calmness, while the Western approach emphasizes motion, muscle tone, and strength. Explicit instructions are provided for more than 70 exercises with over 300 black-and-white photographs.

Garrison, Robert, and Michael Mannion. *Pharmacist's Guide to Over-the-Counter and Natural Remedies.* Garden City Park, NY: Avery, 1999. 368pp. $6.95 (paper).

The authors hope that their book will serve as "a bridge that will help you make informed choices between the familiar drugstore medications and the available herbs, vitamins, minerals, and other natural substances that can be used for medicinal purposes." Some 50 pages are devoted to a discussion of guidelines and precautions concerning the self-treatment of symptoms and advice on selecting over-the-counter products. The bulk of the book, however, consists of an A-to-Z Guide to Common Conditions detailing both OTC and natural remedies for the self-treatment of 75 common conditions such as colds and coughs, and constipation. Each entry contains a short description of the problem followed by suggestions as to OTC and natural remedies. Dosages and warnings are included. The entry for insomnia, by way of example, lists OTC products such as diphenhydramine hydrochloride and natural products such as kava, amantra, melatonin, and valerian. Simple and easy to understand.

Greely, Hugh P., and Anne M. Banas. *The Directory of Complementary & Alternative Medicine.* Marblehead, MA: Opus Communications, 2000. 530pp. $149 (paper).

The authors' objective is "to clarify the confusing CAM (Complementary and Alternative Medicine) field by providing descriptive information about the therapies to help facilities and consumers understand the scope of CAM in existing quality standards for CAM." For each of the more than 100 therapies listed, capsule information is supplied on practitioners, education and training requirements, licensing, certification, professional associations, and practice sites together with a short description of each therapy. The arrangement used for the entries follows with minor modification, the classification scheme for CAM therapies of the NIH National Center for Complementary and Alternative Medicine. The truncated description of each therapy together with basic information relating to training certification and relevant professional associations do not, however, serve "to clarify the confusing CAM field" nor to "encourage health providers to offer the most safe and effective health care alternatives."

Hadady, Letha. *Personal Renewal: Your Guide to Vitality, Allure, and a Joyful Life Using Healing, Herbs, Diet, Movement, and Visualizations.* New York: Harmony, 1998. 304pp. $23.

Hadady, an herbalist and certified acupuncturist, endeavors to bring the ancient world of Asian healing home and "make it American." The objective of her book is "to give you as an individual what you need in order to feel fully alive." The book has five parts: Part One shows how to discuss your original self; Part Two, "Damage Control," offers ways to recondition your face and hair with natural remedies and prevent illness and work-related pains; Part Three covers ways to get into shape and lose weight safely and effectively through the use of herbs, special teas, massage and essential oils; Part Four, "Energy, Vitality, and Sexuality," involves use of aphrodisiac herbs and hormonal massage; Part Five, "Longevity and Spirit," shows how herbal and homeopathic products can help you get in touch with your own wealth of feelings and memories. In sum, a somewhat mystical blend of traditional Chinese medicine, Tibetan medicine, and herbalism.

Hale, Teresa. *The Hale Clinic Guide to Good Health: How to Choose the Right Alternative Therapy.* Woodstock, NY: Overlook Press, 1998. 250pp. $34.95.

Teresa Hale is the founder of the prestigious Hale Clinic in London and has been involved in research projects on complementary medicine. Over 30 different treatments are available from the 100 practitioners based at the clinic. Past patients include the late Princess Diana, Arnold Schwarzenegger, and Tina Turner. The emphasis is on combining orthodox (allopathic) and complementary medicine. Fifty common ailments are described in this book, such as hiatal hernia, phobias, and infertility. For each complaint there is a description of the orthodox approach, alternatives such as acupuncture, homeopathy, and colonic hydrotherapy, followed by the Hale approach that provides interpretation and recommendations. Profiles are provided for some 30 alternative treatments including Buteyko, a revolutionary new breathing therapy introduced to the Western world by the Hale Clinic. The excellent color photographs, quality of the paper, and attractive presentation of the textual matter make this a truly outstanding and delightful book to read.

Hassman, Howard A. *Alternative Treatments for Common Conditions.* St. Louis, MO: Quality Medical Publishing, 2000. 191pp. $16.95 (paper).

Hassman, an osteopath, shows how four disciplines—nutrition, homeopathy, acupressure, and herbal therapeutics—can be used to treat some 75 medical conditions. Medical disorders, with short descriptions averaging about two pages in length, are listed alphabetically indicating what homeopathy, herbal medicine, acupressure, and nutrition can offer by way of treatment. While offering a multidisciplinary approach, little by way of explanation and guidance is supplied.

Ivker, Robert S., Anderson, Robert A., and Trivieri, Larry. *The Complete Self-Care Guide to Holistic Medicine: Treating Our Most Common Ailments.* New York: Tarcher/Putnam, 1999. 502pp. $27.50.

Two practitioners of holistic medicine and a medical writer describe proven self-care approaches for treating over 60 conditions ranging from chronic sinusitis to vaginitis. Each condition is addressed from the perspective of mind, body, and spirit, the multiple factors contributing to the condition, and "a variety of treatment options to either improve it, cure it, or prevent it from recurring." The emphasis throughout is on self-care. Five introductory chapters deal with healing the body, healing the mind, healing the spirit, a wellness self-test, and action steps to establish healthy habits. For each disease, the authors supply information with respect to prevalence, anatomy and physiology, symptoms and diagnosis, conventional treatment, risk factors and causes, emotional and social factors, and holistic treatments. Informative but poorly organized with a highly confusing formatting of the textual material. A better buy is Gale Maleskey's *Nature's Medicines: From Asthma to Weight Gain, From Colds to High Cholesterol—the Most Powerful All-Natural Cures* (Rodale, 1999).

Krohn, Jacqueline, and Francis Taylor. *Finding the Right Treatment: Modern and Alternative Medicine: A Comprehensive Guide to Getting the Best of Both Worlds.* Point Roberts, WA: Hartley & Marks, 1999. 494pp. $24.95 (paper).

This book represents an ambitious attempt to integrate alternative health care with modern medical practice by a physician and allergy technician, respectively, both of whom are homeopaths. Part One discusses the essentials of modern medicine (pharmaceuticals, lab tests, hospitals, and emergency room surgery, radiology, and vaccinations); Part Two describes alternative medicine disciplines (naturopathy, chiropractic, homeopathy, Ayurvedic medicine and Chinese medicine) and alternative therapies (bodywork, herbs, diet, nutritional supplements, aromatherapy, light therapy, sound therapy, and Bach flower remedies); Part Three details common health problems and contrasts the approaches of modern medical treatment with alternative treatment. This juxtaposition of mainstream and alternative medicine, the major portion of the book, falls flat in that the arrangement is muddled with no uniform captions that would enable the reader to make simple comparisons. The text is difficult to read and is buried within multiple headings that lack uniformity. One wishes for better formatting and the use of tables to show comparisons. Despite the title, no assistance is provided in "finding the right treatment." Disappointing.

Kugler, Hans, and Chase Revel. *Amazing Medicines the Drug Companies Don't Want You to Discover.* New York: Berkley Books, 1999. 390pp. $6.99 (paper).

After denouncing the "widespread greed" of doctors, fraud and bribery by drug companies, the FDA's "Gestapo tactics against vitamins," bill padding by doctors, and the overprescribing of drugs, the authors review the evidence of natural alternatives for the treatment of a variety of ailments such as memory loss, prostate disorders, arthritis, heart disease, and ulcers. Apart from the muckraking attitude towards doctors, a serious attempt is made to review the available evidence for the alternative treatment of major diseases—"our research team examined 266 research projects conducted by over 500 medical scientists worldwide." Twenty pages of references are included. The concluding message is that the "healthiest doctors take six

times the RDA of vitamins and minerals—and so should you." A good source of information on many alternative products such as DHEA, melatonin, hypericum, chromium picolinate, carotenes, coenzyme Q10, MSM, and more.

Lane, I. William, and Susan Baxter. *Immune Power: How to Use Your Immune System to Fight Disease—From Cancer to AIDS.* Garden City Park, NY: Avery, 1999. 188pp. $11.95 (paper).

After explaining the basics of the immune system (how the immune system works, vaccination, and cellular specifics), Lane describes "Civil War–Autoimmune Disorders"—immune malfunction through damage, malnutrition, genetic defects, and the development of allergies and asthma. The main thrust of the book is to promote the use of MGN-3 (Arabin-Oxylan compound), a rice brand product that has an extraordinary effect on the immune system, in particular in strengthening the natural killer (NK) cells that are the body's primary natural defense against tumors and viral disease. Lane and Baxter quote evidence that MGN-3 is effective in the treatment of cancer and AIDS and go so far as to assert that, "if MGN-3 can indeed halt HIV progression, as these results indicate it might, then we are on the brink of a major clinical breakthrough." Nine pages of references are supplied but many do not relate to the peer-reviewed research literature. Lane is the author of *Sharks Still Don't Get Cancer* (Avery, 1996).

Marti, James E. *The Alternative Health & Medicine Encyclopedia.* 2nd edition. Detroit: Visible Inc. Press, 1997. 462pp. $17.95 (paper).

This is a second edition of a book originally published in 1995. The first edition presented more than 200 alternative therapies for more than 50 common medical disorders. This expanded and revised edition adds more than 100 new therapies for 20 additional disorders. The basic approach is the same in that, "while the old paradigm viewed the body basically as a machine, the new paradigm focuses on the interconnectivity of body, mind, emotions, social factors, and the environment in determining health status." Typical therapies covered include homeopathy, naturopathic medicine, and hydrotherapy. Separate chapters deal with the use of vitamins, minerals and trace elements, and botanical medicines. The alternative medicine approach to stress-related disorders, drug abuse and addiction, mental health, common male health problems, female health problems, cancer, heart disease, and aging is described. There are also detailed lists of resources. This is a highly readable, encyclopedic compilation of basic facts on a wide variety of alternative medicine therapies but with no attempt at the critical evaluation supplied by

Barrie Cassileth's *The Alternative Medicine Handbook* (Norton, 1998).

Monson, Nancy. *Smart Guide to Boosting Your Energy.* New York: Wiley, 1999. 181pp. $10.95 (paper).

Loosely based upon the concept of energy inherent in Chinese medicine and Ayurveda, this guide presents an assortment of techniques and tips to "boost energy, vim, vigor, vitality, pep, zip, zoom, and oomph." In addition to countering energy zappers and depleters, Monson advocates a combination of nutrition, exercise, lifestyle strategies, vitamins, minerals, herbal supplements, and alternative energy fixers such as essential oils and aromatherapy, flower essences, color therapy, and reflexology. Ephedra, super blue-green algae, and Kombucha are not recommended. "Hot" energy-boosting supplements recommended include ginseng, bee pollen, ginger, carnitine, and creatine. A highly readable admixture of tips, advice, and exhortations with many "smart sources" (resource organizations).

Murray, Michael, and Joseph Pizzorno. *Encyclopedia of Natural Medicine.* Revised 2nd edition. Rocklin, CA: Prima Publishing, 1998. 946pp. $24.95 (paper).

This is an updated, revised book originally published in 1991. Murray and Pizzorno, naturopathic physicians and educators, define naturopathy as a system of health-oriented medicine that stresses maintenance of health and prevention of disease in contrast with the traditional, allopathic, disease-oriented system. Naturopathic physicians are trained to seek the underlying cause of a disease rather than simply to suppress the systems. Naturopathy draws upon nutritional therapy, natural diet, herbal medicine, Ayurveda medicine, and Chinese medicine. Part One explains the cornerstones of good health; Part Two shows how key body systems can be enhanced through detoxification, immune support, and stress management; and Part Three discusses how naturopathic medicine is used to treat some 70 specific health problems. In each instance, the authors describe the condition and identify causes, therapeutic considerations, goals of therapy, and the use of dietary and lifestyle modification, nutritional supplements, and botanical medicines. The text is greatly enhanced by the liberal use of headings such as "Quick Review" and "Treatment Summary," together with informative diagrams and tables. This is a substantial contribution to the literature of alternative medicine in that it moves beyond simple description to a discussion of therapeutic approach and methods.

Null, Gary. *The Complete Encyclopedia of Natural Medicine: A Comprehensive A-Z Listing of Common and Chronic Illnesses and Their Proven Natural Treatments.*

New York: Kensington Books, 1998. 612pp. $35.

Null, a prolific author on alternative medicine topics, offers a "kind of second opinion for today's health care consumer . . . that is like a breath of fresh air. The idea here is to look at things differently and to see how we can incorporate nature, and what's natural, into a new healing paradigm." Spanning some 80 chapters arranged alphabetically by medical condition, Null describes causes, symptoms and alternative treatments that can profitably be employed. The final part of the book consists of patients' testimony of the success achieved in the use of enzyme therapy, hypnotherapy, Rolfing, QiGong, and other therapies. Among the claims made are zinc supplements can help eating disorders; valerian root is an effective nerve tonic; cayenne is a popular arthritis remedy; cabbage juice can prevent stomach and colorectal cancer. Extravagant, uncritical, and undocumented.

Null, Gary. *Get Healthy Now: A Complete Guide to Prevention, Treatment and Healthy Living.* New York: Seven Stories Press, 1998. 1,088pp. $65.

This is an expensive encyclopedic compilation of alternative approaches to staying healthy. The book is divided into 13 parts: Part One covers nutrition; Part Two deals with taking charge of your health (detoxification, weight management, use of herbs); Part Three discusses mental health and psychological well-being; Part Four outlines musculoskeletal fitness; Part Five is devoted to foot and leg care; Part Six covers heart, blood, and circulation; Part Seven deals with allergy and environmental illness; Part Eight provides an overview of cancer treatment and prevention; Part Nine considers chronic conditions; Part Ten pinpoints women's health; Part Eleven is devoted to matters of concern to men; and Part Twelve discusses health, beauty, and longevity. A final section, consisting of some 200 pages, is intended as a resource guide listing the names, addresses, and telephone numbers of practitioners arranged by specialty—homeopathy, chelation therapy, orthomolecular medicine, acupuncture, clinical ecology, and naturopathy—and by state. Apart from quoting a number of authorities, there is no bibliography, list of references, information resources, or identification of the information sources used.

O'Neill, Hugh. *The Doctors Book of Home Remedies for Preventing Disease: Tips and Techniques So Powerful They Stop Diseases before They Start.* Emmaus, PA: Rodale Press, 1999. 637pp. $29.95.

This is a new edition of a book originally published in 1991 and remains a fascinating compilation of plain, homespun remedies for a wide variety of aches, ailments and illnesses—no prescription required, no high-tech tests, and no surgical interventions! Each problem discussed is accompanied by many helpful suggestions: for bad breath, brush your tongue, cleanse your palate, minimize milk products, don't use mouthwash; for postnasal drip, identify the troublemaker, make your bed mite-free, become a house-roving vacuum virtuoso. Some 130 illnesses and medical problems are discussed based on information supplied by medical experts. A lucid compendium of sensible and practical advice on a large number of conditions.

****Pelletier, Kenneth. *The Best Alternative Medicine: What Works? What Does Not?* New York: Simon & Schuster, 2000. 449pp. $26.

Pelletier, the author of the classic *Mind as Healer, Mind as Slayer* (Dell, 1977) and director of the NIH-funded complementary and alternative medicine program at Stanford, describes the increasing popularity of complementary medicine in terms of the complex matrix of cultures, philosophies, traditions, and techniques involved. Pelletier challenges "the polarized, dogmatic thinking that often surrounds the conflict between conventional medicine and CAM. Both of these medical traditions need to be evaluated objectively using the best research available." Of some considerable importance is the fact that upwards of 80 percent of conventional medicine lacks an adequate basis in research. Adopting evidence-based medicine as the basic model of inquiry, Pelletier seeks the middle ground. Based upon an extensive search of the international literature and of multiple databases, Pelletier examines CAM treatments including mind/body medicine, traditional Chinese medicine, acupuncture, European herbs, homeopathy, and naturopathy in terms of "What Works," "What Does Not Work," and "What's In the Works" (current research). One section lists CAM therapies by medical condition treated. More than 50 pages of references provide the documentation for Pelletier's evaluations. This is a magnificent, insightful, and balanced review of CAM that is conceivably the best single book on the subject to date. Outstanding.

**Quick Access Consumer Guide to Conditions, Herbs & Supplements.* Newton, MA: Integrative Medical Communications, 2000. 434pp. $24.95 (paper).

Based on the text of *Quick Access Patient Information on Conditions, Herbs & Supplements* (Integrative Medical Communications, 2000), this volume is almost identical but without the exhaustive "Quick Reference Guide" provided in the patient education version. The arrangement and content is substantially the same—monographs of more than 100 conditions in terms of signs, symptoms, diagnosis and treatment options (traditional and alternative); monographs for some 40 herbs with details of composition, available forms, dosages, precautions, and inter-

actions; and supplements monographs for several dozen vitamins, minerals, trace elements, and micro-nutrients. This is a most attractive and informative consumer-friendly digest of the vast *Integrative Medicine Access: Professional Reference to Conditions, Herbs & Supplements* (Integrative Medical Communications, 2000). Designed for home use. Very Good.

Root-Bernstein, Robert, and Michele Root-Bernstein. *Honey, Mud, Maggots, and Other Medical Marvels: The Science Behind Folk Remedies and Old Wives' Tales.* New York: Houghton, 1997. 279pp. $24.

A husband and wife team extol the virtues of ancient folk remedies that sound utterly preposterous today in view of the fact that we have lost touch with the wisdom of the past. Bloodletting, bathing in mineral springs, cleansing with urine, and using maggots to clean wounds all seem to have no value in an era of medical breakthroughs. Flippant rejection of many millenia of accumulated knowledge exacts its price. Ancient techniques of contraception and use of abortifacients are the starting points for the development of new and improved birth control methods. Likewise, honey is now used in burn therapy in modern hospitals; fresh urine is sterile and can be used as a therapeutic agent to fight infection and inflammation (urotherapy); saliva possesses antimicrobial agents; maggots have use in treating gangrene; and clay can be ingested as a survival food (geopharmacy). This is a serious attempt to place these folk remedies in perspective. Robert and Michele Root-Bernstein (a physiologist and a historian, respectively) write in a light, humorous vein and seem to clinch their argument by pointing out that apes and other mammals tend to dose with the same medicinal plants used in human folk medicines. A unique book that makes for delightful reading.

****Shealy, C. Norman. *The Illustrated Encyclopedia of Healing Remedies.* Boston: Element Books, 1998. 496pp. $14.95.

This book is a comprehensive discussion of the origins of eight alternative therapies—Ayurveda, Chinese herbal medicine, herbalism, aromatherapy, homeopathy, flower remedies, vitamins, and minerals. In each instance, coverage includes the background and history of the therapy together with how it works, information on visiting a practitioner, and data on specific remedies used with dosages and precautions. Part Two of the book consists of a description of 20 common ailments associated with body systems such as the digestive system, urinary system, and eyes. Each description indicates symptoms, treatment (herbalism, aromatherapy, homeopathy, etc.) and cautions. Part Three is a reference section that provides a glossary, list of further readings and useful addresses. A short summary of the contents does not do justice to this book. The color photographs, diagrams, and imaginative use of sidebars are of superlative quality. An excellent book worthy of coffee-table status. Outstanding.

Shealy, C. Norman (consulting editor). *The Complete Illustrated Encyclopedia of Alternative Healing Therapies.* Boston: Element Books, 1999. 383pp. $29.95 (paper).

Like other volumes in this Complete Illustrated Encyclopedia series, this book is superbly illustrated with high-quality color photographs and diagrams that are both informative and aesthetically pleasing. The therapies described are arranged in three categories—energy therapies (acupuncture, Qigong, polarity therapy, therapeutic touch), physical therapies (massage, chiropractic, relaxation techniques), and mind and spirit therapies (group therapies, light therapy, autogenic training). For each therapy described, detailed information is given on origins, how the therapy is performed, the orthodox view of the therapy, precautions, and a "pathfinder" (page references to ailments in which the therapy has been found useful). A final section describes common ailments and relevant alternative therapies contrasted to mainstream medical treatment. A concerted attempt is made to show how alternative therapies can be used in conjunction with conventional treatment. The subject coverage is far from complete in that there is no mention of herbal medicine, homeopathy, and reflexology. This appears to be an expanded version of Shealy's *The Illustrated Encyclopedia of Healing Therapies* (Element Books, 1998).

Taub, Edward. *Doctor Edward Taub's Seven Steps to Self-Healing Pack.* New York: Dorling Kindersley, 1996. 160pp. $24.95.

This "pack" consists of a book that discusses the "healing force" (illness begins in the mind and the mind controls the body), a "Pyramid of Human Aspiration" (a pyramid that folds into a three-dimensional reminder of the seven simple steps to total wellness), 15 questionnaires to evaluate wellness and to assess what is causing imbalance in the body, and pledges to sign in order to commit oneself to ascend the pyramid of human aspiration. In addition, there are four meditation audiotapes that focus on corresponding written meditations in the book. The "Wellness Action Plan," detailed in the book, involves a seven-step program embracing the Einstein Energy Diet, enjoyable exercise, meditation, de-addiction, self-esteem, forgiveness, and love. The Einstein Energy Diet assumes that all life is energy and that food energy turns into the substance of the body and provides fuel for it to function. Fruit and vegetables provide optimal energy while candy and sweets do not sup-

ply lasting energy. Taub's total program is designed to create balance by stimulating your healing force and reviving the innate ability of the body to heal itself. In this manner, the healing force can overcome illness, conquer addictions, and reverse stress. A novel combination of text, questionnaires, pledges, and audiotapes.

Weil, Andrew. *Ask Dr. Weil: Common Illnesses.* New York: Ivy Books, 1997. 87pp. $2.99 (paper).

This slender and compact book draws upon the content of the Ask Dr. Weil Web site (http://www.pathfinder.com/drweil) and Weil's full-length books such as *Spontaneous Healing* (Knopf, 1995), and *Eight Weeks to Optimum Health* (Knopf, 1997). Questions and answers deal with common concerns such as athlete's foot, herpes, hives, styes, swimmer's ear, and yeast infections. In all instances, the approach advocated involves alternative remedies such as herbal medicine, acupuncture, and dietary modification. Simple and to the point.

Weil, Andrew. *Eight Weeks to Optimum Health: A Proven Program for Taking Full Advantage of Your Body's Natural Healing Power.* New York: Knopf, 1997. 276pp. $23.

Dubbed the guru of alternative medicine, Weil presents a comprehensive week-by-week program for enhancing and protecting lifelong health. His main point is that "health is wholeness and balance, and inner resilience that allows you meet the demands of living without being overwhelmed." Moreover, "optimal health brings with it a sense of strength and joy." The prescription for achieving optimal health includes fine-tuning current eating habits, walking, stretching and exercise, the addition of four antioxidant supplements (vitamin C and E, selenium, and mixed carotenes), breathing exercises, visualization, elimination of toxins from the diet, and avoidance of environmental hazards such as ultraviolet rays. Using illustrative case histories, Weil offers a visionary and highly persuasive plan for personal development and wellness.

Woodham, Anne, and David Peters. *Encyclopedia of Healing Therapies.* New York: Dorling Kindersley, 1997. 336pp. $39.95.

A highly attractive, coffee-table-quality book that describes and illustrates the different approaches of complementary medicine. While introductory chapters describe holistic medicine, its rise in popularity, and its emphasis on wellness and well-being, the bulk of the book consists of a visual guide to over 90 widely used complementary therapies with information on their history and how they work, what to expect at a consultation, research and scientific evidence, self-help techniques, and compatibility with conventional medicine. Using high-quality photographs and illustrations, the book offers concise and informative descriptions of a wide variety of touch movement therapies, medicinal therapies, mind and emotive therapies, and diagnostic techniques. A final section includes an extensive array of treatment options for over 200 mental, physical, and emotional health problems.

Zand, Janet, Allan Spreen, and James B. Lavalle. *Smart Medicine for Healthier Living: A Practical A-Z Reference to Natural and Conventional Treatments for Adults.* Garden City Park, NY: Avery, 1999. 657pp. $21.95 (paper).

> This book follows Zand's previous work, *Smart Medicine for a Healthier Child: A Practical A-Z Reference to Natural and Conventional Treatments* (Avery, 1994). The major sections are identical: "Elements of Health Care (The Nuts and Bolts of Conventional and Natural Treatment)"; "Common Health Problems (Disorders from A-Z with Recommendations for Conventional and Natural Treatments)"; and "Therapies and Procedures (Techniques for Using Conventional and Natural Treatments)." A novel—and highly valuable—feature of the book lies in the juxtaposition of conventional treatments and alternative therapies. The authors show how conventional treatment can be supplemented by nutritional supplements, dietary modification, herbal medicine, homeopathy, and acupressure in the treatment of more than 300 diseases and disorders. For each condition, conventional treatment is outlined together with detail on alternative treatments. For example, for varicose veins, in addition to sclerotherapy and stripping, try vitamin C and E supplements, butcher's broom, ginkgo biloba, hawthorn, horse chestnut, Bach flower remedies, homeopathy, and aromatherapy. Zand and colleagues outline the essentials of integrative medicine written in lay terms.

Acupuncture

Degraff, Deborah A. *The Body Owner's Manual: An Acupuncturist's Teachings on Health and Well-Being.* New York: Berkley Books, 1998. 339pp. $13 (paper).

> DeGraff invites the reader to enter into the world of medicine as a healing art and to look at the body in a different way by listening to and trusting in your body. Blending East and West, Degraff aims at empowering the reader through an understanding and knowledge of self-care skills in order to live in a state of balance and harmony. Part One of her book discusses the basics of self-care with an excellent introduction to traditional Chinese medicine; Part Two consists of a self-care dictionary showing self-care practices

recommended for a variety of problems such as low back pain, bronchitis, and sinus infections; Part Three is devoted to stories of healing that portray the healing experience of 10 of Degraff's patients. This is an exquisitely sensitive and insightful book that stresses the wisest guidance comes from inside yourself and an awareness of the state of your Qi (life force). Splendid!

Aromatherapy

Dodt, Colleen K. *The Essential Oils Book: Creating Personal Blends for Mind & Body.* Pownal, VT: Storey Communications, 1996. 152pp. $12.95 (paper).

> The application of pure essential oils in one's life can bring about significant benefit and change. Aromatherapy is the use of pure essential oils to enhance the quality of body, mind, and spirit. Dodt, an herbalist, describes the properties and applications of a wide assortment of essential oils in terms of benefits, suggested uses, recipes, and cautions. Separate chapters deal with blending equipment and supplies, recipes for producing home aroma (dishwashing, freshening carpets, and creating a bedroom of flowers), aromatic recipes for essential beauty (bath salts, shampoos, and rinses for baths), and other uses for essential oils—traveling, caring for the elderly and sick, and pet care. An attractive introduction to the olfactory magic of essential oils.

Edwards, Victoria H. *The Aromatherapy Companion: Medicinal Uses, Ayurvedic Healing, Body-Care Blends, Perfumes and Scents, Emotional Health and Well-Being.* Pownal, VT: Storey Books, 1999. 281pp. $19.95 (paper).

> Edwards invites the reader to join her "for a walk along the scented path and to share my lifelong enchantment with nature's gifts of ethereal sense and sublime colors." Using clever illustrations, charts, and boxes, Edwards lucidly explains the origins of aromatherapy, essential oils and their properties, safety and toxicity guidelines, basic aromatherapy applications, how to create your own blends, and aromatherapy for children, teenagers, pregnancy, menopause, and successful aging. One chapter is devoted to aphrodisiacs—effect of pheromones, creating romance with aroma, "scentual" bathing, loving touch, and love potions. Recipes are provided for a blend to attract love, a blend to bring a lover back, and a blend to stimulate erotic longing. A fascinating and delightful book on aromatherapy. Great for browsing.

Fitzsimmons, Judith, and Paula M. Bousquet. *Seasons of Aromatherapy: Hundreds of Restorative Recipes and Sensory Suggestions*. Berkeley, CA: Conari Press, 1998. 235pp. $18.95.

The authors introduce the reader to the joy of using essential oils for therapy and indulgence in that aromas entice and exhilarate, educate, and heal. In addition to the pleasing smell, the real beauty of aromatherapy is that the essences work on a cellular and physical level and in the emotional, intellectual, spiritual, and aesthetic areas of your life. Using a starter kit of 12 oils (chamomile, eucalyptus, lavender, rosemary, peppermint, etc.), the authors show how to prepare recipes suited to each season and month. This "scentsational" book is packed with shopping tips, recipes, step-by-step directions, and helpful suggestions for creating pleasant and relaxing potions.

*Lawless, Julia. *The Complete Illustrated Guide to Aromatherapy: A Practical Approach to the Use of Essential Oils for Health and Well-Being*. Boston: Element Books, 1997. 224pp. $24.95 (paper).

Lawless, in a book characterized and enhanced through the use of profuse color photographs and illustrations, defines five areas of aromatherapy specialization—simple aromatherapy for home use; cosmetic aromatherapy; perfumery and the psychotherapeutic use of oils for the effects of their odors on the mind; massage using essential oils; and medical and clinical aromatherapy, where essential oils are used to treat medical complaints. The major portion of the text covers medical aromatherapy that details how aromatic remedies can be applied to disorders of the skin, circulatory system, respiratory system, nervous system, and so on. An index of essential oils profiles dozens of oils with reference to quality, appearance, and scent; its general actions; and ways it is used. Like other books in this Element Books series, the textual material is greatly enhanced through the use of splendid graphics. Good.

Naylor, Nicola. *Discover Essential Oils*. Berkeley, CA: Ulysses Press, 1998. 112pp. $8.95 (paper).

This is a volume in the Ulysses Discover Handbook series. Essential oils are contained in the glands, sacs, veins, and glandular hairs concentrated in different parts of plants. Oil massage is the usual form of treatment because the essential oil is quickly absorbed through the skin and carried by the blood around the body. Essential oils may also be given by professional aromatologists as intramuscular injection. Therapeutic use at home may involve baths (sitz, hand, and foot), compresses, inhalations, ointments, lotions, and creams as well as massage treatment. Naylor, a British aromatologist, offers a concise explanation of chemistry, botany, therapeutic use, and the buying and storing of essential oils. Three chapters are devoted to essential oils in health care settings, professional treatment, and case studies. Informative and highly readable.

O'Hara, Gwydion. *The Magick of Aromatherapy*. St. Paul, MN: Llewellyn Publications, 1998. 284pp. $12.95 (paper).

O'Hara, a pagan high priest, attempts to combine both the magical and healing aspects of aromatherapy. The text covers the principles of aromatherapy, the practice, and the therapeutic blends. One chapter deals with magical blends, formulated for love and lust, success and prosperity, magical empowerment, health, and ritual blends. A most unusual book that details recipes for achieving love and prosperity in addition to healing.

Price, Shirley. *Practical Aromatherapy: How to Use Essential Oils to Restore Vitality*. London: Thorsons, 1999. 226pp. $12 (paper).

While offering much useful information on essential oils, techniques of aromatherapy, massage, and Swiss Reflex Therapy (a treatment technique devised by the author based on reflexology), Price, a British aromatherapist, fails to present an organized and coherent explanation. Several useful chapters detail how to prepare oils for massage and provide recipes together with a table of essential oils and a therapeutic index. Not as informative or well organized as Julia Lawless's *The Complete Illustrated Guide to Aromatherapy* (Element, 1997).

Rechelbacher, Horst. *Aveda Rituals: A Daily Guide to Natural Health and Beauty*. New York: Owl/Holt, 1999. 266pp. $22 (paper).

Twenty years ago, Rechelbacher founded Aveda by creating pure, plant-based beauty products. Aveda is now an international company that has created over 700 plant-based products for hair, skin, and body, which are sold in salons and spas. In this book, Rechelbacher outlines the wisdom of Ayurveda, aromatherapy, and other medicinal traditions and, on a highly personal note, shares a menu of rituals, touching upon nurturing the inner spirit, meditation, cleansing, skin care, personal beauty, and massage. With over 125 color photographs, the text takes the high road to health and well-being stressing the interconnectiveness of beauty, health, mind, body, and spirit. Contains a glossary of essential oils and list of resources.

Rose, Jeanne. *375 Essential Oils and Hydrosols*. Berkeley, CA: Frog Ltd., 1999. 245pp. $14.95 (paper).

Rose profiles 375 different substances used in aromatherapy. The major portion of Rose's book is devoted to providing an introduction to aromatherapy and botany, detailing the family, habitat, and growth, components, scent, properties, indications, and uses of essential oil plants such as blue sage, gardenia, and oregano. Also included are essays on evergreens, lavender, chamomile, essential oils of the Old Testament, and descriptions of distilleries and the distillation process. Much of the writing is esoteric and obscure: "Hydrosols are the real aromatherapy. They can also be considered the homeopathy of aromatherapy; as herbs are to homeopathy, so essential oils are to hydrosols. Hydrosols represent the true synergy of herbalism and aromatherapy."

Walters, Clare. *Aromatherapy: The Illustrated Guide.* Boston, MA: Element Books, 1998. 144pp. $19.95 (paper).

This is a beautifully illustrated book with an abundance of full-color photographs showing the historical origins of aromatherapy, how it works, preparation, and chemical components of essential oils, properties, the art of massage (a fundamental technique in aromatherapy), aromatherapy in the home, visiting a therapist, and aromatherapy for women, children, and the elderly. More than one-half of the book consists of a "Materia Medica" containing profiles of 36 of the oils most commonly and safely used in aromatherapy. For each oil, basic information is provided for attributes and characteristics, properties (method of extraction, chemical constituents, aroma), uses through the ages, home use, and health notes. A delightful book, rich in informative detail.

Alternative Medicine . . .

African Americans

Reese, Sara Lomax, and Kirk Johnson (editors). *Staying Strong: Reclaiming the Wisdom of African-American Healing.* New York: Avon, 1999. 341pp. $14 (paper).

Reese, the publisher of *HealthQuest* magazine, states that her book is "filled with information that will motivate, inspire, educate, and empower." Her intent is to explain to African Americans how to use alternatives to mainstream medicine in order to heal body, mind, and spirit. Reese outlines the principles of "whole living" that reflects a way of life that celebrates community, commitment, balance, interconnections, and self-sufficiency. Whole living is natural, spiritual, respects many healing traditions, and looks at the complete person. Part One explains how alternative healing methods can help you live a fuller, healthier life; Part Two explains key alternative healing methods such as acupressure, chiropractic and reflexology; Part Three,

"Help Yourself," describes holistic approaches to three dozen health problems. The text is lucid, highly informative, and packed with helpful, practical advice.

Walker, Marcellus A., and Kenneth B. Singleton. *Natural Health for African Americans: The Physicians' Guide.* New York: Warner, 1999. 348pp. $14.99 (paper).

The authors, both physicians and practitioners of complementary and alternative medicine, start with the conviction that as a group, African Americans suffer disproportionately from serious chronic illnesses including heart disease, cancer, stroke, and diabetes. They state that, "we have seen firsthand the limitations and failures of conventional, Western medicine in the treatment of African Americans. We have seen too many members of our community die prematurely of preventable and controllable diseases . . . our decades of experience working with African Americans have taught us that the best approach to overall health is a combination of conventional, mainstream medicine and natural or 'alternative' healing techniques." Their book reflects a holistic approach dealing with living with stress, dietary modification, detoxification, weight control, exercise, nutritional supplements, and overcoming addictions. A redefinition of what it means to be healthy by two African American physicians, both board certified in internal medicine. Contains lists of recommended readings, organizations and Web sites. Insightful.

Aging

Bland, Jeffrey S., with Sara H. Benum. *Genetic Nutritioneering.* Los Angeles: Keats, 1998. 272pp. $16.95 (paper).

This book attempts to show how diet, lifestyle, and environment influence genetic expression and health as we age. Healthy aging, the authors contend, is controlled not only by genetic inheritance but also by how we communicate with our genes through diet and lifestyle. The Human Genome Project proves that more important than genetic inheritance is the phenotype—the result of gene expression and environment—as opposed to genotype. After explaining "how diet communicates with your genes," Bland and colleagues describe how to prevent and control diabetes, arthritis, cancer, and other diseases. A final chapter discusses "how to transform your genetic destiny." This is a book of more interest as an explanation of the relationship of genetic inheritance to diet, lifestyle, and environmental exposure than as a prescription for change. Stimulating and provocative reading.

Conkling, Winifred. *Stopping Time: Natural Remedies to Reverse Aging.* New York: Dell, 1997. 414 pp. $5.99 (paper).

Stop the clock by using a holistic approach to overall health! Four major types of natural healing are considered—herbal medicine, nutrition supplements, homeopathy, and acupressure. Part One of the book describes growing old naturally; Part Two shows how to gray gracefully (with nutrition, weight control, relaxation); while Part Three outlines the alternative approach to some three dozen ailments contrasting conventional care with the natural approach. A somewhat pedestrian presentation.

Dollemore, Doug, and Prevention Health Books for Seniors (eds.). *The Doctors Book of Home Remedies for Seniors: An A-to-Z Guide to Staying Physically Active, Mentally Sharp and Disease-Free.* Emmaus, PA: Rodale, 1999. 578pp. $27.95.

This is a compilation of proven remedies that draw upon, as in other Rodale books, interviews with highly qualified medical specialists and practitioners of alternative medicine. Focusing on the health concerns of people over 60, useful and practical information is assembled in relation to medical problems that commonly affect older Americans. Topics covered include angina, back pain, foot pain, gout, lowered sexual desire, phlebitis, and sciatica. Each topic covered, averaging about three pages in length, features a description of the problem, "Try This First" (self-care tips), "Other Wise Ways," "When to See a Doctor," and "Advice on Managing Your Meds" (medications). The first part of the book provides sensible strategies for staying well with respect to exercise, diet, accident prevention, and staying mentally sharp. A simple, somewhat pedestrian, but eminently useful book.

Null, Gary. *Gary Null's Ultimate Anti-Aging Program.* New York: Kensington Books, 1999. 498pp. $29.95.

Throw out your calendar and forget about chronological age! The message conveyed is quite simple—no one needs to simply accept a decline in vitality, be it wrinkles and balding, gray hair, or osteoporosis and loss of muscle mass and tone. Based on an analysis of 5,000 studies and experience with more than 1,000 volunteers, Null advocates the adoption of a vegetarian diet and other dietary changes involving no cheese, milk, yogurt, foods treated with pesticides/herbicides, caffeine, or chocolate, and the liberal use of vitamins, nutrients, and herbs. An 83-page chapter consists of testimonials from people who have adopted Null's program. An extensive bibliography lists research studies. Unfortunately, details of the program are buried in a mass of theoretical speculation, argumentative discourse, and extraneous detail. Diffuse and difficult to read.

Ullis, Karlis, with Greg Ptacek. *Age Right: Turn Back the Clock with a Proven, Personalized Antiaging Program.* New York: Simon & Schuster, 1998. 319pp. $23.

Antiaging expert Ullis offers a personalized program for those who think that growing old is anything but graceful. Four key factors are associated with aging—energy, sex, lifestyle, and biomechanical motion-and there are three aging pathways—mind, body, and spirit. Ullis shows how to discover your aging pathway and how to build an antiaging regimen that addresses one's individual strengths and weaknesses. Specific recommendations are provided on nutrition, exercise, and antiaging supplements, including an "antiaging cocktail." One chapter details an "Antiaging Medicine Chest" that recommends a variety of vitamins, minerals, hormones, antioxidants, and herbs. This is a most complicated program explained in terminology that approximates the complexity and detail of a professional textbook. Not very useful for most medical consumers.

Anxiety

Bloomfield, Harold H. *Healing Anxiety with Herbs.* New York: HarperCollins, 1998. 344pp. $23.

Bloomfield notes that 65 million Americans suffer annually from anxiety and insomnia and that one out of every two people will experience some form of mild to moderate anxiety during their lifetime. The remedy is not addictive tranquilizers and sleeping pills. In many cases, states Bloomfield, the best and safest remedies are natural herbs that have far fewer, if any, of the plaguing side-effects of benzodiazepine tranquilizers. Hypericum (St. John's wort), valerian root, gingko biloba, and kava all show great promise in relieving anxiety and insomnia. Sedative herbs such as California poppy, Reishi mushrooms, and chamomile can induce calmness and relaxation. Separate chapters are devoted to herbs in traditional medicine, herbal scents (aromatherapy), and "flower power" (Bach flower remedies). This book remains a most informative summary of new developments in the use of botanical medicines to treat anxiety and insomnia.

Bourne, Edmond. *Healing Fear: New Approaches to Overcoming Anxiety.* Oakland, CA: New Harbinger, 1998. 398pp. $16.95 (paper).

Bourne, a psychotherapist, maintains that "anxiety arises fundamentally from a state of disconnection—a disconnection of each individual from self, significant others, environment, community, society, and spirituality." His emphasis is on "healing" rather than on "applied technology." Healing is best achieved in combination with cognitive behavioral therapy and medication. Separate chapters deal with relaxation and exercise, nutrition, addressing personality issues, developing your "observing self," letting go, learning to love, and acquiring courage. The approach advocated is to complement and not replace conventional treatment of anxiety. This book reflects holistic concepts and values and the importance of the spiritual dimension in recovery. A somewhat technical discussion.

Arthritis

Adderly, Brenda D., and Chanteil Miller. *The Arthritis Cure Fitness Solution.* Washington, DC: LifeLine Press, 1998. 173pp. $19.95.

This book goes a step beyond the use of glucosamine sulfate and chondroitin as advocated in Jason Theodosakis's *The Arthritis Cure: The Medical Miracle That Can Halt, Reverse, and May Even Cure Osteoarthritis* (St. Martin's Press, 1997). Adderly and Miller provide an easy-to-follow four-week plan to improve flexibility, increase strength, enhance aerobic stamina, and improve quality of life. Explicit instructions, with good black-and-white photographs, are given for developing an exercise program and fitness plan. A clear statement of the importance and value of exercise in the achievement of perfect health.

Conkling, Winifred. *Natural Medicine for Arthritis.* New York: Dell, 1997. 304pp. $5.99 (paper).

This is a comprehensive review of the natural approaches that can both ease the pain and improve the condition of the joints without recourse to toxic medications that can be both confusing and potentially dangerous. The natural approach advocated involves the use of dietary modification, vitamins and minerals, exercise, herbal medicine, acupressure, homeopathy, hydrotherapy, and a number of other complementary treatments such as copper bracelets, DMSO, reflexology, TENS units, and yoga. A useful summary of what complementary medicine can offer in the treatment of arthritis. Inexpensive.

Holt, Stephen, and Jean Varilla. *The Power of Cartilage.* New York: Kensington Publishing, 1998. 269pp. $14 (paper).

Holt, a physician, states that "from this book, you will learn how cartilage may be used to stop or prevent the pain of arthritis, speed wound healing, alleviate the miseries of psoriasis, boost immune function, and whether it figures in the fight against cancer." With much background detail, Holt and Varilla review the health benefits of cartilage in the treatment of a wide variety of diseases, pointing out that cartilage can modulate or inhibit the angiogenesis that can promote tumor growth. Shark cartilage can also be an effective therapy in the treatment of arthritis and sports injuries. Although attempting to be objective in discussing the untold merits of cartilage, Holt and Varilla lapse into enthusiastic endorsement: "shark cartilage has a history of more than six years of safe and effective use with over 400 million doses sold for bone and joint health."

****Horstman, Judith. *The Arthritis Foundation's Guide to Alternative Therapies.* Atlanta: Arthritis Foundation, 1999. 285pp. $24.95 (paper).

Does your doctor talk to you about alternative therapies for arthritis? Can alternative medicine help? In a world where hucksters abound, do Ayurveda, homeopathy, Qi Gong, copper bracelets, and so on, work? This official publication of the Arthritis Foundation, compiled with the assistance of a board of medical editors and consultants, offers excellent summaries of a wide variety of therapies and alternative healing systems; massage and body works; acupuncture and acupressure; mind, body, and spirit; herbs and supplements; and miscellaneous therapies (bees, bracelets, lasers, and magnets). In addition to informative digests, the book offers highly valuable explanations and guidance as to what complementary medicine can and cannot do, definition of terms such as complementary medicine, alternative medicine, holistic medicine and integrative medicine, what to do before you commit to alternative therapy, how to avoid ripoffs, and how to work with your doctor and complementary medicine provider. In addition, an extensive listing of relevant books, journals, Web sites, and organizations is provided. This is an eminently successful attempt on the part of the Arthritis Foundation to "lay the information down in front of you, not to tell you what to do." The basic message is: "read about a therapy, learn all that you can, and talk to your doctor before trying any new treatment." Outstanding.

Lahita, Robert G. *The Arthritis Solution: The Newest Treatments to Help You Live Pain-Free.* New York: Avon, 1999. 243pp. $5.99 (paper).

This is an excellent source of up-to-date information, not readily available, on the new anti-inflammatory family of drugs called Cox-2 inhibitors that are more specific in their action than other nonsteroidal anti-inflammatory drugs (NSAIDS) such as aspirin, ibuprofen, and naproxin (the Cox-1 inhibitors). Cox-2 inhibitors now used to reduce pain and swelling also appear to have fewer side effects than the current NSAIDS. Lahita, a physician at New York Medical College, places the Cox-2 inhibitors within the context of other treatments available such as NSAIDS, salicylates, corticosteroids, analgesics, and disease modifying antirheumatic drugs (DMARDS). Two chapters deal with the future of arthritis treatment and living with arthritis. This is a highly informative explanation of current treatments for rheumatoid arthritis made even more valuable by the inclusion of a glossary, list of resources (books, Web sites, support organizations, magazines and newsletters and government publications), and a bibliography. Valuable and inexpensive.

Theodosakis, Jason, Brenda Adderly, and Barry Fox. *Maximizing the Arthritis Cure: A Step-by-Step Program to Faster, Stronger Healing During Any Stage of the Cure.* New York: St. Martin's Paperbacks, 1999. 302pp. $6.50 (paper).

This is an inexpensive paperback version of a book originally published in a hardcover edition in 1998. The major point made is that the symptoms of osteoarthritis can be relieved, halted, reversed, and in many cases cured by following a program that includes taking glucosamine and chondroitin sulfate. One chapter details other nutritional substances and minerals that may add to the impact of glucosamine and chondroitin. These include SAM-e, hydrolyzed collagen, and Cox-2 inhibitors. A simple and persuasive prescription for relief from arthritis pain.

Weatherby, Craig, and Leonid Gordin. *The Arthritis Bible: A Comprehensive Guide to Alternative Therapies and Conventional Treatments for Arthritic Diseases.* Rochester, VT: Healing Arts Press, 1999. 244pp. $14.95 (paper).

This is a very readable attempt to find the middle ground between the slavish followers of a therapeutic cookbook approach (despite the fact that the patient is growing worse) and "the holistic and alternate" armies announcing famous victories that have never taken place. Weatherby and Gordin summarize what is known about rheumatic diseases and show the role played by conventional drugs, dietary therapies, vitamins and minerals, traditional herbs, nutraceutical remedies from nature (emu oil, bovine tracheal cartilage), antibiotic therapy, homeopathic remedies, and folk medicine. One chapter is devoted to the cartilage therapy "revolution," covering glucosamine, chondroitin, gelatin, and Boswella herb. This book is a serious attempt to separate the credible from the laughable.

Back Pain

Credit, Larry P., Sharon G. Hartunian, and Margaret J. Nowack. *Relieving Sciatica: Using Complementary Medicine to Overcome the Pain of Sciatica.* Garden City Park, NY: Avery, 1999. 133pp. $10.95 (paper).

Sciatica is a painful symptom under the category of low back pain. The pain of sciatica is felt along the course of the sciatic nerve, which runs from the low back into the buttock area, down the back of the thigh and the inner leg, and extends as far down as the foot. After explaining the symp-

toms and causes of sciatica and the approach of conventional medicine, Credit and colleagues turn to a consideration of what 15 complementary medicine options can offer. These options include Alexander technique, foot reflexology, rolfing, and the Trager Approach. Under each option, details are provided as to how it views and treats sciatica, relevant research, estimated cost and duration, health insurance coverage, credentials and education of practitioners, and further sources of information. End-of-book material includes a glossary, overview of research issues, trends in health insurance, and bibliographic notes. A concise and practical summary.

Mitchell, Deborah. *Natural Medicine for Back Pain.* New York: Dell, 1997. 192pp. $5.99 (paper).

A book for those who have tried conventional back-pain treatments and have had little or no success. Mitchell offers a smorgasbord of natural therapies including acupuncture, chiropractic, hypnosis, massage, meditation, therapeutic touch, and yoga. Part Two, the major part of the book, describes in some detail 38 therapy options that are effective in acute or chronic back pain. A useful chart shows which natural therapy can be used to treat acute pain, methods of prevention and maintenance, treatment of chronic pain, and pain control. Each therapeutic option is explored from several angles—how to treat yourself or, if needed, how to find an appropriate practitioner; what to expect from various therapists and practitioners; and what kind of results you can expect to achieve. Part Three summarizes what can be expected from conventional treatment: prescription and OTC drugs, injection therapy, TENS units, and surgery. Contains a glossary, a list of resource organizations, and suggestions for further reading. An inexpensive purchase, packed with a large amount of useful information.

Breast Cancer

Falcone, Ron. *Natural Medicine for Breast Cancer.* New York: Dell, 1997. 174pp. $5.99 (paper).

Falcone's major emphasis is on primary prevention based on diet, immunity enhancement, positive attitude, and an overall healthy lifestyle. The "medicines" prescribed include vitamins and other supplemental therapies, homeopathic herbal and plant remedies, food and diet programs, massage, and mind-body techniques. In a chapter entitled "Coping with Chemotherapy," Falcone argues that toxic therapy serves to weaken rather than strengthen immunity. Special nutrients useful for reducing the side effects of chemotherapy include the antioxidant vitamins A, C, and E, and the B-complex. A sensible and simple statement as to how natural medicines can complement rather than replace the conventional treatments of surgery, chemotherapy, and radiation.

Cancer

Bognar, David. *Cancer: Increasing Your Odds for Survival: A Resource Guide for Integrating Mainstream, Alternative, and Complementary Therapies.* Alameda, CA: Hunter House, 1998. 300pp. $15.95 (paper).

This is a book based on the PBS documentary series *Cancer: Increasing Your Odds for Survival,* narrated by Walter Cronkite. Bognar, a producer and writer, lost his partner to breast cancer. Moving on from his tragic loss, Bognar offers a "comprehensive overview of topics essential to increasing survival odds," including a discussion of "treatments, complementary therapies, latest developments, commentary, organizations, and resources pertinent to surviving cancer." Rather than duplicating the coverage of other cancer books, Bognar, in a highly personalized manner, examines cancer survival rates, second opinions, availability of state-of-the-art treatments, key points for survival, choosing an alternative treatment, what body-mind interventions can offer, psychological aspects, spirituality, and action steps for your "healing journey." Insightful interviews with a number of experts such as Joan Borysenko, Lawrence LeShan, and Bernie Siegel are included, together with a listing of comprehensive cancer centers, support groups, cancer organizations and programs, and Web sites. A book that is frank, supportive, and infused with hope.

Diamond, John, and W. Lee Cowden. *Cancer Diagnosis: What To Do Next.* Tiburon, CA: AlternativeMedicine. com, 2000. 360pp. $14.95 (paper).

At the outset of the book, the statement is made that "many of the treatments described in this book are, by definition, alternative, they have not been investigated, approved, or endorsed by any government or regulatory agency." Cancer care, according to the authors, will be advanced by word of mouth "as each cancer patient recovers their health, thanks to alternative medicine, and tells a friend and the family doctor, this will transform Western medicine." The allegation is made that powerful economic forces, including pharmaceutical companies and agencies such as the FDA and NIH, "want health care to stay exactly the way it is because they're thriving under it." In this manner, the politics of cancer have an overriding influence on the science of cancer. Despite these extravagant claims, the book has major value in that it offers a lucid description and analysis of the role of alternative medicine in the treatment of cancer with much detail on nutritional considerations, herbal cancer treatment, the new cancer

pharmacology, boosting the immune system, enhancing metabolism, and physical support and energy support therapies. An appendix lists resources for cancer patients and an endnotes section contains 28 pages of references to the professional literature. An eloquent statement of what alternative medicine has to offer to the cancer patient. "Give your doctors a copy of this book and insist they read it."

Gaynor, Mitchell L., and Jerry Hickey, with William Fryer. *Dr. Gaynor's Cancer Prevention Program.* New York: Kensington Books, 1999. 316pp. $24.

Gaynor's approach has been labeled as "a potent blend of science, nutrition, spiritual awareness, and hope." Gaynor, a board certified oncologist, claims that "with the help of this book, you will most probably be able to protect yourself from cancer for the full length of a long life." Prevention is based on the use of phytonutrients that, if taken in sufficient quantity, can free us from the fear of cancer by dramatically lowering our probability of ever contracting it. In a chatty, highly readable style the authors discuss foods, compounds, enzymes, nutrients, vitamins and minerals that have antioxidant activity in the body. Separate chapters are devoted to nutrient antioxidants, Omega-3 oils, soy and genistein, amino acids, garlic, fiber, and green tea. This is an eminently reasonable and cogently argued case for the activation or inactivation of your genes by the food you eat.

****Gordon, James S., and Sharon Curtin. *Comprehensive Cancer Care: Integrating Alternative, Complementary, and Conventional Therapies.* Cambridge, MA: Perseus Publishing, 2000. 314pp. $37.95.

Gordon, a physician, was the first chairman of the Advisory Council of the NIH Office of Alternative Medicine, and is currently chairman of the White Commission on Alternative Medicine and the director of the Center for Mind-Body Medicine (CMBM); Curtin is a patients' advocate. Their book is based on the two groundbreaking conferences on Comprehensive Cancer Care sponsored by the CMBM in conjunction with the National Cancer Institute, American Cancer Society, and the National Center for Complementary and Alternative Medicine. The result is a supportive and reliable guide to complementary and alternative therapies for cancer interspersed with scientific explanations and descriptive case histories of actual patients. Here can be found authoritative explanations of the Gerson diet, Dr. Burzynski's antineoplastins, Dr. Nicholas Gonzalez's program of dietary therapies, together with lesser known therapies such as Cooley's toxins, Newcastle virus, and Sun's "soup." The authors offer hopeful and supportive guidelines for readers to integrate conventional, complementary and alternative cancer therapies. More than 80 pages of appendix material lists relevant organizations, retreats, and wellness programs for people living with cancer, Internet resources, notes, and a bibliography. Outstanding.

Issels, Josef. *Cancer: A Second Opinion.* Garden City Park, NY: Avery, 1999. 216pp. $12.95 (paper).

Issels, who died in 1998, was a controversial German doctor who achieved documented cancer cures utilizing unconventional, alternative therapies, and who maintained that those who believe that the localized tumor comes first and is then followed by generalized illness are wrong. Instead, Issels holds that cancer is a generalized illness of the body that first causes systemic illness and only afterwards the tumor. In this manner, the tumor is a symptom of the illness. Issels explains the case for whole-body treatment and shows how his system of treatments combines basic, causal therapy and specific tumor therapy. Basic causal therapy involves elimination of all causal factors such as dental and tonsilar foci, abnormal intestinal flora, and treatment of secondary damage to restore normal function of organs and organ systems. An appendix includes case histories and x-rays of patients cured by Issels. There is an extensive bibliography of mainly German publications. Definitely a highly contrarian view of cancer treatment.

Labriola, Dan. *Complementary Cancer Therapies: Combining Traditional and Alternative Approaches for the Best Possible Outcome.* Roseville, CA: Prima, 1999. 340pp. $18.95 (paper).

A naturopathic physician intends his book "for those who wish to treat their cancer (or that of a loved one) using a well-coordinated combination of conventional and natural therapies." Labriola attempts to bridge the gap between conventional and alternative medicine for the patient with cancer. The best of both worlds, "with the cooperation of your oncologist and natural medicine provider," involves not using nonconventional medicines during the "protected zone"—during the time-period and in the part of the body where the conventional treatment does its work. This is an unusual and valuable book in that the major focus is on techniques of combining conventional and alternative therapies to reduce the risk of complications, minimize side effects, and ensure maximum efficacy.

Mitchell, Deborah. *The Broccoli Sprouts Breakthrough: The New Miracle Food for Cancer Prevention.* New York: St. Martin's Paperbacks, 1998. 165pp. $4.99 (paper).

Mitchell claims that eating "as little as one-quarter ounce of broccoli sprouts daily could reduce your chances of getting cancer by 20 percent, 30 percent, and even as much as 50 percent." Sprout power stems from sulforaphane, a substance that belongs to a group of chemoprotectors known as phytochemicals. The combination of glucosinolate and sulforaphane gives broccoli their superior cancer-fighting ability. A major portion of the book shows how to incorporate broccoli sprouts into the diet in a tasty manner. Two weeks of menus and recipes are supplied that use broccoli sprouts. One chapter details other cancer-fighting foods such as grains, cereals, roots, tubers, plantains, and vegetables.

Moss, Ralph W. *Herbs Against Cancer: History and Controversy.* Brooklyn, NY: Equinox Press, 1998. 300pp. $16.95 (paper).

This is not a book of instructions for cancer patients on how to treat them themselves. Instead, Moss offers "a work of historical and critical analysis based on 'friendly skepticism.'" Moss states that he is "neither promoter nor denigrator" of herbal usage against cancer. Ten chapters cover history and treatments. Separate chapters are devoted to controversies around the world—curaderm (Australia), Pau d'Arco (Brazil), oleander (Turkey), aloe vera (United States). This is a scholarly and cautionary guide to what herbal medicine can offer in the treatment of cancer.

Shamsuddin, Abul Kalam M. *IP6: Nature's Revolutionary Cancer-Fighter.* New York: Kensington Books, 1998. 144pp. $5.99 (paper).

Shamsuddin, a pathologist at the University of Maryland, argues that the B vitamin inositol and its derivative IP6—a natural component of grains such as rice, corn, wheat, and legumes such as soybeans—are anti-cancer nutrients. According to Shamsuddin, IP6 causes a consistent, reproducable and statistically significant reduction in cancers that affect tissues and organs including the colon, prostate, and liver. Moreover, IP6 can prevent kidney stone formation and reduce two key risk factors for heart disease: serum cholesterol and triglycerides. The attempt to describe the research basis for IP6 falls flat while the text is excessively technical and difficult to understand.

*Simon, David. *Return to Wholeness, Embracing Body, Mind, and Spirit in the Face of Cancer.* New York: Wiley, 1999. 275pp. $24.95.

Simon, a physician, outlines the innovative holistic mind-body approach developed at the Chopra Center for Well-Being of which Simon is medical director. Deepak Chopra states in his foreword that "David (Simon) reminds us that facing our mortality offers a window into our immortality. A reservoir of energy, creativity, and vitality resides within us all, and the very practical tools offered in this book enable us to tap into its healing waters." Based upon his experience in personally supporting hundreds of patients facing cancer, Simon discusses nutritional healing, the miracle and mythology of vitamins and minerals, the wisdom of herbs, sensual healing, emotional healing, and being holistically specific (approaching common cancers from a mind-body perspective). A major point made is that you—the real you—does not have cancer and that the essential nature of who you are is beyond illness. An excellent and compassionate approach to healing—lyrical and uplifting. Good.

Stopping Cancer Before It Starts: The American Institute for Cancer Research's Program for Cancer Prevention. New York: Golden Books, 1999. 329pp. $25.

The American Institute for Cancer Research (AICR) is the only national cancer charity focusing on the link between diet, nutrition, and cancer. Rejecting the notion that cancer is "a toss of the genetic dice," the research compiled by AICR shows a direct and undeniable link between cancer and diet. This practical handbook offers a comprehensive plan for cancer prevention involving increased physical activity, better food choices, and the benefits of a vegetarian diet. Often, minor and incremental changes can add up to a big change in one's overall health. Major emphasis is placed on nutrition with five chapters devoted to achieving the best nutrition for cancer prevention. Eating healthier, staying physically active, watching one's weight, and not smoking is not a complicated recipe for good health.

Williams, Penelope. *New Cancer Therapies: The Patient's Dilemma.* Buffalo, NY: Firefly, 2000. 328pp. $16.95 (paper).

Williams, a cancer survivor, tells the stories of cancer sufferers forced to hide their alternative treatments from their closed-minded conventional doctors. She states that her book "is not a tirade against establishment medicine or a paean of praise for all alternative cancer therapies." Instead, her intent is to offer a "gentle plea for cessation of hostilities between the two camps," focusing on the personal dilemma for patients and not medical debate. Much of the content is based upon the author's experience in interacting with staff and patients at the Immuno-Augmentative Therapy (IAT) clinic in Freeport, Grand Bahama. Williams offers an insightful and sensitive view of what it is like for a patient to access and utilize unconventional, alternative treatment. This is a fascinating look at the underground world of alternative cancer treatment in the Bahamas, Mexico, Canada, and elsewhere.

Children

Gladstar, Rosemary. *Rosemary Gladstar's Herbal Remedies for Children's Health.* Pownal, VT: Storey Communications, 1999. 75pp. $8.95 (paper).

Gladstar (herbalist, mother, and grandmother) believes that all children benefit from a close association with nature and from the use of herbs and the ancient tradition of herbalism. Moreover, herbs provide tremendous benefits for children's health. "Children's bodies are sensitive and respond naturally and quickly to the healing energies of herbs. Cuts, burns, bee stings, colds, and runny noses become opportunities for you and your children to see how effectively herbal remedies work." Gladstar describes a children's herbal medicine chest, basic herbal preparations with suggested dosages for children, and herbal remedies for common childhood ailments in the form of teas, powders, oils, salves, pastes, and syrups. Catnip tea is useful for teething, blackberry root tea for diarrhea, garlic and mullein flower oil for ear infections, and so on. In addition to imparting fascinating information concerning natural remedies, Gladstar writes sensitively and insightfully: "girls and boys—gender isn't relevant—are often found looking at the flowers, lost in play for hours in the gardens, enchanted by the pollen-covered insects and butterflies lazing on the launching pads of freshly opened blossoms."

Sawyer, Joan, and Roberta MacPhee. *Head Lice to Dead Lice.* New York: St. Martin's Paperbacks, 1999. 176pp. $5.99 (paper).

Emergency: what do you do if you have head lice (go directly to page 89!). Sawyer and MacPhee open their book with a letter from the "Lice Ladies" that details their personal experience with head lice in their children: "I grabbed a flashlight and shone it on the spot that Talia pointed out. There it was! A louse!! I grabbed it with my fingernails and ran shrieking upstairs to where my unsuspecting husband lay sound asleep in bed." In a humorous vein, the authors discuss the increasing number of treatment failures with Nix, Rid, and Kwell (the most commonly used OTC pediculicides). The chemical warfare approach is noneffective. Instead, Sawyer and MacPhee advocate a five-step "battle plan" involving use of a pediculicide (optional), applying olive oil as a smothering agent, cleaning the environment, combing out the lice and nits with the oil in the hair, and checking for any remaining nits. An excellent discussion of a "lousy" subject offering an alternative (olive oil) to the use of harsh chemicals.

White, Linda B., and Sunny Mavor. *Kids, Herbs, and Health.* Loveland, CO: Interweave Press, 1998. 272pp. $21.95 (paper).

White, a mother of two and a physician, and Mavor, a professional herbalist, offer practical, natural solutions for your child's health from birth to puberty. Herbal medicines, they claim, are often better for children in that they can both ease symptoms and get at the root of the imbalance that causes the illness. Their book is arranged by medical problem such as ear infection, flu, colic, asthma, coughs, and so on. For each ailment, such as colds, White and Mavor discuss both conventional approach methods (OTC cold medications, for example) and alternatives in the form of saline nose drops, echinacea, lemon balm, herbal steams, "runny nose tea," and so on. Each section indicates when to call a doctor. Contains plenty of folk remedies such as "Grandma's Headache Remedies" that work and homemade expectorant syrup for stubborn, dry coughs. Practical and reader-friendly.

Common Cold and Flu

Bruning, Nancy Pauline. *Natural Medicines for Colds and Flu*. New York: Dell, 1998. 216pp. $5.99 (paper).

Veteran medical journalist Bruning addresses her book to the millions who suffer from colds and flu each year and who wish to relieve symptoms without side effects. Conventional medicines offer little in the way of prevention and over-the-counter medications may do more harm than good. The holistic, alternative approach advocated involves the use of food as medicine, vitamins and mineral supplements, herbs, homeopathy, and mind-body medicine. A final chapter, "Putting It All Together," succinctly outlines specific programs using all the natural therapies described to stop a cold at the first sign, to shorten the duration and lessen symptoms in the middle of one, and to lessen your chances of getting sick in the first place. An excellent digest of what alternative medicine can do to prevent and relieve colds and flu. Deserves to be expanded into a larger book.

Sahelian, Ray, and Victoria Dolby Toews. *The Common Cold Cure: Natural Remedies for Cold and Flu*. Garden City Park, NY: Avery, 1999. 167pp. $9.95 (paper).

How to boost your immune system and beat the bugs forever lurking on the hand you shook, the doorknob you turned, and the keypad at the bank machine. After outlining conventional treatment ("prescriptions that appease the patient"), Sahelian and Toews discuss the gold-medal infection fighters—vitamin C, zinc, and echinacea. Other herbs that can support the immune system and fight infection include astragalus, elderberry, ginseng, and mullein. One chapter offers a listing of practical ways to conquer a cold and fight a flu, 10 picks for avoiding a cold, how to

boost immunity with vitamins and mineral supplements, immediate actions to be taken, and a plan of attack if the flu virus invades. A final chapter gives a breakdown, symptom by symptom, of many natural ways to lessen discomfort when in the throes of an upper respiratory infection. An informative handbook packed with many helpful suggestions to alleviate the misery of colds and flu.

Trubo, Richard. *The Natural Way to Beat the Common Cold and Flu: A Holistic Approach for Prevention and Relief*. New York: Berkley Books, 1998. 162pp. $6.50 (paper).

While there is no miracle cure or magic bullet for the common cold, there are plenty of strategies to make the experience more tolerable. These include consuming vegetables rich in antioxidants, nutritional supplements, and herbs such as echinacea, goldenseal, astragalus, licorice, eucalyptus, garlic, and ginger. Separate chapters discuss complementary therapies such as homeopathy, how to minimize stress, and the adoption of a cold-free lifestyle. There is no index.

Depression

Carrigan, Catherine. *Healing Depression: A Holistic Guide*. New York: Marlowe, 1999. 257pp. $15.95 (paper).

Carrigan outlines a new approach that integrates spiritual, nutritional, physical, and psychological factors that contribute to depression. Carrigan's text is the result of 18 years' experience of using psychiatric drugs, plus one year withdrawing from those drugs, and another year recovering from the effects of the drugs. The book is divided into six parts: Part One describes how to get started; Part Two discusses the medical connection (allergies, metabolic and digestive deficiencies); Part Three analyzes the role of stress; Part Four deals with nutrition; Part Five outlines the use of vitamins, minerals, and other supplements; and Part Six covers habits of mind. Extensively utilizing a question-and-answer technique, Carrigan overloads her textual explanation with excessive personal narrative that blunts the force of her message. A diffuse and somewhat muddled presentation.

Strohecker, James, and Nancy Shaw Strohecker (editors). *Natural Healing for Depression: Solutions from the World's Great Health Traditions and Practitioners*. New York: Perigee, 1999. 338pp. $15.99 (paper).

Depression rarely has a single cause and requires a holistic approach to its understanding and treatment. Depression always involves both mind and body, the individual person, and the environment in which the person lives. Complete recovery requires that many paths be undertaken. The authors bring together contributions from nine nationally recognized experts in the major fields of complementary and alternative medicine to present a comprehensive and holistic vision of depression. Five of the contributors are experts in the major systems of traditional medicine–Ayurveda, Chinese medicine, herbal medicine, homeopathy, and naturopathic medicine. Three contributors are experts in mind/body medicine, nutritional medicine, and spiritual medicine. The final contributor, a psychiatrist, represents the true integrative approach by blending Western medicine with nutritional medicine, herbs, and leading-edge psychiatry. This is a comprehensive, holistic, and integrative view of depression that goes well beyond the narrow psychopharmacological approach. Appendixes list recommended readings, Internet sites, quick references to therapies, and relevant organizations. Among the authors represented in this volume are Joseph Pizzorno and Hyla Cass.

Diabetes

Guthrie, Diana W., with Richard A. Guthrie. *Alternative and Complementary Diabetes Care: How to Combine Natural and Traditional Therapies.* New York: Wiley, 2000. 244pp. $14.95 (paper).

The emphasis of the Guthries (a holistic nurse and a physician respectively) is on how to use alternative medicine as an adjunct to conventional diabetes care. Much attention is paid to positive thinking, dealing with conflict, relaxation, nutrition, and the role of herbs in changing blood glucose levels. So much of the content of the book is devoted to description of herbal medicine and other alternative treatment options that the application of natural therapies to diabetes is lost. A poorly focused book.

Mitchell, Deborah. *Natural Medicine for Diabetes.* New York: Dell, 1997. 192pp. $5.99 (paper).

A panoramic look at what 20 complementary and alternative methods can do in managing diabetes. The natural therapies discussed address four key areas: nutrition, exercise, stress reduction, and the mind/body connection. All of the healing approaches are meant to complement a patient's current diabetes management program. Part One explains the essential facts of diabetes; Part Two summarizes 20 complementary therapies such as herbal medicine, homeopathy, and nutritional supplements; Part Three describes conventional medical therapy in the form of insulin, diabetes, pills with glucagon, and medical interventions for diabetic complications. Mitchell offers a mixture

of hope, answers, and tools to help diabetics take control of their diabetes.

Eye Care

Grossman, Marc, and Glen Swartout. *Natural Eye Care: An Encyclopedia: Complementary Treatments for Improving and Saving Your Eyes.* Los Angeles: Keats Publishing, 1999. 196pp. $16.95 (paper).

Two optometrists trained in Chinese medicine, acupuncture, and naturopathic medicine attempt to integrate the full range of alternative therapies as they apply to vision and vision disorders. Chapters devoted to major eye disorders such as glaucoma, macular degeneration, cataracts, and dry eyes describe both the standard Western medical approach to treatment, and alternative medicines such as herbal remedies, acupressure points, nutritional modification, vision therapy, and homeopathy. Holistic treatment for glaucoma includes, for example, the use of vitamins, acupressure, herbal remedies, homeopathic preparations, and even marijuana. Emphasis is placed on prevention and health maintenance in that eye tissue places tremendous demands on all body systems. The authors advocate complementary rather than alternative treatments. The book is well documented and offers many helpful suggestions for improving overall eye care.

Fibromyalgia and Chronic Fatigue Syndrome

Skelly, Mari, and Andrea Helm. *Alternative Treatments for Fibromyalgia and Chronic Fatigue Syndrome: Insights from Practitioners and Patients.* Alameda, CA: Hunter House, 1999. 270pp. $15.95 (paper).

This book serves a dual purpose: to explain fibryomalgia and chronic fatigue syndrome from the viewpoint of symptoms, diagnosis, and treatment, and to outline alternative methods of treatment including nutrition, Chinese medicine, spirituality, massage and physical therapy, osteopathy, chiropractic and craniosacral therapy, and so on. Through the liberal use of patients' stories and practitioners' commentary, Skelly and Helm succeed admirably in showing how to draw upon a wide range of healing options. Contains list of resources, organizations, newsletters and Web sites, together with a glossary.

Gastrointestinal Health

Berkson, D. Lindsey. *Healthy Digestion the Natural Way: Preventing and Healing Heartburn, Constipation, Gas, Diarrhea, Inflammatory Bowel and Gallbladder Dis-*

eases, Ulcers, Irritable Bowel Syndrome, Food Allergies, and More. New York: Wiley, 1999. 256pp. $16.95 (paper).

Berkson, a chiropractor and nutritionist, reviews what can go wrong with the normal process of digestion and describes the symptoms and causes of specific digestive conditions such as heartburn, diarrhea, inflammatory bowel disease, and gallbladder disease. In each instance, corrective action is suggested relying on self-help techniques, dietary modification, exercise, mind-body and breathing techniques, and reflexology. Berkson argues that it is preferable to try natural alternatives before turning to drugs and surgery. "Natural remedies are essential tools to help you take sensible responsibility." A clear statement of the alternative approach to gastrointestinal problems.

Jensen, Bernard. *Doctor Jensen's Guide to Better Bowel Care: A Complete Program for Tissue Cleansing through Bowel Management.* Garden City Park, NY: Avery, 1999. 244pp. $14.95 (paper).

Based on six decades of experience, Jensen endeavors to raise bowel consciousness by showing how digestive malfunction can cause toxins to build up in the intestines, which in turn can make the entire body ill. After reviewing common bowel disorders, Jensen details his seven-day cleansing program, which involves cleansing drinks, laxatives, colemas (a special kind of enema that is more thorough in its internal cleansing of the bowel), supplements, and rectal implants. Twelve pages of instructions are provided detailing the procedures and operation of the colema. A seven-week building and replacement program is designed to follow the seven-day cleansing program. The essential point made by Jensen is that the immune system can only be strengthened in a clean body with a minimal amount of accumulated toxic material. Ten pages of gruesome color photographs are included showing the putrefactive debris that issued from individuals who undertook the seven-day cleanse. Graphic!

Nicol, Rosemary. *Irritable Bowel Syndrome: A Natural Approach.* Berkeley, CA: Ulysses Press, 1999. 229pp. $13.95 (paper).

Irritable Bowel Syndrome (IBS) (a.k.a. spastic colitis, mucus colitis, "tense tummy") is a general term for a group of common intestinal tract disorders affecting some 20 to 30 percent of the inhabitants of Western nations. Nicol provides a clear explanation of the causes and symptoms of IBS, the role of stress, and the mainstream antidotes—reducing stress, controlling feelings, learning to relax, exercising, and so on. The alternative approach to alleviating IBS involves the use of homeopathic remedies, medicinal herbs, naturopathy, osteopathy, hypnotherapy, Chinese

medicine, Ayurveda and biofeedback. A final, comprehensive chapter discusses foods to be avoided, together with dietary suggestions and bland recipes. A useful, well-balanced book, packed with much practical advice.

Trenev, Natasha. *Probiotics: Nature's Internal Healers.* Garden City Park, NY: Avery, 1998. 250pp. $12.95 (paper).

Probiotics, Trenev explains, are the friendly bacteria that live and work in your gastrointestinal tract and constitute your first line of defense against illness and disease. The friendly bacteria are *Lactobacillus acidophilus, Bifido-bacterium, bifidum,* and *Lactobacillus bulgaricus.* Part One of the book includes information on the great impact that friendly bacteria and diet have on good health and on their antibiotic, antiviral, and anticancer capabilities. Part Two opens with some general guidelines on taking probiotics and is followed by an A-to-Z listing of common illnesses and conditions that can result from bacteria deficiency. Recommended probiotic regimens are detailed. Strong advocacy of the mustering and deployment of your bacterial army.

Trickett, Shirley. *Candida: A Natural Approach.* Berkeley, CA: Ulysses Press, 1999. 196pp. $11.95 (paper).

When candida and other harmful yeasts proliferate, they block the sites of the bowel where the enzymes necessary for the breakdown of food inhabit. This results in poor digestion, food intolerance, bloating, and altered bowel habits. An overgrowth of candida in the colon can also inhibit the absorption of essential nutrients, thereby creating vitamin and mineral deficiencies. After portraying the symptoms and discomforts of candida, Trickett (a British nurse) shows how to manage the food intolerances that cause candida. Separate chapters deal with foods needed to heal, guidelines for a strict candida diet, and how to get started. Also included are 47 pages of recipes for quick meals, special-occasion cooking, and yeast-free breads.

Trickett, Shirley. *Irritable Bowel Syndrome and Diverticulosis: A Self-Help Plan.* London, UK: Thorsons, 1999. 228pp. $11 (paper).

How to achieve harmony in the bowel and relieve the chronic constipation, diarrhea, gas, and discomforts associated with irritable bowel syndrome (IBS). After discussing symptoms (sluggish bowel, hyperactive bowel, confused bowel), Trickett discusses causes and the relationship of IBS to the nervous system, stress, hormones, candida albicans, food intolerance, and prescribed drugs. Self-help methods suggested include relaxation, exercise, vitamins, and minerals. The final part of the book describes what complementary medicine can contribute in the form of homeopathy, therapeutic massage, colonic irrigation, reflexology, shiatsu, and aromatherapy. This is a comprehensive review of IBS with many helpful suggestions. Since Trickett is a British nurse, it is not surprising that the list of addresses and references is almost exclusively British.

Webster, David. *Acidophilus Colon Health: The Natural Way to Prevent Disease.* New York: Kensington Books, 1999. 157pp. $10 (paper).

"If your colon is alkaline due to secretions from pathogens harbored there, toxins and their insidious by-products are already building up. They are like termites eating away at your foundation." A healthy colon is the body's first line of defense against disease. Acidophilus, a beneficial bacteria that lives in the healthy colon, plays a critical role in the strength of this protection. When antibiotics or other drug therapy destroy the resident acidophilus, the colon becomes susceptible to pathogens, yeasts, parasites, and viruses. To reestablish healthy colon flora, Webster recommends the use of edible-grade, sweet dairy whey in the daily diet. If this fails, the Webster Implant Technique (WIT) can be used—involving the implanting of a specific human strain of acidophilus culture to jump-start the colon's own acidophilus colony. An appendix lists where to purchase WIT recommended products, and an 11-page listing of references is included. A book that argues that this whey is the way to go!

Headaches and Migraine

Bic, Zuzana, and L. Francis Bic. *No More Headaches, No More Migraines: A Proven Approach to Preventing Headaches and Migraines.* Garden City Park, NY: Avery, 1999. 134pp. $10.95 (paper).

How to become headache-free through a combination of good nutrition, physical activity, and stress management. One of the most important headache triggers is the level of lipids and fatty acids in the blood. Fat levels are affected by the same things that can trigger headaches—lack of physical activity, emotional upset, inadequate sleep, stress, and poorly balanced nutrition. The lifestyle modification advocated to prevent headaches and migraines involves a balanced diet low in fat and refined sugar and high in complex carbohydrates, together with a regimen of physical activity and techniques to reduce stress. A final chapter introduces ways of measuring your progress at home without special training. A natural alternative to the use of drugs to control headaches and migraines.

Finnigan, Jeffry. *Life Beyond Headaches.* Olympia, WA: The Finnigan Clinic, 1999. 125pp. $14.95 (paper).

Finnigan, a chiropractor, intends his book to be "a self-actualization catalyst." His basic assumption is that "with the Life-Force, your body has the potential to produce all the hormones and chemicals known, and unknown, at the right time in the right amount. Your body then distributes these substances to the right places, without side effects as long as we haven't interfered with the process." The "Six Foundational Keys to Health Amplification" that must be turned on involve air, food and water, exercise, sleep, positive mental attitude, and a healthy nervous system. One chapter specifically addresses headache. The title of the book is a misnomer in that the bulk of the content is devoted to advancing the theory of the Six Foundational Keys ("linchpins" of health).

Heart Disease

DeFelice, Stephen L. *The Carnitine Defense: A Nutraceutical Formula to Prevent and Treat Heart Disease, the Nation's #1 Killer.* New York: Rodale/St. Martin's, 1999. 266pp. $23.95.

Nutraceuticals are foods and dietary supplements with disease-fighting properties. DeFelice, an endocrinologist and clinical pharmacologist, argues that the "Carnitine Defense" is a combination of nutraceuticals, an elixir or mixture of natural molecules that will help prevent destructive heart disease. Carnitine increases use of fat in the body as an energy source at the cellular level. It also inhibits damaging fatty buildup in the heart and other tissues and lessens heart risks, especially of heart attacks stemming from coronary artery disease. DeFelice explains what carnitine does, the mechanism of protection involved, where you can buy it and how much to take. The carnitine elixir advocated contains, in addition to carnitine, vitamin E, folic acid, vitamin B6, vitamin B12, magnesium, chromium, and alcohol. Do not wait until definitive studies are performed, urges DeFelice, because "many lives would unnecessarily be lost due to heart attacks during the many years that it would take to complete the studies." Somewhat surprisingly, DeFelice argues that there is "no need to conduct double-blind studies." Informative and controversial.

Goldberg, Burton, and the editors of *Alternative Medicine Digest. Alternative Medicine Guide to Heart Disease.* Tiburon, CA: Future Medicine Publishing, 1998. 293pp. $18.95 (paper).

The basic message conveyed is "Hold the Angioplasty . . . Cancel the Bypass," avoid heart attack, and reverse stroke damage. Goldberg maintains that heart disease is one of the most preventable chronic degenerative diseases. The therapies advocated build upon dietary modification, exercise, and lifestyle habits. The effective treatments described include chelation therapy ("scrubbing the arteries"), hyperbaric oxygen therapy, nutritional supplements, herbal medicines, amino acids, coenzyme Q10, magnet therapy, and so on. Posing the rhetorical question, "why haven't I heard about these treatments?" Goldberg suggests that the answer lies in politics and greed. "The U.S. medical monopoly (has) . . . a literal investment in keeping nonpatentable and inexpensive treatments from the public." Widespread use of chelation and hyperbaric oxygen therapies "would cut deeply into the conventional medical profit pie." This is a fascinating compilation of theory, fact, hype, speculation, anecdotal evidence, and sometimes plausible explanation. Highly readable.

Heller, Richard F., Rachael F. Heller, and Frederic J. Vagnini. *The Carbohydrate Addict's Healthy Heart Program: Break Your Carbo-Insulin Connection to Heart Disease*. New York: Ballantine, 1999. 352pp. $24.95.

The logic is simple: too much insulin in the blood, hyperinsulinemia, can lead directly to heart disease, high blood pressure, insulin resistance, diabetes, and excessive weight gain. Insulin levels can rise as a result of foods rich in carbohydrates—not just starches, snacks and sweets—but also low-cal foods. Carbohydrate craving can wreak havoc in the body, drive up insulin levels, and can seriously compromise one's health. The authors offer a balanced, back-to-basics, scientifically-based program to correct the insulin imbalance that can trigger craving for high-carbohydrate foods. The Program advocated involves two stages, the "Basic Plan" and "Heart Health-Enhancing Options." Each plan in turn involves multiple guidelines. This is a very complicated and complex description replete with a host of plan stages, steps, and guidelines. For those that are skeptical, the authors recommend that you "try our eating program for three days. You might be in for the biggest surprise of your life."

Holt, Stephen. *The Natural Way to a Healthy Heart: Lessons from Alternative and Conventional Medicine*. New York: Evans, 1999. 328pp. $19.95.

Holt offers "a marriage of conventional medicine and natural options for cardiovascular health." His emphasis is on the promotion of cardiovascular wellness and a reduction of risk factors. An exclusive focus on lowering cholesterol is counterproductive: "In the absence of a nutritional program to improve general health, it is not always safe, nor is it cost effective, to reduce cholesterol by excluding cholesterol intake in the diet and/or prescribing synthetic drugs that lower fats (cholesterol in the blood)." This is an excellent, informative discussion of the keys to prevention, culprits such as cholesterol, triglycerides and homocysteine, importance of weight control, role of nutrition, use of soy

and healing plants (ginkgo, hawthorn, ginseng, green tea), and a "CardioPlan" to cardiovascular health. An excellent, sensible, and balanced approach to cardiovascular health, blending conventional and alternative approaches.

Keane, Maureen, and Daniella Chace. *What to Eat If You Have Heart Disease: Nutritional Therapy for the Prevention and Treatment of Cardiovascular Disease*. Lincolnwood, IL: Contemporary Books, 1998. 223pp. $14.95 (paper).

Two nutritionists describe the cardiovascular system as a "living river" that nourishes the cells that make up our bodies. The authors do not recommend anything radical—just a whole-foods diet moderately low in fat and rich in fruits and vegetables, that is augmented by a basic food supplement program. Part One explains the medical problems involved in heart disease (atherosclerosis, dyslipidemias, hypertension, heart failure); Part Two shows how to get started with a basic diet plan, a recovery diet, a low-fat diet, a diet for hypertension, and a heart failure diet. Appendixes list a glossary, references, and mail-order resources. Readers will probably find the diet plans more useful and less intimidating than the technical discussion of the cardiovascular system and the chemistry of lipids.

McCully, Kilmer S. *The Homocysteine Revolution: Medicine for the New Millenium*. New Canaan, CT: Keats, 1999. 192pp. $16.95 (paper).

The major point made is that homocysteine, a byproduct of metabolism, is a better indication of risk of heart disease than high cholesterol. Elevation of blood homocysteine results in atherosclerosis in that arteries are damaged by the injurious effect of homocysteine on cells and tissues of the arteries. The homocysteine theory considers atherosclerosis to be the result of dietary imbalance from potential deficiencies of vitamin B6, B12, and folic acid, while the cholesterol approach incriminates the toxicity of dietary fats in the development of vascular disease. After explaining the causes of atherosclerosis and the role of homocysteine, McCully (a pathologist) moves beyond cholesterol to implicate homocysteine in the causation of a number of other chronic diseases including cancer. A highly persuasive book, totally convincing, and well documented.

McCully, Kilmer S., and Martha McCully. *The Heart Revolution: The B-Vitamin Breakthrough That Lowers Homocysteine, Cuts Your Risk of Heart Disease, and Protects Your Health*. New York: HarperCollins, 1999. 234pp. $24.

This book covers much of the same ground as the same author's *The Homocysteine Revolution: Medicine for the New Millenium* (Keats, 1999). The basic point made is the same:

that it has never been scientifically proven that fats and cholesterol cause atherosclerosis or that lowering the amount of fat and cholesterol in our diets will reduce the risk of developing heart disease. Instead, McCully advances the homocysteine theory of heart disease—when there is too much homocysteine in the blood, arteries are damaged and plaque forms. This results from a deficiency of B vitamins—namely B6, B12, and folic acid. In a very revealing foreword, Michelle Stacey, the author of "The Fall and Rise of Kilmer McCully," (*New York Times Magazine*, 9 August 1997) describes how McCully lost his job, laboratory, and funding at Massachusetts General Hospital due to his espousal of the homocysteine theory. "Many people had invested heavily in the cholesterol theory, and few wanted to hear it challenged." Furthermore, "the cholesterol bandwagon was loaded up and ready to go." Pharmaceutical companies have a vested interest in keeping cholesterol and its expensive drug treatments in the forefront of cardiac treatment. McCully makes a powerful, well-documented statement that demands attention. Gripping and compelling reading.

Sachs, Judith. *Natural Medicine for Heart Disease*. New York: Dell, 1997. 255pp. $5.99 (paper).

In addition to nutrition, exercise and stress reduction techniques, a vast array of other natural remedies can be employed: herbs, homeopathy, yoga, breathing, meditation, biofeedback, and more. These alternative methods are less expensive, noninvasive and, when used appropriately, have no side effects. Many claims are made: you can lower your blood pressure with cayenne pepper; folic acid reduces homocysteine, a toxic amino acid that creates arterial lesions; T'ai Chi may be the most effective therapy to remove the emotional triggers in a highly stressed person; safe plant enzymes found in soy products are more effective than heparin; and more. Separate chapters are devoted to the benefits of herbs, homeopathy, Chinese and Ayurvedic medicine, and other complementary treatments such as chelation therapy and reflexology. Clearly written with a decided contrarian tone.

Hepatitis

Roybal, Beth Ann. *Hepatitis C: A Personal Guide to Good Health*. 2nd edition. Berkeley, CA: Ulysses Press, 1999. 151pp. $13.95 (paper).

This is an updated and revised edition of a book originally published in 1997 that offers a comprehensive guide to the "silent epidemic" of hepatitis C. Roybal summarizes existing knowledge with respect to the nature of the virus, causes, modes of transmission, symptoms, diagnostic tests, treatment, and options. Two chapters deal with alterna-

tive treatments (herbal medicine, Ayurveda, homeopathy, and naturopathic medicine), the role of diet (nutritional supplements, antioxidants), and the beneficial effects of exercise. An extensive glossary defines technical terms used in the text and there is a listing of resources, organizations, support groups, and references. Detailed, informative, and highly useful.

Hypertension

Mann, Samuel J. *Healing Hypertension: Uncovering the Secret Power of Your Hidden Emotions*. New York: Wiley, 1999. 244pp. $24.95.

This book is a study of the mind-body relationship of hypertension. Mann, a hypertension specialist, rejects the notion that the cause of essential hypertension is unknown. Mann's point is that getting angry or tense can undoubtedly elevate blood pressure but it does not cause hypertension. Instead, "it is our hidden emotions, the emotions we do not feel, that lead to hypertension and many other unexplained physical disorders." In some people, hypertension is genetic while in others it is driven by hidden emotions. Mann shows how to determine if hidden emotions play a role and outlines how persons can foster the healing process through support groups, therapy, and a sense of connectiveness with others. To correct overdiagnosis and overtreatment of hypertension, one chapter is devoted to the correct use of medication. This is an intriguing book that tends to underestimate the difficulty involved in unraveling the mind-body connection.

Immunity

Chitow, Leon. *Antibiotic Crisis, Antibiotic Alternatives*. London, UK: Thorsons/HarperCollins, 1998. 233pp. $19.95.

A British author (a naturopath and osteopath) draws attention to the alarming spread of antibiotic-resistant bacteria such as the superbug *Staphylococcus aureus* now resistant to almost all antibiotics except highly potent, highly toxic forms of antibiotics which can themselves cause serious side effects. Antibiotic misuse is rampant. People demand antibiotics and doctors commonly comply. The solution lies in immune enhancement through lifestyle modification; detoxification (fasting for health); and the use of supplements, herbs, hydrotherapy, and acupuncture. If you have to take antibiotics, then foods and substances should be consumed to develop probiotics—the friendly bacteria that can restore the natural balance and population levels of friendly bacteria in the body. Despite the alarmist title, this is an entirely reasonable and highly persuasive book warning against the extravagant and profligate misuse of antibiotics.

McKenna, John. *Natural Alternatives to Antibiotics.* Garden City Park, NY: Avery, 1998. 188pp. $12.95 (paper).

The massive overprescription and misuse of antibiotics has led to a growing number of serious health concerns. Today's stronger antibiotics can totally destroy beneficial intestinal bacteria, leading to bowel disorders and depressed immunity. McKenna maintains that it is possible to treat infections without antibiotics, although accepting the fact that antibiotics may sometimes be needed. The natural alternatives advocated include herbs that fight infection (echinacea, wild indigo, myrrh, garlic, wormwood), homeopathic remedies, nutritional supplementation (immune-enhancing vitamins and minerals), and bacterial supplementation ("Healthy Flora, a Healthy Body"). The major point made is that the best alternative to antibiotics is to maintain your health to ensure that antibiotics will not be needed.

Mitchell, Deborah. *Natural Medicine for Super Immunity.* New York: Dell, 1998. 240pp. $5.99 (paper).

How to give a boost to your immune system, naturally and safely, without the use of drugs or other medical interventions through diet, herbs, nutritional supplements, body therapies, mind-body approaches, and detoxification programs. Separate chapters deal with common immune disorders and diseases, foods for optimal health, supplemental nutrition, healing herbs, body therapies such as acupuncture and massage, and mind-body boosters (biofeedback, meditation, and detoxification). This is a somewhat simplified presentation characterized by dramatic language: "there are battles raging within you . . . 24 hours a day, your internal army fights to protect and maintain your health against countless invasions and invaders."

Menopause

Gittleman, Ann Louise. *Super Nutrition for Menopause.* Garden City Park, NY: Avery, 1998. 226pp. $10.95 (paper).

Gittleman, a nutritionist and former director of the Pritikin Longevity Center, outlines a nutrition program that can prevent and control the unpleasant symptoms associated with the natural life change of menopause. While the uncomfortable symptoms associated with menopause such as hot flashes and mood swings can be connected to lower hormonal output, this should not lead to the misconception that menopause is a pathological process. The cumulative effects of long-term nutrient deficiencies and negative life-

style habits have been blatantly ignored. A vital and balanced diet supplemented with vitamins, minerals, essential fatty acids, and herbs that reinforce the body's glandular system can provide natural relief from menopausal discomforts without the risks inherent in hormone replacement therapy. Three detailed chapters outline an exercise and nutrition program with planning and recipes.

Laucella, Linda. *Hormone Replacement Therapy: Conventional Medicine and Natural Alternatives: Your Guide to Menopausal Health-Care Choices.* 3rd edition. Los Angeles, CA: Lowell House, 1999. 237pp. $16.95 (paper).

This is an update of a 2nd edition published in 1994. Using a question-and-answer format, Laucella (a writer and editor) attempts to present women with a wider range of choices when dealing with hormone replacement therapy. These choices include non-drug treatments such as acupuncture, homeopathy, naturopathy, aromatherapy, Chinese medicine, and herbs. This new edition contains a new chapter on perimenopause together with updated information on menopause and women's menopausal health care options. Laucella shows how lifestyle changes can enhance a women's health with or without hormone replacement therapy, how self-help techniques can minimize the discomforts of menopause, and what complementary medicine has to offer.

Liew, Lana, with Linda Ojeda. *The Natural Estrogen Diet: Healthy Recipes for Perimenopause and Menopause.* Alameda, CA: Hunter House, 1999. 212pp. $13.95 (paper).

Phytoestrogens are a diverse group of plant-derived substances that have estrogenic activity in animals. The most commonly studied phytoestrogens include the isoflavenoids, lignans, and coumestans found in high amounts in soy beans, flaxseed, and alfalfa. Phytoestrogens have an estrogenic effect similar to those seen in patients treated with hormones. For those who cannot, or do not wish to take hormones, there are alternatives. Liew (an Australian physician) and Ojeda (a pioneer in women's health care) discuss a variety of foods that are rich in naturally occurring plant estrogens that can work to minimize menopausal systems while also benefiting the bones and heart, and possibly curbing the risk of breast cancer. In particular, soy products are a rich source of potent isoflavones, a subclass of plant estrogens. One chapter is devoted to explaining how to integrate natural estrogens into your life. The bulk of the book consists of recipes for appetizers, snacks, soups, main courses, and desserts. How to manage menopausal symptoms the natural way!

Murray, Frank. *All About Menopause: Phytoestrogens and Red Clover: Frequently Asked Questions.* Garden City Park, NY: Avery, 1998. 93pp. $2.99 (paper).

The safe and natural way to ease hot flashes, help prevent osteoporosis, night sweats, vaginal dryness, and cope with other menopause-related problems lies in the use of phytoestrogens (plant estrogens). The typical Western diet, relying heavily on processed foods, is deficient in phytoestrogens. Hormone replacement therapy is not the answer. Instead, phytoestrogens provide a significant level of estrogenic activity in the body. Phytoestrogens include flavanones, isoflavones, lignans, coumestans, chalcones, flavanols, and flavones. Very high levels of all estrogenic isoflavones are found in red clover, which appears to be a safe source of phytoestrogens for those who lack the time or desire to eat legumes regularly. Red clover supplements are readily available. The question-and-answer format provides answers to what to look for in buying red clover supplements, when to expect results, and possible side effects. An attractive approach to menopause management that avoids the complications and risks of synthetic hormones. Contains a glossary and index.

Rushton, Anna, and Shirley A. Bond. *Natural Progesterone: The Natural Way to Alleviate Symptoms of Menopause, PMS, and Other Hormone-Related Problems.* London, UK: Thorsons, 1999. 162pp. $15 (paper).

Natural progesterone has been neglected and ignored for more than 40 years in favor of the less effective, more toxic synthetic substitutes (progestins). Rushton and Bond maintain that progesterone is a totally essential hormone whose role has been sadly underemphasized and undervalued by the medical profession. The authors claim that natural progesterone, available in transdermal creams and sublingual tablets, can significantly reduce symptoms such as weight gain, heavy bleeding, and mood swings, as well as providing protection against osteoporosis and heart disease. Separate chapters deal with the use of natural progesterone in the fertile years, and in menopause, cancer, and osteoporosis. This is a British book that lists mainly U.K. resources in an appendix. Progesterone products are available without a prescription in the United States but can only be obtained in the United Kingdom by prescription.

Nutrition

Abravanel, Elliot D., and Elizabeth King Morrison. *Doctor Abravanel's Body Type Diet and Lifetime Nutrition Plan.* Revised edition. New York: Bantam, 1999. 365pp. $13.95 (paper).

This is a revised edition of a book originally published in 1993. In a foreword to this new edition, Abravanel states that he has been "concerned over the past 10 years or so by the significant number of readers who have not been able to determine their body type to their own satisfaction." Consequently, the "Body Type Checklist" has been revised to assist readers in finding their correct body type. The "Body Type Diets" have also been modified to meet today's scientific nutritional standards. The basic principle remains the same—that each person has a distinct body type determined by the dominant gland (adrenal, thyroid, pituitary, or, for some women, gonadal) that determines body shape and build, preferred foods, energy patterns, and how fat is deposited in the body. Accordingly, weight loss and maintenance diets that work well for adrenal types are not suitable for thyroid types, and so on. Menu plans with recipes are presented for each body type. A peculiar blend of research in endocrinology and traditional morphological types combined with nutritional supplementation and exercise.

Balch, Phyllis A., and James F. Balch. *Prescription for Dietary Wellness Using Foods to Heal.* Garden City Park, NY: Avery, 1998. 318pp. $16.95 (paper).

The authors describe power foods for longevity, energy, the immune system, healing specific disorders, and "brain food." The powerful prescription forces specified include fresh vegetables, fruits, sea vegetables, whole grains, nuts, seeds, beans, legumes, soybean products, and herbs. The phytochemicals contained in many of these foods show potent anticarcinogenic activity. Part One reviews the nutritional powerhouse contained in foods; Part Two offers a comprehensive explanation of individual foods; while Part Three lists almost 300 kitchen-tested recipes spanning some 100 pages. A most informative discussion of what constitutes healthy eating.

Becker, Gail L. *Savvy: A Shopper's Guide to Brand-Name Dietary Supplements.* New York: Dell, 1997. 472pp. $6.50 (paper).

A dietitian offers a compact reference resource that answers most questions about dietary supplements—how to select them, rules of thumb in buying supplements, safety factors, and dosages. Simply defined, dietary supplements are substances that can be consumed to add to the nutrients obtained from the foods that you eat. The bulk of the book consists of dietary supplement information chapters showing the brand name, retail price, serving size and amount, percentage met of the RDI, USP standard and expiration date, availability (drugstore, supermarket, direct mail order, etc.), and other characteristics. More than 100 charts detail vitamins, minerals, herbals, and botanicals, and specialty products. Appendix material contains manufacturer contact information, a glossary of terms, and recommended readings. Highly informative, but the value of the book is reduced by the difficulty in locating information in massive charts that are poorly arranged and formatted.

Challem, Jack, Burton Berkson, and Melissa Diane Smith. *Syndrome X: The Complete Nutritional Program to Prevent and Reverse Insulin Resistance.* New York: Wiley, 2000. 272pp. $24.95.

The hallmark of Syndrome X is a resistance to insulin, the hormone that enables the body to use the energy stored in the food we eat. If you have insulin resistance together with high cholesterol, high triglycerides, high blood pressure, or too much body fat, you have Syndrome X. The authors maintain that Syndrome X is primarily a nutritional disease caused by eating the wrong types of foods. In a somewhat alarmist manner—"you are about to be engulfed in one of the largest disease epidemics ever to strike North America," Challem and colleagues outline a nutritional program to counter Syndrome X involving the use of key supplemental vitamins, minerals, herbs, and vitamin-like nutrients that can be used to jump-start or fine-tune your body's defenses. Chief among these supplements is alpha lipoic acid, "The Master Nutrient." Nine "Anti-X" diet principles are described together with an Anti-X diet and recipes.

Craig, Selene Y., and the editors of *Prevention* Magazine Healthbooks. *The Complete Book of Alternative Nutrition: Powerful New Ways to Use Foods, Supplements, Herbs, and Special Diets to Prevent and Cure Disease.* Emmaus, PA: Rodale Press, 1997. 283pp. $19.95.

This is a highly readable and practical guide to the healing power of food. Part One reviews a wide range of alternative diets such as macrobiotics, the Ornish program, the Pritikin Plan, and fasting that are highly beneficial; Part Two, the Alternative Pharmacy, reviews alternative supplements (amino acids, enzymes, spirulina) and herbal nutrition—"where kitchen meets pharmacy;" Part Three describes the role of nutrition in healing arthritis, cancer, diabetes, migraines, and so on; Part Four consists of a detailed chart showing the diets, herbs, and supplements that can help prevent or reverse specific conditions or diseases. Once again, as in other volumes in this Rodale series, the editors have digested the cumulated wisdom and advice of a wide array of professionals—medical doctors, researchers, nutritionists, naturopaths, doctors of Oriental medicine, and so on. An attractive and informative book.

Firshein, Richard N. *The Nutraceutical Revolution: Twenty Cutting-Edge Nutrients to Help You Design Your Own Perfect Whole-Life Program.* New York: Riverhead Books, 1998. 371pp. $24.95.

Nutraceuticals are nutrients that have the capacity to act like medicines. Firshein maintains that nutrition can literally save lives. Twenty chapters describe an assortment of supplements, vitamins, herbs, minerals, amino acids, and phytochemicals. These include fish oil, coenzyme Q10, tyrosine, quercetin, black cohosh, and saw palmetto. Soy can help balance hormones and prevent cancer; fish oil seems to work wonders with chronic inflammatory disease; black cohosh is a remedy for PMS; lutein is useful in treating macular degeneration and other eye diseases; and so on. Detailed documentation is provided for each chapter. An index of ailments is supplied that lists useful nutraceuticals for treating common medical conditions such as arthritis and urinary tract infections. Far reaching claims based upon the belief that the future of medicine lies in nutraceuticals.

***Mortimore, Denise. *The Complete Illustrated Guide to Nutritional Healing: The Use of Diet, Vitamins, Minerals, and Herbs for Optimum Health.* Boston: Element Books, 1998. 256pp. $24.95 (paper).

An excellent book, utilizing splendid color photographs and illustrations, for those who wish to improve their health by nutritional means. Nutritional healing is defined as a practical way of overcoming illness and promoting health naturally without the use of toxic drugs. Nutritional healing bases its success on five ground rules of dietary change for restoring the body's health—correcting faulty digestion, decreasing toxic overload of rich and overprocessed food, releasing healing energy for elimination of toxins, rebalancing the intestinal bacteria to improve absorption of vitamins, minerals, and amino acids, and identifying and supporting weakened, overburdened organs through correct supplementation. Part One of the book covers basic principles of nutritional healing; Part Two details optimum nutrition; Part Three shows how to assess your health and diet in terms of food, allergies, pollution, and stress; Part Four describes nutritional healing for common ailments; Part Five discusses nutrition and female health; and Part Six consists of appendices detailing food combining and specific diets—the Detoxification Diet, Hypoallergenic Diet, and so on. An outstanding book like other books in this Element Book series, packed with useful information at the same time as being aesthetically pleasing. Excellent.

Napier, Kristine. *Eat to Heal: The Phytochemical Diet and Nutrition Plan.* New York: Warner, 1998. 282pp. $5.99 (paper).

Napier, a dietitian, announces that "your kitchen is about to become your medicine cabinet—not only big in size, but mighty in the power it has to give you energetic, great health." Nutrition can now be used to prevent, manage, and perhaps delay, the premature onset of chronic disease. Phytochemicals (plant chemicals) add a whole new dimension to the nutritional goodness of fruit, vegetables, and grains. Napier explains the myriad health benefits conveyed by phytochemicals. Separate chapters show how phytochemicals and other nutrients work together, phytochemicals listed by food groups, and phytochemicals that fight specific diseases. Other chapters contain recipes and suggest where to buy fruits, vegetables, grains, and legumes. The author does not, however, clearly describe and explain what phytochemicals are.

Weil, Andrew. *Eating Well for Optimum Health: The Essential Guide to Food, Diet, and Nutrition.* New York: Knopf, 2000. 307pp. $25.

Following up on his *Spontaneous Healing* (Knopf, 1995) and *Eight Weeks to Optimum Health* (Knopf, 1997), Weil now turns his attention to nutrition and diet. As a starting point, Weil states his "conviction that healthy and delicious food are not mutually exclusive; the concept of 'eating well' must embrace both the health-promoting and pleasure-giving aspects of foods." Weil introduces little here that is controversial. Instead, he offers a number of basic propositions—we have to eat to live, eating is a major source of pleasure, eating is an important focus of social interaction, how we eat reflects and defines our personal and cultural identity, and so on. After discussing the basic facts concerning fats, carbohydrates, minerals, and vitamins, etc., Weil presents his Optimum Diet with weekly menus. Recipes are given for soups, salads, appetizers, fish, vegetables, pasta, rice, potatoes, and desserts. In all, a very readable and entertaining discussion of the basics of nutrition but entirely lacking in the often contrarian advice offered in Weil's other books. Bland reading!

Osteoporosis

Germano, Carl, with William Cabot. *The Osteoporosis Solution: The New Therapies for Prevention and Treatment.* New York: Kensington Books, 1999. 203pp. $22.

Germano (a dietitian) and Cabot (an orthopedist) reject the "Tums" theory that holds that calcium replacement is the nutritional "be-all and end-all" of treating osteoporosis. Instead, they show that the dietary supplement ipriflavone prevents bone loss and improves bone density as effectively as any drug such as calcitonin and estrogen replacement therapy. Isoflavones, found naturally in soy, have been successfully used as phytoestrogens to reduce bone loss without the detrimental effects of estrogen. The authors advocate bone health through nutritional intervention.

Girman, Andrea, and Carol Poole. *Preventing Osteoporosis with Ipriflavone.* Roseville, CA: Prima, 2000. 235pp. $14.95 (paper).

This is a book that aims to give ipriflavone, a dietary supplement derived from natural substance found in soybeans, the notice that it deserves. According to Girman and Poole, numerous scientific studies have proved that ipriflavone protects against the bone loss that leads to osteoporosis. In contrast with conventional therapies, including the use of Fosamax, Evista, and other hormones, ipriflavone has few side effects. Separate chapters are devoted to the scientific evidence, how ipriflavone works, and its safety record. The authors also identify the many health benefits of soybeans (from which ipriflavone is derived) especially for women during or after menopause. There are 25 pages of references to the scientific literature.

Pain

Movig, Dianne. *Healing the Pain: Medical, Alternative and Self-Help Options for Pain Relief.* Lincolnwood, IL: Publications International, 1998. 256pp. $4.99 (paper).

Patients are not expected to stoically bear pain and it is no longer considered an unavoidable companion to illness, injury, and surgery. This compact book outlines 16 options for pain management ranging from conventional treatments such as prescription and nonprescription medication and nerve blocks to alternative treatments such as acupuncture, chiropractic, and herbs. Each description covers an average of eight pages. The second half of the book discusses various illnesses that cause pain (arthritis, cancer, gout, headache) and the treatment methods that can bring relief. A simple summary.

PMS

DeAngelis, Lissa G., and Molly Siple. *SOS for PMS: All-Food Solutions for Premenstrual Syndrome.* New York: Plume, 1999. 276pp. $15.95 (paper).

DeAngelis and Siple, two dietitians, maintain that a "wonderful assortment of fresh, unrefined, unprocessed foods can help restore body chemistry and prevent PMS." Irritability, anxiety, mood swings, nervous tension, bloating, headaches, and fatigue can be lessened through diet. More than 100 easy-to-cook recipes incorporate a rich mixture of vitamins, minerals, fresh and dried fruit, fish, vegetables and salads, meat and poultry, and grains.

Marshel, Judy E., and Anne Egan. *PMS Relief: Natural Approaches to Treating Symptoms*. New York: Berkley Books, 1998. 296pp. $6.99 (paper).

The authors maintain that it is not necessary to suffer from the discomforts of bloating, fluid retention, weight gain, swollen breasts, food cravings, mental cramps, and PMS. A healthy diet, proper vitamins, minerals, herb supplements, and lifestyle factors play a critical role in eliminating the symptoms of PMS. The "PMS Design for Health Program" advocated involves avoiding foods that trigger symptoms and substituting foods rich in phytoestrogens, potassium, B-vitamins, and complex carbohydrates. Exercise can also reduce PMS symptoms. One chapter details how massage and acupressure can relieve PMS. But the explanation of PMS is far from clear and the solutions advocated do not appear to match the symptoms.

Mitchell, Deborah. *Natural Medicine for PMS*. New York: Dell, 1998. 224pp. $5.99 (paper).

Mitchell, a medical writer, advances the case for the use of natural medicine in treating the cyclical, metabolic disturbances of premenstrual syndrome (PMS) that affects millions of women. Several introductory chapters are devoted to explaining the female menstrual cycle and the symptoms and causes of PMS. The natural therapies advocated include diet and exercise, vitamins and mineral supplementation, stress reduction, use of European and Chinese herbs, homeopathy, acupressure, and yoga. Three specific programs are outlined, with combinations of elements best suited to an individual patient's constellation of symptoms. Several appendixes list relevant resource organizations, sources of tapes, remedies, and other natural medicine supplements and suggested readings. A compact well-written alternative approach to PMS.

Pregnancy and Childbirth

Goldberg, Linda, Ginny Brinkley, and Janice Kukar. *Pregnancy to Parenthood: Your Personal Step-By-Step Journey through the Childbirth Experience*. Garden City Park, NY: Avery, 1998. 342pp. $12.95 (paper).

"If you want to be a participant, not a spectator, in the birth of your baby, this is your playbook." The authors intend their book to be used in conjunction with early pregnancy, childbirth preparation, breastfeeding, and new mothers' classes. Clearly and concisely, they provide a month-to-month breakdown of the physical changes to expect during pregnancy, the emotional aspects, do's and don'ts of sex during and after pregnancy, nutritional and exercise plans, care of the newborn, and infant feeding. A most supportive book with good photographs and cartoons illustrating the text that moves well beyond the traditional medical approach to pregnancy and childbirth.

**Marti, James E., with Heather Burton. *Holistic Pregnancy and Childbirth*. New York: Wiley, 1999. 287pp. $16.95 (paper).

This book, according to the authors, "was written to help you make your pregnancy and childbirth the most beautiful experience of your life." The holistic approach advocated is more likely to result in a more comfortable pregnancy, a shorter labor, and a joyful delivery of a perfectly healthy baby. In choosing the holistic approaches recommended, three basic criteria were used—every procedure should be holistic so that pain relief should stimulate the body to produce its own natural painkillers; every procedure must be noninvasive and safe for the mother and baby; every procedure must be effective and focus on the prevention of discomfort and complications rather than merely treating the disorders once they develop. The arrangement of the book is chronological with separate chapters for each month of pregnancy. Typical approaches advocated include acupuncture, aromatherapy, homeopathy, meditation, and nutritional supplements. Individual chapters cover monitoring physical changes; choosing a holistic caregiver; preparing a holistic "birth plan," designing an optimal exercise program; practicing a daily relaxation program of yoga, breathing, and meditation; adopting holistic approaches to bonding, postpartum recovery, and breastfeeding; and preventing common baby discomforts during the first week of a child's life. A most lucid, sensitive, and supportive book. Very good.

Wesson, Nicky. *Enhancing Fertility Naturally: Holistic Therapies for a Successful Pregnancy*. New York: Healing Arts/Inner Traditions, 1999. 191pp. $14.95 (paper).

After explaining infertility in terms of causes, emotional effects, and typical medical and surgical fertility treatments (drugs, IVF, GIFT, and other techniques), Wesson switches her attention to the benefits of alternative therapies such as acupuncture, cranial osteopathy, Chinese herbal medicine, homeopathy, hypnotherapy, and reflexology. The text is sprinkled with case histories attesting to the effectiveness of alternative therapies. The book is characterized by a very diffuse writing style and lack of supporting data. Unconvincing.

Prostate Problems

Falcone, Ron. *Natural Medicine for Prostate Problems*. New York: Dell, 1998. 188pp. $5.99 (paper).

Falcone reviews the traditional treatment for prostate diseases such as benign prostatic hypertrophy (BPH), prostatitis, and prostate cancer. Standard treatments involve surgery, laser ablation, and microwave thermotherapy. The major part of the book is devoted to a discussion of the many natural medicines such as therapeutic diets, high-dose vitamins, adjuvant vaccine programs, herbal therapies, homeopathy, massage, and hydrotherapy that can be used alongside traditional therapy. Separate chapters deal with sex and the prostate, complementary approaches to treating prostate cancer, and how to put a complementary program into practice. Falcone fails, however, to prevent a balanced picture and does not clearly show how alternative treatments can supplement traditional treatments.

Preuss, Harry G., and Brenda Adderly. *The Prostate Cure: The Revolutionary, Natural Approach to Treating Enlarged Prostates.* New York: Crown, 1998. 251pp. $23.

By age 50, one-half of normally virile men have some symptoms of benign prostatic enlargement (BPH) and by age 70, 70 percent of men have the problem. Typical symptoms include frequency, dribbling, incontinence, bladder infections, and difficulty in urinating. In two chapters, Preuss and Adderly review the standard treatment options such as surgery (prostatectomy, TURP, TUIP, and TUNA) and medical options (Hytrin, Proscar, saw palmetto, and pygeum africanum). The "revolutionary" approach advocated involving the use of Cernitin, a flower pollen extract, offers a safe, natural and effective way to treat the symptoms of BPH. A seven-step proactive program outlined involves working with your physician for a proper diagnosis, taking Cernitin to reduce symptoms, regular exercises, maintaining ideal body weight, eating a diet healthful for proper functioning of the urinary tract, fighting anxiety and depression; and taking yourself lightly. Twenty-eight pages of bibliographic notes are included at the end of the book, together with a glossary. Useful as an overview of the multiple treatment options for coping with BPH.

Respiratory Ailments

Hale, Teresa. *Breathing Free: The Revolutionary 5-Day Program to Heal Asthma, Emphysema, Bronchitis, and Other Respiratory Ailments.* New York: Harmony Books, 1999. 281pp. $23.

Hale, the founder of one of London's leading alternative health clinics, points out that overbreathing, or hyperventilation, starves the body and brain of something it needs more than oxygen—carbon dioxide. Conventional medicine has never fully addressed the causes or effects of hyperventilation. When we hyperventilate, we take in too much air and breathe out too much precious carbon dioxide, which means that the body is unable to absorb the small but essential amount of oxygen it needs. The extraordinary notion that asthma is caused by hyperventilation is based upon the pioneering work of Professor Konstantin Buteyko, a Russian doctor. Hale provides a detailed explanation of Buteyko's technique and offers the reader detailed instructions for following her "Breath Connection" program. This program involves dietary and lifestyle changes together with breathing exercises. The techniques for the breath connection are clearly explained. This is a book that will especially appeal to the parents of asthmatic children.

Sexuality

Bonnard, Marc. *The Viagra Alternative: The Complete Guide to Overcoming Erectile Dysfunction Naturally.* Rochester, VT: Healing Arts Press, 1999. 224pp. $14.95 (paper).

The use of Viagra (sildenafil) has been associated with heart attacks, hypertension, color-blindness, and other health problems. Taking Viagra can end up accentuating the greater underlying problem of which erectile dysfunction (ED) was a symptom. After reviewing the use of traditional treatments for ED and the promise of future drugs, Bonnard (a psychiatrist specializing in sex therapy) advocates usage of herbal remedies such as ginkgo biloba, ginseng, garlic, and Bach flower remedies, together with dietary and lifestyle changes involving yoga, meditation, and relaxation exercises. Bonnard offers a detailed and informative explanation of the many aspects of ED but does not present a coherent and clear description of natural remedies.

Roybal, Beth Ann, and Gayle Skowronski. *Sex Herbs: Nature's Sexual Enhancers for Men and Women.* Berkeley, CA: Ulysses Press, 1999. 323pp. $14.95 (paper).

Why use expensive Viagra? Sex herbs offer natural alternatives that can boost sexual desire, pleasure, and fulfillment for both men and women. Moreover, herbs can also aid health conditions that might otherwise inhibit sex. Widely available herbs include Daminiana (a Mexican remedy known to produce an aphrodisiac effect), Yohimbe (rumored to be used in the United States by male porn stars to help maintain erections during film production), and Fo-ti (used in Chinese medicine to increase sexual desire and drive). Separate chapters detail herbs used to increase sexual pleasure and desire; to relieve prostate problems, impotence, menopause, and PMS; and to improve overall well-being. While providing much detail on dozens of herbs, no guidance is given on how to select the most appropriate herbs for a specific use, and there is an almost total absence of dosing instructions beyond "follow the instructions on the product's label." The details supplied with respect to "cautions" are generalized and nonspecific. Stimulating reading but not a very practical guide.

Sachs, Judith. *Sensual Rejuvenation: Maintaining Sexual Vigor Through Midlife and Beyond.* New York: Dell, 1999. 244pp. $5.99 (paper).

Sachs, a well-known sex educator, takes a new look at midlife sexuality and asserts that sex at midlife can be better than it has ever been. Her objective is to outline "an easy-to-follow program to revamp your sex life using up-to-the-minute research from psychologists, sexologists, and physicians, tapping into techniques culled from conventional sex therapy as well as alternative and complementary medicine." The book's coverage is extensive and somewhat superficial, discussing a myriad of topics such as use of replacement hormones to rejuvenate your sex life, natural sex aids (vitamins, minerals, herbs), aromatherapy, fantasy, phone sex, erotic books and films, sex in cyberspace, masturbation, suggested "repertoire of pleasure techniques," erectile dysfunction, vasectomy and prostatectomy, and more. A grab-bag of potent reading.

Taylor, Susan. *Sexual Radiance: A 21-Day Program of Breathwork, Nutrition, and Exercise for Vitality and Sensuality.* New York: Harmony, 1998. 243pp. $23.

This is a woman's book! Taylor, with a doctorate in nutritional biochemistry, believes that sexual radiance (sex appeal) is the combination of physical vitality and the free flow of sexual energy. The basis for sexual radiance is metabolism and this can be adjusted to "manufacture" sexual energy. The program advocated by Taylor includes a "Vitality Diet," breathing for sexual energy, exercises that energize, and maintenance of a diet plan. Four chapters are devoted to "Energy Systems," the "Art of Tantric Sex," "Divine Orgasms," and the "Mind-Body Response." An interesting blend of biochemistry, yoga, Taoism, tantric sex, nutritional science, and exercise.

Wright, Jonathan V., and Lane Lenard. *Maximize Your Vitality & Potency: For Men Over 40.* Petaluma, CA: Smart Publications, 1999. 256pp. $14.95 (paper).

If hormone replacement therapy works for women, preventing a substantial proportion of such serious age-related conditions such as heart disease and osteoporosis, why would not male sex hormones do the same for men? Wright and Lenard claim that replacing men's testosterone as it de-

clines with age can help stimulate sexuality, prevent atherosclerosis, stroke, and heart attacks, normalize cholesterol and blood sugar, keep the prostate gland healthy, and prevent low-grade "depression." A final chapter details how to obtain natural testosterone creams, gels, and sublingual tablets from compounding pharmacies. These products are virtually undistinguishable from the mass-produced variety. Informative and readable.

Skin Diseases

Lane, I. William, and Linda Comac. *The Skin Cancer Answer.* Garden City Park, NY: Avery, 1999. 137pp. $9.95 (paper).

Depletion of the ozone layer results in the increased incidence of skin cancer. Rejecting the "cut, burn, and poison remedies of allopathic medicines," Lane and Comac wish to trade surgery, chemotherapy, and radiation treatment for a simple, topical application of chemicals derived from plants. Part One of their book offers a very readable look at the skin cancer problem; Part Two outlines the causes and the various types of skin cancer; Part Three looks at the answer—glycoalkaloids. This new approach proposed in the fight against skin cancer was discovered by a veterinarian in Australia. A glycoalkaloid-based topical cream shows promising results in the treatment of basal cell carcinoma. This is a very clear description of the skin problem problem, with excellent color photographs. Lane is an agricultural biochemist; Comac is a freelance writer.

LeVan, Lisa. *The Psoriasis Cure.* Garden City Park, NY: Avery, 1999. 154pp. $13.95 (paper).

Like many of those afflicted by psoriasis, LeVan (a health researcher and educator) discovered that conventional treatments only relieve symptoms and prevent secondary infections. Common treatments such as light therapy, corticosteroids, methotrexate, and cyclosporine often result in multiple, even life-threatening complications that produce no relief. The "Psoriasis Cure" program advocated by LeVan is based upon a combination of dietary modification, use of nutritional supplementation, changes in lifestyle, and pursuit of healthy habits. Separate chapters detail the anti-psoriasis diet—"how to fuel your body's healing process with foods that can lessen your psoriasis symptoms," and "how to beat stress before it beats you." The basic message is—eat to beat psoriasis.

Sports Performance

Burdenko, Igor, and Scott Biehler. *Overcoming Paralysis*. Garden City Park, NY: Avery, 1999. 240pp. $14.95 (paper).

Burdenko, a Russian with a doctorate in sports medicine, now runs a water and sports therapy institution in Boston. Biehler broke his spine in a motorcycle accident that left him paralyzed from the waist down. After treatment from Burdenko, Biehler can now move his legs underwater and continues to improve. The Burdenko Method uses water as a modality for exercise. People who are handicapped or injured can regenerate the natural healing process in their bodies through exercise. The book is divided into three parts: Part One provides information about recovering from an injury with the proper rehabilitation and conditioning and how the Burdenko method can be used to help natural healing through the use of water as a therapeutic modality; Part Two describes wheelchair exercises that can be used on land; Part Three illustrates 100 water exercises with drawings and step-by-step instructions. Emphasis is placed on positive thinking, diet therapy and pain management. Clearly written and eminently hopeful.

Dorfman, Lisa. *The Vegetarian Sports Nutrition Guide: Peak Performance for Everyone from Beginners to Gold Medalists*. New York: Wiley, 2000. 270pp. $16.95 (paper).

Dorfman argues that "contrary to popular belief, vegetarians are more than granola-eating former hippies and picky eaters who pore over food labels checking for meat and animal by-products." Her objective is to describe how to maximize the benefits of a vegetarian diet for specific athletic needs. Part One of the book explains food's impact on physical activity and sports (the best "fuels"—carbohydrates, proteins, fats, vitamins, minerals and phytochemicals); while Part Two details how to supplement the "Sports Machine" to achieve plant-based peak performance. Dorfman offers a wide assortment of tasty vegetarian recipes, menus, and suggestions. An appendix spotlights the nutritional profiles (one-day food diaries and nutritional analysis) of 17 world-class athletes. An excellent summary of the nutritional requirements of vegetarian athletes.

Hatfield, Frederick C., and Frederick C. Hatfield II. *Nature's Sports Pharmacy: A Natural Approach to Peak Athletic Performance*. Lincolnwood, IL: Contemporary Books, 1999. 230pp. $14.95 (paper).

A book not about herbs for curing or preventing disease but rather one with a focus on herbs and combinations of herbs in light of their potential use by athletes. The Hatfields list and describe herbs for improving digestion and assimilation of foods, improving energy levels for training and competition, developing the ability to adapt to the stresses of intense training, adopting nutritional strategies for increasing muscle mass, and enhancing mental concentration and sleep. An extensive 35-page glossary of herbal and nutritional terms is also provided, together with a summary of important herbal tonic recommendations. An informative introduction to athletic nutrition and the best herbal substances for peak athletic performance.

Weight Management

Cooper, Jay with Kathryn Lance. *The Body Code: A Personalized Wellness and Weight Loss Plan Developed at the World Famous Green Valley Spa*. New York: Pocket Books, 1999. 242pp. $24.

Genes determine our blood type, hair texture, and eye color, and also assign to each person a unique metabolic type—the rate at which we burn calories and store fat. Each type has an ideal exercise regimen. The four types—Warrior Adrenal, Nurturer-Ovarian, Communicator-Thyroidal, and Visionary-Pituitary—are similar to the dosha types of Ayurvedic medicine. Cooper outlines the exercise, and the body motion, and nutrition guidelines followed at his Green Valley Spa in southern Utah. This is a program for taking control of your metabolism according to your genetic type. An innovative mixture of nutrition and genetics!

Mitchell, Deborah. *Natural Medicine for Weight Loss*. New York: Dell, 1998. 223pp. $5.99 (paper).

To believe that over 100 million obese people in the United States actually will themselves to be overweight, or that they are happy about it, is implausable and defies logic. Instead, Mitchell asserts that obesity is a metabolic and endocrine disorder. Several different genes and 10 different hormones are associated with being overweight. "Losing weight is not about willpower," states Mitchell, "it's about taking advantage of the natural herbs, nutrients, and techniques that can help in losing weight and maintaining the loss." The formula advocated is in the form of an equation: Good Dietary Habits + Enjoyable Exercise + Positive Mind-Body Reinforcement + Nature's Helpers = Permanent Weight Loss. Rejecting fad diets, diet drugs, and yo-yo dieting, Mitchell offers food plans and shows how to use chromium picolinate and other thermogenic agents, herbal forms of Phen-Fen, herbal appetite suppressants, amino acids, and touch therapies to reduce the desire for food. One chapter discusses where to turn for help. An attractive, cogent, and persuasive alternative to the mainstream treatment of obesity.

Women

Coutinho, Elsimar M., and Sheldon J. Segal. *Is Menstruation Obsolete? How Suppressing Menstruation Can Help Women Who Suffer from Anemia, Endometriosis, or PMS.* New York: Oxford University Press, 1999. 190pp. $24.

> This is a contrarian view of menstruation. The authors argue that menstruation is not the natural state of women and that it actually places them at risk of several conditions of varying severity. While menstruation may be culturally significant, it is not medically meaningful. Menstrual suppression can lead to an improvement of women's health. Among the menstrual cycle-related disorders are dysmenorrhea, myoma, endometriosis, and PMS. Suppression can be achieved either through surgical methods (hysterectomy, endometrial resection, ovariectomy), or less drastically through the use of oral contraceptives. The major conclusion reached is that freeing women of menstruation significantly reduces the risk of life-threatening disease such as ovarian and uterine cancers. Bleed no more—the loss of blood is absolutely needless! Coutinho, a Brazilian, was the discoverer of Depo-Provera; Segal is an embryologist and endocrinologist. Fascinating and provocative reading, literate and persuasive.

Harrar, Sari, and Sara Altshul O'Donnell. *The Woman's Book of Healing Herbs: Healing Teas, Tonics, Supplements, and Formulas.* Emmaus, PA: Rodale Press, 1998. 494pp. $29.95.

> Two editors of *Prevention* magazine point to the fact until the early part of the twentieth century, herbalism was the primary system of healing in the United States. Now, there is the beginning of a stampede back to the green pharmacy as people rush to purchase echinacea, garlic, ginkgo and kava. This comprehensive book is divided into nine parts: Part One describes our herbal heritage; Part Two lists 53 top healing herbs for women; Part Three details teas, tinctures, decoctions, baths, compresses, poultices, and liniments; Part Four describes aromatherapy and flower essences; Part Five shows how to stay healthy with herbs; Part Six discusses the healing power of herbs; Part Seven lists herbs for beautiful skin, hair, and nails; Part Eight describes herbs for emotional healing; and Part Nine offers a herbal resource guide—botanical names of the healing herbs and where to buy herbs and herbal products. Combines lucid textual material with excellent color photographs.

Hudson, Tori. *Women's Encyclopedia of Natural Medicine: Alternative Therapies and Integrative Medicine.* Los Angeles: Keats, 1999. 358pp. $24.95.

> Hudson, a naturopathic physician, describes in detail natural treatment protocols used to treat gynecological problems such as amenorrhea, abnormal uterine bleeding, fibrocystic cysts, genital herpes, heart disease, menopause, and osteoporosis. Major emphasis is placed on the use of nutrtional supplements, botanicals, and additional natural therapies. A balanced picture is achieved in that each chapter, while outlining a natural approach, also details treatment by conventional medicine. Highlights gentle, natural, naturopathic solutions to women's health problems. Well organized and highly readable.

Kenley, Joan, with John C. Arpels. *Whose Body Is It Anyway? Smart Alternatives and Traditional Health Choices for Your Total Well-Being.* New York: Newmarket Press, 1999. 335pp. $24.95.

> Kenley, a psychologist and wellness coach, presents a balanced picture of major health issues confronting women—hormonal changes, hot flashes, incontinence, heart disease, breast cancer, fibroids, hysterectomy, osteoporosis, and weight problems. Throughout the book, standard therapies are contrasted with alternative and complementary treatment options. One chapter summarizes what alternative treatment therapies such as Ayurveda and Chinese medicine can accomplish. Appendix material includes a diagnosis questionnaire, glossary, list of resources, professional organizations, and references. Clearly written and printed in large type that makes for easy reading.

Null, Gary, and Barbara Seaman. *For Women Only: Your Guide to Health Empowerment.* New York: Seven Stories Press, 1999. 1,572pp. $75.

> This is a massive compilation of practical, philosophical, and spiritual information on women's health with due attention paid to feminism, activism, and consumerism relating to a wide variety of health issues of concern to women. Part One, authored by Gary Null, consists of descriptions of alternative treatment solutions for 39 medical problems such as breast cancer, eating disorders, herpes, menstrual cramps, migraines, and sexual dysfunction. In each instance, Null outlines alternative approaches such as homeopathy, imagery, Ayurveda, naturopathy, and so on. Part Two, authored by Seaman, tackles the health empowerment of women and includes extracts, reprints, and interviews of dozens of contributors such as Germain Greer, Erica Jong, Susie Orbach, Gloria Steinem, and Shere Hite. Apart from the medical detail presented by Null, the most interesting part of this book is that assembled by Seaman covering topics such as motherhood, sex and orgasm, rape, women and white coats, genital mutilations, self-helpless gynecology, lesbian health, and so on. Fascinating reading!

Ojeda, Linda. *Her Healthy Heart: A Woman's Guide to Preventing and Reversing Heart Disease Naturally.* Alameda, CA: Hunterhouse, 1998. 336pp. $14.95 (paper).

The idea that women are immune to heart disease is a myth. Heart disease kills more women than all types of cancer combined. The primary focus of Ojeda's book is on the prevention of heart disease through diet and nutritional supplements rather than on diagnosis and treatment. After identifying risk factors unique to women, Ojeda discusses cholesterol, importance of low fat diets, fiber and proteins, the use of super-supplements—antioxidants, B vitamins, minerals—healing foods and herbs, and healthy behavior for the heart. One chapter is devoted to choosing and taking supplements. A 32-page list of references is appended. A simple and sensible explanation directed to women.

Sultenfuss, Sherry Wilson, and Thomas J. Sultenfuss. *A Woman's Guide to Vitamins, Minerals and Alternative Healing.* Lincolnwood, IL: Contemporary Books, 1999. 324pp. $15.95 (paper).

The authors (a medical writer and dermatologist respectively) stress the vital role that vitamins, minerals, herbs, and alternative healing play in maintaining an efficiently working female system. Their book, based upon a review of the scientific literature on vitamins, minerals, and herbs, is intended to "arm women with enough information to make intelligent decisions on nutritional choices, vitamins and mineral supplements, and medical options for optimal health. Part One is an overview of vitamins and minerals; Part Two consists of the inside story on nutritional supplements; Part Three deals with topics of prime concern to women such as menopause, PMS, skin and aging, and weight; Part Four shows how alternative therapies such as acupuncture, chiropractic, and osteopathic medicine can help women; while Part Five provides recommendations for vitamins and mineral intake. There are almost 50 pages of bibliographic notes. While digesting much research data, the presentation is somewhat unfocused and unsystematic.

Viagas, Belinda Grant. *Natural Healthcare for Women.* Tucson, AZ: Fisher Books, 1999. 240pp. $12.95 (paper).

Viagas, a British naturopathic physician, structures her book "like a walk through a woman's life, beginning in childhood and then following the hormonal trail through to old age." Separate chapters deal with girls, puberty, menstruation, sexual maturity, fertility, pregnancy, birth, baby care, menopause, and growing older. The natural care advocated includes the use of herbs, relaxation, exercise, massage, and nutrition. A generalized and somewhat diffuse discussion.

Wallis, Lila A., with Marian Betancourt. *The Whole Woman: Take Charge of Your Health in Every Phase of Your Life.* New York: Avon, 1999. 528pp. $17.50 (paper).

A professor of medicine at Cornell Medical College (Wallis) laments the lack of understanding of the differences in treating women. Women's health is very different from men's health, not only because of different hormones but because women's lifespan does not follow the linear pattern of men's health. Wallis and Betancourt (a medical writer) discuss women's health concerns chronologically according to four life phases: adolescence (ages 12-20), adulthood (ages 20-45), perimenopausal phase (ages 45-65), and postmenopausal phase (ages 65 and up). Drawing upon her nearly 50 years of practicing medicine, Wallis offers an information-rich compendium of valuable advice on matters of basic concern—fitness, contraception, STDs, pregnancy, menopause, heart disease, osteoporosis, and so on. An excellent information resource.

Ayurvedic Medicine

Atreya. *Ayurvedic Healing for Women: Herbal Gynecology.* York Beach, ME: Samuel Weiser, 1999. 241pp. $14.95 (paper).

The classics of Ayurveda state that all diseases begin with three humors—vata, pitta, and kapha. Ayurveda determines a person's individuality by determining which of the three natural forces dominate one's organism. After describing the female anatomy according to Ayurveda, Atreya explains imbalances and the disease process, and the effects of plants and foods on the body. The Ayurvedic method of treating gynecological problems such as premenstrual and menstrual difficulties involves correcting chronic imbalances in the digestive, nervous, and endocrine systems through the use of powdered plants, roots, fruits, seeds, and occasionally flowers. Atreya provides herbal formulas for treating a wide variety of ailments such as cysts, fibroids, vulvodynia, pelvic inflammatory disease, and endometriosis. The ultimate goal, according to Atreya, is not health but peace—health will come when there is peace in the soul and in the mind. An intriguing, alternative approach to women's health concerns.

Chopra, Deepak. *Healing the Heart: A Spiritual Approach to Reversing Coronary Artery Disease.* New York: Harmony, 1998. 152pp. $18.

A prescription showing how to reduce the risk factors for coronary disease by following an individually tailored regimen based upon the principles of Ayurveda. Chopra, a prolific author of books on mind-body medicine, explains that Ayurveda expresses the similarities and differences among people in terms of three metabolic types known as doshas: vata dosha, pitta dosha, and kapha dosha. Corresponding to the body types, Chopra offers prescriptions for diet, exercise, and lifestyle that best suit the individual and maintain balance of the mind-body system. Specific suggestions relating to appropriate meditation, exercise, massage, and nutrition are given and contrasted with the current strategies used in traditional Western medicine. A simple and clear exposition of how Ayurveda approaches coronary artery disease.

Godagama, Shantha. *The Handbook of Ayurveda: India's Medical Wisdom Explained.* Boston: Journey Editions, 1998. 128pp. $14.95 (paper).

Ayurvedic medicine is based on the concept of three doshas (bodily energies)—vata, pitta, and kapha. Each person's dominant dosha is established at conception and determines not only physical appearance but also any predisposition to particular conditions and disorders. The aim of Ayurveda, Godagama explains, is to bring the doshas into balance. The role of the Ayurvedic doctor is to assess the effects of the doshas and to counter the influence of those which are harmful. Godagama, a consultant at the prestigious Hale Clinic in London, admirably succeeds in explaining the fundamental elements of Ayurveda, food and diet, the recommended Ayurvedic lifestyle to restore and maintain harmony, treatments, and plants and remedies. Of particular interest is a description of what happens during a visit to an Ayurvedic clinic. The lucid text is enhanced by the inclusion of excellent artwork, diagrams, illustrations, and color photographs. A truly holistic approach to healing.

***Warrier, Gopi, and Deepika Gunawant. *The Complete Illustrated Guide to Ayurveda: The Ancient Healing Tradition.* Boston, MA: Element Books, 1997. 192pp. $24.95 (paper).

Ayurveda is the oldest complete medical system in the world with recorded origins going back about 3,500 years. Utilizing lavish full-color photographs and illustrations, the authors explain the basic tenets, aims and methods of Ayurveda, the five elements (panchamahabhutas), the three doshas or bioenergetic forces that determine one's prakrti or physical constitution, and the three gunas or psychic forces that determine mental and spiritual health. Two detailed chapters are devoted to diagnosis in Ayurveda and treatment that consists of drugs (ausadha), diet (anna), and

practices (vihara), prescribed jointly or separately. This is a splendid, profusely illustrated text that presents a comprehensive picture of modern Ayurveda. Warrier and Gunawant are Ayurvedic practitioners. Excellent.

Curanderismo

Avila, Elena, with Joy Parker. *Woman Who Glows in the Dark: A Curandera Reveals Traditional Aztec Secrets of Physical and Spiritual Health.* New York: Tarcher/Putnam, 1999. 337pp. $24.95.

Curanderismo is derived from the Spanish word *cura*, which means *to heal* or *to be a priest*. It is medicine and spirituality practiced simultaneously. Curanderismo uses whatever works—herbs, counseling, soul retrieval, psychodrama, rituals, spiritual cleansings, and even referral to medical doctors. It represents a blending of African medicine, Spanish medicine, and Aztec medicine. On a very personal level, Avila (a psychiatric nurse) describes her apprenticeship to a master curandera in Mexico, who taught her how to use herbs, massage, psychological counseling, rituals, and other tools in the treatment of both physical and emotional ailments. One reviewer notes that Avila is "a wise and courageous woman who restores our souls to our bodies and our bodies to sacred earth through her profound teaching of ancient ways in modern times." A sensitive and mind-expanding exploration of curanderismo.

Diet Therapies

Gittleman, Ann Louise. *Super Nutrition for Men.* Garden City Park, NY: Avery, 1999. 253pp. $10.95 (paper).

Gittleman maintains that innovative nutrition can protect the prostate, heal the heart, supercharge sex, reduce hair loss, and help individuals to overcome addictions. The diet plan that works for most men is the 40/30/30 plan pioneered by Barry Sears. This involves 40 percent of total calories to be derived from carbohydrates (bread, pasta, potatoes), 30 percent from natural and unprocessed fats (such as butter and olive oil), and 30 percent from protein (including low-fat cottage cheese, eggs, fish). Many men can expect to increase lean muscle mass on this program in as little as 30 days, while trimming body fat to the ideal range of 14–18 percent. Sample menus are supplied for "super nutrition" at home and away from home.

Katahn, Martin, with Jami Pope. *The T-Factor 2000 Diet.* New York: Norton, 1999. 462pp. $24.95.

Every year between 80 and 100 million people in the United States go on a weight-loss diet. About 95 percent of them ultimately fail to reach and maintain their goal. Analysis of the reasons why some have succeeded proves, according to Katahn, that "one way or another, successful people have discovered and continued to follow the weight management principles that were introduced in the original T-Factor Diet 10 years ago." Permanent weight loss requires that the dieter make a permanent reduction in the fat content of the diet consumed. The T "stands for two processes involved in metabolism—thermogenesis, and the thermic effects of food and exercise." The diet advocated shows how to increase thermogenesis—how to burn extra calories and prevent them ending up in your fat cells. Separate chapters deal with putting the T-Factor 2000 diet to work, what to expect, the T-Factor rotation plan, the vegetarian T-Factor diet, recipes, and testimonials. An appendix supplies the scientific background. Contains much theory and extraneous material. Katahn is a psychologist; Pope is a dietitian.

Ross, Julia. *The Diet Cure: The 8-Step Program to Rebalance Your Body's Chemistry and End Food Cravings, Weight Problems, and Mood Swings—Now!* New York: Viking, 1999. 390pp. $23.95.

Ross promises that "this is not going to be like any diet book you have ever read . . . your body needs help. Years of dieting, psychotherapy, and the best pep talks about accepting your body as is can't help much when what you really need is a biochemical overhaul." Ross, the director of Recovery Systems and an outpatient treatment program, believes that amino acids are the key to the "Diet Cure." These amino acids are stronger than willpower and more effective and safer than Prozac and Phen-Fen. Eight steps are outlined to overcome the physical, bodily handicaps that can lead directly to food cravings, emotional eating, low energy and weight gain. These steps are correcting brain chemistry imbalances; ending low-calorie dieting; balancing unstable blood sugar; repairing low thyroid function; overcoming addictions to foods to which you are allergic; calming hormonal activity; eradicating yeast overgrowth; and fixing fatty acid deficiency. Separate chapters are devoted to shopping for master plan supplies, menus, meal ideas, and recipes. A detailed prescription by a pioneer in the field of nutritional psychology.

Twigg, Stephen. *The Kensington Way.* New York: Dutton, 1999. 275pp. $22.95.

Twigg, a British holistic health practitioner, has spent the past 20 years helping some of the world's most wealthy, famous, and powerful people (including the late Princess Diana) look after their health and appearance. Fleeing from fish sticks and french fries, Twigg embraces "Food Combining" ("the greatest diet in existence") that has a simple rule—don't allow protein-rich foods to be in your stomach with starch- or sugar-rich foods. To avoid a multitude of medical problems, correct food combining is essential. Twigg provides explicit instructions on correct combining. The "Kensington Way Master Plan" utilizes a rich assortment of affirmations, checklists, eating records, schedules, eating patterns, strategies, timing tips, and more. There are some 50 pages of recipes for the Kensington cook. This is a very complex and complicated program that necessarily involves a massive amount of time and patience to achieve the claimed benefits of food combining.

Enzyme Therapy

Cichoke, Anthony J. *The Complete Book of Enzyme Therapy.* Garden City Park, NY: Avery, 1998. 492pp. $19.95 (paper).

Enzymes are basic to the process of digestion, as well as to nutritional absorption, tissue repair, immune system function, and regulation of the aging process. Any significant depletion of these vital enzymes in our bodies can have a detrimental impact on our well-being. The essential theory advanced is that our bodies are enzyme-depleted by an "over-processed" national diet and a growing amount of enzyme-depleting chemicals found in our food supply and environment. Initiating an enzyme-rich diet results in the enzymes striking back against disease. Part One of the book explains enzymes and what they do; Part Two shows how enzyme therapy can be used to treat over 150 disorders from acne to yeast infections; while Part Three presents other complementary therapies that can be incorporated into a treatment program. Cichoke also introduces his "EASE" (Enzyme Absorption System Enhancers) method of healing. Appendix material contains a glossary, a list of digestive enzyme products, treatment centers, and a bibliography. This is a highly detailed compilation of data, well-documented and organized. All that you will ever want to know about enzyme therapy.

Faith and Spirituality

Koenig, Harold G. *The Healing Power of Faith: Science Explores Medicine's Last Great Frontier.* New York: Simon & Schuster, 1999. 331pp. $25.

Marrying science and spirituality, Koenig narrates, through the use of case histories, how religious people have stronger marriages, healthy lifestyles, more successfully cope with stress and depression, have stronger immune systems, resist serious cardiovascular disease, and use fewer expensive hospital services than individuals who are not religious. Religious patients with hip fracture recover faster than their nonreligious counterparts, while nonreligious patients with heart disease are three times more likely to die following surgery than their religious counterparts. While the stories of real people presented attest to the important role of religion and spirituality in healing, Koenig fails to provide a synthesis, summary, or explanation of the phenomena he reports. Koenig is the director of Duke University's Center for the Study of Religion/Spirituality and Health.

Hellerwork

Golten, Roger. *The Owners Guide to the Body: How to Have a Perfectly Tuned Body and Mind.* London, UK: Thorsons/HarperCollins, 1999. 183pp. $19.95 (paper).

An illustrated guide showing how to get the best from your body based on the principles of Hellerwork—the dynamic program to improve posture, energy, vitality, and confidence. Joseph Heller trained with Ida Rolf in 1972 and was appointed first president of the Rolf institute. Hellerwork is a synthesis of classic structural integration and personal growth work, which together transforms your relationship with your body and your experience of being alive. Moreover, it helps to integrate body and mind. In essence, Hellerwork is a systematic structural approach to holistic health, based upon an understanding of the relationship of man with a single most powerful force operating on his body throughout life—gravity. Golten, the United Kingdom's leading Hellerwork practitioner, explains both its theoretical basis and how to focus on the simple art of movement, standing, walking, running, breathing, and sitting down. Recommended techniques are presented within the context of understanding the vital principles of human movement.

Herbal Medicine and Phytomedicine

General Works

Bratman, Steven, and David Kroll. *Natural Health Bible: From The Most Trusted Source in Health Information, Here Is Your A-Z Guide To Over 200 Herbs, Vitamins, and Supplements.* Roseville, CA: Prima Health, 1999. 495pp. $19.99 (paper).

The editors claim that their book is "based on science, not opinion, anecdote or folk wisdom," and draws upon European sources of scientific information, where study of herbs

and supplements is part of mainstream medicine. Part One of the book, "Conditions," contains information about some 50 illnesses and health problems. Each entry describes the condition, conventional treatments, and identifies the herbs, supplements, and lifestyle changes that may be of help. Part Two covers over 150 popular natural substances from acidophilus to zinc. The daily requirements, therapeutic dosages, and therapeutic uses are listed for each herb together with the scientific evidence as to safety and efficacy. In each instance, the type of supporting research is noted—double-blind studies, single-blind studies, uncontrolled studies and so on. This is a very informative summary of how herbs can be of use in treating many common ailments.

Bratman, Steven, David Kroll, and Angelo DePalma. *Natural Pharmacist: Natural Health Bible.* Rocklin, CA: Prima, 1999. 512pp. $19.99 (paper).

The authors review the effectiveness of the most popular herbs, vitamins, and supplements. Every claim is reviewed by the authors who reflect expertise in medicine and pharmacology. Their book is divided into two parts: Part One covers 51 conditions with discussion of treatment options; Part Two describes and evaluates 161 herbs and supplements. Information is also supplied on drug-herb and drug-supplement interactions together with a list of references to the studies cited.

Byers, Dorie. *Herbal Remedy Gardens: 38 Plans for Your Health and Well-Being.* Pownal, VT: Storey Books, 1999. 219pp. $16.95 (paper).

Master gardener Dorie Byers offers simple growing instructions for than 20 versatile medicinal herbs such as garlic, chamomile, echinacea, marjoram, and valerian. For each herb described, a sidebar identifies optimal growing conditions, optimal zones for growing, common propagation, types of plants, and usage. Gardens are suggested for special health needs such as "Decongestant Gardens," "Eye Care Gardens," "Healthy Heart Gardens" and so on. The "Cold and Flu Garden" described contains peppermint, catnip, cayenne, thyme, rosemary, yarrow, and garlic. Instructions are provided for growing herbs from seeds and for starting herbs from seedlings. One chapter details garden maintenance. This is an unusual book that offers great appeal to those who wish to engage in healthy gardening.

Cass, Hyla. *All About Herbs: Frequently Asked Questions.* Garden City Park, NY: Avery, 1999. 96pp. $2.99 (paper).

Answers basic questions about popular herbs—how much to take and when to take them. Questions and answers are organized in short chapters devoted to echinacea, garlic, ginkgo, ginseng, kava, milk thistle, St. John's wort, and saw palmetto. Herbs have become, according to Cass, the latest "discovery" in the United States despite the fact that American doctors have dismissed their value in favor of expensive prescription drugs. A final chapter outlines how to select herbal products such as tablets, capsules, teas, tinctures, or raw herbs. A simple and concise introduction to the subject.

***Fetrow, Charles W., and Juan R. Avila. *The Complete Guide to Herbal Medicines.* Springhouse, PA: Springhouse, 1999. 618pp. $21.95.

Fetrow and Avila, clinical pharmacy specialists and educators, believe that herbal medicines are here to stay and that those proven to be safe and effective deserve to be considered valid treatment options. To discern fact from myth, Fetrow and Avila have adapted their earlier *Professionals Handbook of Complementary and Alternative Medicine* (Springhouse, 1998) for popular use. The resulting book presents both the scientific facts and the folklore on more than 300 commonly used herbal medicines. Entries are arranged alphabetically and contain the product's commonly used name, general description, common dosages, side effects, interactions, important points to remember, why people use the herb, what the research shows, and selected references. Entries average about two pages in length. Information is also provided for a select number of nonherbal medicines such as bee pollen, chondroitin, coenzyme Q10, and melatonin. This is an excellent, informative, and authoritative source on herbs now in widespread use—ginseng, St. John's wort, kava, etc. Excellent.

Foster, Steven. *101 Medicinal Herbs, an Illustrated Guide.* Loveland, CO: Interweave Press, 1998. 101pp. $19.95 (paper).

Here is a splendid, concise guide to herbs based upon contemporary scientific research authored by a respected authority on herbal health. In view of the fact that it is bewildering to shop for herbs and sift through multiple products prepared in the form of tinctures, capsules, and tablets, Foster offers the consumer a quick reference guide to the 101 herbs most often sold as dietary supplements to support natural health. Each herb entry, averaging two pages in length, contains common and botanical names, historical uses, health conditions and herbal actions (what it is used for), forms of the herb typically available, dosages, and cautions. A "Therapeutic Cross-Reference List" is intended as a quick guide to symptoms and conditions for the listed herbs which have clinically proven effects. The lucid text is accompanied by high-quality color photographs. A detailed bibliography and glossary are included. Informative and authoritative.

Foster, Steven, and Varro E. Tyler. *Tyler's Honest Herbal: A Sensible Guide to the Use of Herbs and Related Remedies.* 4th edition. Binghamton, NY: Haworth Herbal Press, 1998. 442pp. $39.95.

This is a new, updated edition of a 1993 book. Like its predecessor, the 4th edition is a summary of basic scientific information on the botany, chemistry, and pharmacology of herbal drugs and medicinal plants. Included are new monographs on a number of herbs such as butcher's broom, capsicum, evening primrose oil, feverfew, ginger, and pau d'arco. Tyler, the dean of American herbalism, errs on the side of conservatism, insisting that herbs be assessed from a scientific viewpoint. Blue cohosh, he states, should not be used for self-treatment, while garlic should not pose any health risks—"eat leeks in March and wild garlic in May, and all the year after physicians may play." Authoritative, based on scientific evidence.

*George, Stephen C. *The Doctor's Book of Herbal Home Remedies: Cure Yourself with Nature's Most Powerful Healing Agents: Advice from 200 Experts on More Than 140 Conditions.* Emmaus, PA: Rodale, 1999. 596pp. $29.95.

The bulk of this hefty compilation consists of an A-to-Z guide to the medicinal value and application of dozens of herbal remedies based upon the collective wisdom of some 200 medical doctors, physicians, professional herbalists, and other experts. The arrangement is by some 140 medical conditions. Each listing includes a description of the problem, "Fast Facts," and applicable herbs. For osteoporosis, try horsetail, nettle, oats, dandelion, and soy; for urinary tract infections, use goldenrod, pipsissewa, marshmallow, cleavers, and cranberry. Remedies are suggested for pets in addition to humans. Back-of-the-book material includes a guide to the safe use of herbs and essential oils, and where to find the best herbs. Good.

Grifith, H. Winter, with Cynthia Thomson. *Healing Herbs: The Essential Guide.* Tucson, AZ: Fisher Books, 1999. 328pp. $12.95 (paper).

Since Dr. Griffith died in 1993, this book is presumably authored by Cynthia Thomson, who is listed as a technical consultant. Thomson is a dietitian. Information is presented in chart form for more than 210 herbs. Each chart indicates the name of the herb, parts used for medicinal purposes, known effects, possible additional effects, warnings and precautions, toxicity, adverse reactions, side effects, overdose symptoms, dosages, and storage. Relative contraindications are specified—consult your doctor if you're pregnant, breastfeeding, and treating infants and children. Telegraphic summaries of essential facts that may not satisfy many who require more explanation.

Harrar, Sari, and Sara Altshul O'Donnell. *The Woman's Book of Healing Herbs: Healing Teas, Tonics, Supplements, and Formulas.* Emmaus, PA: Rodale Press, 1999. 495pp. $18.95 (paper).

In this profusely illustrated book with many color photographs and drawings, the editors describe our herbal heritage, 50 top healing herbs for women, how to make herbal medicines at home (teas, tinctures, poultices, liniments, infused oils, salves, and ointments), herbal tonics, herbs for beautiful skin and hair, herbs for emotional healing, and an A-to-Z guide to common medical problems with suggested herbal remedies. This is a splendid book characterized by lucid text and excellent illustrations and photographs. Reliable, balanced, and practical.

Hobbs, Christopher. *Herbal Remedies for Dummies.* Foster City, CA: IDG Books Worldwide, 1998. 352pp. $19.99 (paper).

Hobbs, a fourth generation botanist and co-founder of the American Herbalists Guild, is highly qualified to serve as a tour guide to the world of herbal medicine for the millions of people who do not respond to traditional health care. Part One of his book orients the reader to the fascinating world of herbs ("so what are herbal remedies anyway?"); Part Two describes how to grow, process, store, and cook with herbs; Part Three ("the Part of Tens") offers 10 reasons to take herbs, 10 power herbs to take daily, and 10 great teas to make. A symptoms guide of nearly 100 pages lists suggested remedies and supportive programs for dozens of symptoms such as indigestion and insomnia, indicating herbal remedies, herbal formulas, and healthy habits. Appendixes supply a "Herb Talk Glossary," herbal dosage guide, and a listing of resources. The clever use of icons, as in other "Dummies" books enhances the text. Eminently readable—a great reference source for both browsing and rapid lookup.

Hoffman, David. *The Complete Illustrated Holistic Herbal: A Safe and Practical Guide to Making and Using Herbal Remedies.* Rockport, MA: Element Books, 1997. 256pp. $24.95 (paper).

Books on herbal medicine are often characterized by colorful photographs and illustrations. This book is no exception. More than 200 commonly used herbs are illustrated with information on the part of the herb used, collection (harvesting), constituents, and actions. One section of the book offers advice on how to harvest and store herbs, with easy instructions showing how to prepare herbal tinctures, creams, capsules, and pills. A "Therapeutic Index" indicates which herbs might be useful for particular diseases together with a suggested herbal medicine chest for the home. Another section, "Systems of the Body," looks in detail at each system of the body and the patterns of disease for which they are susceptible, and identifies the herbs that can help restore and heal the body. A concerted, and largely successful, attempt is made to place herbs within a holistic framework by not merely listing herbs but rather examining the action of herbs in the context of the various systems of the body taking into account feelings, mind, and spirit. A delightful and highly informative book.

Keville, Kathi, with Peter Korn. *Herbs for Healing: A Drug-Free Guide to Prevention and Cure.* New York: Berkley, 1998. 523pp. $7.99 (paper).

A book dedicated to "everyone who strolls down the path of natural healing. May it be lined with healing herbs and lead to health and happiness." The authors urge that the reader should think of herbalism in a new light. Do not simply replace a drug with a handful of herb pills! Their book is a compact and densely packed handbook that shows how to use herbs for health and healing; the many types of herbal preparations (tinctures, compresses, poultices, salves, etc.); how herbs can help in pain, depression, digestion, urinary and respiratory tract disorders; herbal remedies for women, men, and children; herbals for first aid; aromatherapy; skin and health care; cooking for health; and how to use herbs safely. Appendixes list common and botanical names. A bibliography and list of resources is included. Inexpensive, easy-to-use, and highly informative.

Lininger, Skye, and others. *The Natural Pharmacy.* Rocklin, CA: Prima, 1998. 447pp. $19.99 (paper).

Lininger, a nutrition-oriented chiropractor, offers a comprehensive work assembled by a team including Lininger, a group of naturopaths, and several medical doctors. Their goal is "to create a book that stressed the integrated approach to self-care, to create a tool that would let readers assess the pluses and minuses of the use of vitamins, minerals, herbs, homeopathic remedies, and other nutrients for the most common and troublesome health conditions." The subject matter is arranged in four sections—conditions, nutritional supplements, herbs, and homeopathic remedies. The conditions section, covering several dozen specific conditions, offers a useful checklist at the end of each condition that serves as a useful reminder of what nutrients, herbs, and homeopathic remedies might be useful. This feature refers the reader to relevant information to be found in the other sections. In the herb section, the active ingredient is described (if known) together with the available forms and dosages. A serious attempt has been made to refrain from making any statements without providing scientific documentation in the form of footnotes. There are 47 pages of references appended. The book is a printed version of *HealthNotes On-Line,* a database used by many health food stores and pharmacies.

Lobay, Douglas. *Amazing Natural Medicines: A Modern and Scientific Guide to the Use of Diet, Vitamins, Minerals and Botanical Medicines in the Treatment of Disease.* Kelona, British Columbia: Apple Communications, 1998. 185pp. $13.95 (paper).

Lobay, a Canadian naturopathic physician, outlines natural methods of boosting your immune system, building healthy bones, controlling high blood pressure, fighting infection, healing stomach ulcers, treating depression, preventing strokes, promoting weight loss, and so on. The natural method advocated involves the use of botanical medicines, nutritional supplementation, and dietary modification. This is an unsystematic and uncritical review of the value of naturopathic medicine. Most of the references listed are to publications of the 1980s and earlier.

Loe, Theresa. *The Herbal Home Companion.* New York: Kensington Books, 1997. 224pp. $14 (paper).

A general, easily understandable introduction to herbs in the garden (starting and maintaining an herb garden), herbs in the kitchen (tips on using the garden's bounty), and herbs in the home (herbal cosmetics, scenting the home, and herbal treasures such as pressed herb candles). While providing a good, overall introduction to the wide variety of herbs, the book is of minimal value in terms of therapeutic use.

Maleskey, Gale, and the editors of *Prevention* Health Books. *Nature's Medicines: From Asthma to Weight Gain, from Colds to High Cholesterol—The Most Powerful All-Natural Cures.* Emmaus, PA: Rodale Press, 1999. 688pp. $31.95.

Maleskey and a team of 15 researchers review more than 95 vitamins, minerals, herbs and other natural supplements that are in common use. The information presented is based upon interviews with highly qualified health authorities, including medical doctors and practitioners of alternative medicine. Part One explains what you need to know about supplements; Part Two, "The Powerhouse of Nature's Medicines," is an A-to-Z guide to the healing power of effective natural medicines such as feverfew, ginger, and selenium; Part Three provides authoritative advice on the use of supplements in treating common diseases. By way of example, the section on breast cancer discusses the use of antioxidants, estrogen-lowering herbs (phytoestrogens), red clover and flaxseed, while the chapter on osteoarthritis describes the use of glucosamine sulfate, and devil's claw. A concerted attempt is made to present a balanced presentation, replete with multiple cautions and warnings.

**McCaleb, Robert, Evelyn Leigh, and Krista Morien. *The Encyclopedia of Popular Herbs: Your Complete Guide to the Leading Medicinal Plants.* Roseville, CA: Prima Health, 1999. 451pp. $29.95.

In view of the paucity of scientific research, how can consumers use herbs intelligently and safely? To facilitate informed decision making, the authors attempt to summarize the strength of the research supporting each herb they discuss. Detailed descriptions are provided for more than 40 herbs in common use. For each herb described, information is supplied with respect to botany, benefits, international status (official acceptance and approved uses in other countries), how it works, major constituents, safety, dosages, standardization, and references to the research literature. A unique feature of the book is the use of a "Five-Star Rating System" that offers a subjective judgment of each herb, taking into account the amount of research, type of research (clinical, laboratory etc), history of use, safety record, and international acceptance. The ratings range from excellent (five stars) to poor (one star). This is a highly useful book that offers significant, practical guidance in the intelligent use of herbs. Truly, in the authors' words, "an herb book for you and your doctor, or if you are a doctor, for you and your patients." Very good.

Mindell, Earl, and Virginia Hopkins. *Prescription Alternatives: Hundreds of Safe, Natural, Prescription-Free Remedies to Restore and Maintain Your Health.* 2nd edition. Lincolnwood, IL: Keats, 1999. 562pp. $19.95 (paper).

This is an updated and expanded edition of a book originally published in 1998. The major point made remains the same in that Mindell argues that "as a general rule, prescription drugs cause imbalances in the body ranging from depletion of vitamins and minerals to constipation and lowered immune function." The objective of this book is to show how the drugs you are taking affect your body, the steps you can take to counter these imbalances, and what alternative treatments are available. Separate chapters are devoted to changing the "pill-popping mindset," how to avoid prescription drug abuse, and how drugs interact with food and drink. Part Two of the book contains 12 chapters that review drugs used for heart disease, digestive disorders, diabetes, eye diseases, and so on. In each chapter, natural alternatives are suggested. For example, natural alternatives to coumadin and heparin for preventing stroke and blood clots are garlic, onions, fish, bioflavonoids, and also nutrition supplements such as magnesium, folic acid, and selenium. The recommendations are based on Mindell's "Seven Core Principles for Optimum Health."

Packer, Lester, and Carol Colman. *The Antioxidant Miracle: Your Complete Plan for Total Health and Healing.* New York: Wiley, 1999. 256pp. $24.95 (paper).

Packer and Colman, enthusiastically make the case for antioxidants that can protect the body from the damage caused by free radicals, which can injure healthy cells and tissues. "By controlling free radicals," they state, "antioxidants can make the difference between life and death, as well as influence how fast and how well we age. . . . Their role in the human body is nothing less than miraculous." Separate chapters detail the protection conferred by lipoic acid, vitamin E, vitamin C, coenzyme Q10, and glutathione. Also discussed are flavonoids, carotenoids, and selenium. Part Four of the book consists of the "Packer Plan"—an "Antioxidant Feast"—with specialized supplement programs for smokers, diabetics, menopausal women, and athletes. This book presents strong and reasoned advocacy of "the miracle" offered by antioxidants. Packer is a professor in the department of molecular and cell biology at the University of California at Berkeley; Colman is a medical writer.

Pederson, Stephanie. *Natural Care Library.* 10 titles. *Echinacea: Amazing Immunity; Ginseng: Energy Enhancer; Ginkgo: Increase Intellect & Improve Circulation Garlic: Immunity Booster & Heart Helper; Kava: Relax Your Muscles & Mind; St. John's Wort: Improving Moods and Immunity; Saw Palmetto: Hormone Enhancer; Vitamin B: Balancing Body & Mind; Vitamin C: Building Flexibility & Fighting Infection; Vitamin D: Making the Most of Minerals; Vitamin E: Protective Antioxidants.* New York: Dorling Kindersley, 2000. 64pp each. $3.95 each (paper).

Each title in this 10-volume series provides a brief description of the herb discussed, medical conditions that it can treat, recommended doses, precautions, and common side effects. However, only 60 percent of the subject content is unique to each title. The remaining 40 percent —dealing with herbal history, science talk, rethinking medications, formula guide, grow it yourself, do-it-yourself remedies, herb glossary, list of herbal organizations, and growing herbs—is common to all 10 titles. While attractive in appearance, with multiple color photographs and drawings together with clear explanation, it is manifest that this 10-title series should have been published as an integral whole at a reasonable price rather than chopped into 10 overlapping pieces for a grand total of $39.50. Dubious marketing!

Perce, Andrea. *The American Pharmaceutical Association Practical Guide to Natural Medicines.* New York: Morrow, 1999. 728pp. $35.

This book is a comprehensive compilation of natural medicines and remedies. Information is provided on more than 300 natural remedies. Reliable data has been derived from medical and botanical databases, research studies, government analyses, and secondary sources. The bulk of the book consists of monographs that conform to a standardized format—primary, scientific, and common names, major characteristics, what it is used for, forms available, dosage, reported efficacy, potential harm, and text citations. Each natural remedy is assigned a numerical rating of one to five that provides a general sense of what to expect in terms of effectiveness. Also included is an index of symptoms with suggested remedies, and an index of remedies. A most comprehensive, well-researched, and well-documented compilation of reliable information presented in a form that is also readily understandable to consumers.

Rister, Robert. *Japanese Herbal Medicine: The Healing Art of Kampo.* Garden City Park, NY: Avery, 1999. 412pp. $19.95 (paper).

Kampo is a unique, ancient system of herbal medicine that has been reborn in modern Japan. The curative art of Kampo combines herbs to relieve carefully defined patterns of symptoms, and to recreate the healthful conditions of balance that existed in the body, mind, and spirit before disease struck. Although Kampo is faithful to the ancient formulas of Chinese medicine and can be used knowledgeably with acupuncture, moxibustion, or therapeutic massage, no other technique is required to enhance Kampo's healing effects. Moreover, Kampo itself is pain-free. Rister explains in Part One of his book the concepts and principles of Kampo, how to buy and use the Japanese medicinal herbs described, and details of Kampo formulas. Part Two of the book is an alphabetical listing of more than 100 disorders that are treatable with Kampo. Each entry contains a brief description of the condition in mainstream medical terms followed by how Kampo views the condition and the treatment options involving both individual herbs and formulas that Kampo has to offer. Two appendixes list sources of Kampo services and products and Japanese medicinal herbs. Also provided are a glossary and a 66-page listing of references. An interesting insight into the ancient art of Kampo.

****Sifton, David (editor). *The PDR Family Guide to Natural Medicines and Healing Therapies.* New York: Three Rivers Press, 1999. 400pp. $23 (paper).

This book, by the publisher of the prestigious PDR, asks "how can you tell a real remedy from a hyped-up fraud?" On a highly cautious note, the introduction points out that many of the healing therapies have yet to pass scientific tests and that "some never will and are dismissed by virtually all knowledgeable observers." On neutral ground, the book "endeavors to clearly label those claims for which there is a generally favorable consensus, and those for which there is no support." The book is divided into five parts: Part One provides an overview of the major types of unconventional therapy available in the United States today; Part Two offers specifics on each individual approach; Part Three is a guide to natural medicines (drawing upon the *PDR for Herbal Medicines*, Medical Economics, 1999); Part Four provides essential information on some 50 vitamins, minerals, and other dietary elements; Part Five, a "Treatment Finder," indexes the most "plausible" therapeutic options by the ailments they address. The descriptions of alternative therapies are highly informative, covering "Consider This Therapy For . . . ," how the treatments are done, what the treatment is intended to accomplish, who should avoid this therapy, side effects, how to choose a therapist, and when to see a conventional doctor. For each alternative therapy, a list of readings and resources is provided. An authoritative compilation that successfully hews to the middle of the road. Outstanding.

Walker, Lynne, and Ellen Paige Hodgson Brown. *The Alternative Pharmacy*. Paramus, NJ: Prentice Hall, 1998. 414pp. $22.

"Nature's Medicine Chest," as advocated by the authors, includes popular herbal and homeopathic remedies that are good to have on hand both for emergency first aid and to treat ailments. These include tea tree oil, peppermint oil, Black ointment, Calendula tincture, and Bacticin drops. The bulk of the book consists of an A-to-Z guide to common ailments and their best treatments. Homeopathic and herbal treatments are contrasted with conventional treatments. Over 200 health conditions are listed alphabetically. Two or three pages are devoted to each health condition. There are 574 references included in an endnotes section. An appendix in the form of the "Natural Remedy Health Advisor" tabulates conditions, remedies, type of remedy (Chinese, herbal, homeopathic, combination, etc.), and directions for use. Walker holds a doctorate in pharmacy and a master's in Chinese herbology and acupuncture; Brown is a former attorney, now active in the field of alternative health. Informative and eminently readable.

Zampieron, Eugene R., and Ellen Kamhi. *The Natural Medicine Chest: Natural Medicines to Keep You and Your Family Thriving Into the Next Millenium*. New York: Evans, 1999. 244pp. $14.95 (paper).

This is a most attractive and enthusiastic attempt to bring the "excitement about the exquisite gifts of Nature from the plant kingdom to the people." Using plants as medicine "brings people back towards an understanding of how they, themselves, fit into the cycle of nature." The text of the book began as a script written for radio broadcast. Zampieron (a naturopath) and Kamhi (the "Natural Nurse") are weekly guests on American Health Network's, "Ask the Family Doctor." After summarizing the history of botanical medicine in Part One, the authors present the "Natural Medicine Chest," short two- to three-page descriptions of the availability and usage of some 40 plants. Part Two contains "Facts about Herbs from the Shaman's Garden" that were gleaned from Kamhi's stay with a curandera (shaman) in southern Mexico. An appendix lists resources including conducted international tours for exploring Chinese medicine and Ayurvedic medicine. A popular, highly readable, though uncritical, summary of the basic facts of botanical medicine.

Alpha-Lipoic Acid

Watson, Cynthia M. *All About Alpha-Lipoic Acid: Frequently Asked Questions*. Garden City Park, NY: Avery, 1999. 96pp. $2.99 (paper).

Alpha-lipoic acid, first isolated in 1951, when taken as a supplement, is used by the body as an antioxidant that can offer powerful protection against free-radical damage to cells. It can also raise cellular levels of glutathione, the body's primary antioxidant. Utilizing a concise question-and-answer format, Watson reviews the benefits of alpha-lipoic acid in relation to the aging process, liver function, diabetes, the nervous system, heart disease, cancer, and immunity. Alpha-lipoic acid is safe and nontoxic in dosages from 100 mg. to 1,200 mg. In very high dosages, such as 1,800 mg. per day, it can be toxic or fatal. A list of 10 references is appended to identify the source of the information presented in the text. Similar to, but not as detailed as Allan Sosin and Beth Lay Jacobs's *Alpha-Lipoic Acid: Nature's Ultimate Antioxidant* (Kensington, 1998).

Andro

Lenard, Lane. *The Smart Guide to Andro: The Safe and Natural Testosterone Precursor for Sex and Athletic Enhancement*. Petaluma, CA: Smart Publications, 1999. 86pp. $6.95 (paper).

Andro (aka androstenedione) received prominence when it was revealed that baseball slugger Mark McGwire was using andro, which was neither illegal nor immoral. Lenard does a great service by bringing together the basic facts by answering 31 essential questions—such as what is andro, does it help grow bigger muscles and stronger bones, is it an anabolic steroid, can it cause heart disease, does it increase sex drive and overcome impotence, should it be banned from competitive sports, and should women use andro? The text is documented by more than 100 references to the research literature. Lenard concludes that "because the sex hormones play such important roles in the body, it would seem prudent to consult with a knowledgeable physician before starting to use androstenedione and then periodically thereafter." An excellent, clearly written digest of essential facts.

Antioxidants

Dolby, Victoria. *All About Green Tea: Frequently Asked Questions*. Garden City Park, NY: Avery, 1998. 96pp. $2.99 (paper).

Dolby considers that green tea offers an incredible array of life-enhancing and even life-preserving properties and that it has real benefits for cancer, immunity, longevity, mental acuity, diabetes, ulcers, osteoporosis, and dental health. Black tea lacks the polyphenols that are associated with the long list of health benefits. Answers most questions associated with green tea as an ancient healing beverage. Contains a glossary and list of references.

*Papas, Andreas. *The Vitamin E Factor: The Miraculous Antioxidant for the Prevention and Treatment of Heart Disease, Cancer, and Aging*. New York: HarperPerennial, 1999. 395pp. $12.95 (paper).

Papas heaps paeans of praise on vitamin E that, he claims, can help prevent heart disease and cancer, strengthen immunity, retard Alzheimer's disease, and be of use in treating cataracts, diabetes, and asthma. Vitamin E is an amazing nutrient and a master antioxidant. Papas, an antioxidant researcher, describes how vitamin E is absorbed, how it works in the body, its role in relation to a number of chronic diseases, where to find vitamin E in foods and how much should be taken (diet versus supplements), and purchasing the best vitamin E products (those that contain all eight components of the vitamin E family—four tocopherols and four tocotrienols. This is an exemplary book that summarizes current research knowledge in a highly understandable manner. Also included are a listing of resources, and an extensive 28 pages of references. Highly informative and educational. Good.

Passwater, Richard A. *All About Antioxidants: Frequently Asked Questions*. Garden City Park, NY: Avery, 1998. 96pp. $2.95 (paper).

Antioxidants work by destroying harmful chemicals in the body called "free radicals." Among the diseases linked to excess free radicals are aging, cancer, heart disease, autoimmune diseases, rheumatoid arthritis, Alzheimer's disease, cataracts, and Parkinson's disease. Passwater explains in question-and-answer format the basics of antioxidants, antioxidants for a healthy heart and cancer prevention, and how to use antioxidants such as vitamins E and C, carotenoids, bioflavonoids, coenzyme Q10, and glutathione. A simple explanation of antioxidant nutrients. Contains a glossary, references, and suggested readings.

Arctic Root

Germano, Carl, and Zakir Ramazanov. *Arctic Root (Rhodiola rosea): The Powerful New Ginseng Alternative*. New York: Kensington Books, 1999. 170pp. $5.95 (paper).

The authors set out to present the scientific evidence, mainly accumulated in Russia, that shows the promise of *Rhodiola rosea* in addressing heart disease, cancer, depression, and in strengthening immunity. In addition to documenting current research, the authors conclude their book with the statement that "*Rhodiola rosea* is probably the only substance to reach the West in significant quantities which is not claimed to be a cure for anything in particular yet may be an important adjunct to health for almost any disease condition. Without a doubt, *Rhodiola rosea* is probably the most successful and versatile of the adaptogens now available." There are 16 pages of references to the scientific literature mainly published in Russia. Reflects far-reaching advocacy.

Arginine

Fried, Robert Woodson C. Merrell. *The Arginine Solution: The First Guide to America's New Cardio-Enhancing Supplement*. New York: Warner, 1999. 244pp. $23.

The "magic bullet," according to Fried and Merrell, is the amino acid L-arginine that is fast emerging as one of the most potent nutraceuticals yet described. It works when the body breaks it down, in the process of releasing a simple gas, nitric oxide (or NO), that plays an important role in bodily systems. Viagra could not have been invented without an understanding of nitric oxide's key role in relaxing the smooth muscles of blood vessels. Arginine-derived nitric oxide (ADNO) relaxes arteries, opens the coronary arteries that supply blood to the heart, helps prevent LDL cholesterol from oxidizing and becoming worse, serves an anticoagulant, and may reduce pregnancy-related hypertension.

After explaining the "Basis for the Nitric Oxide Revolution" and how arginine promotes blood circulation, Fried and Merrell recommend their "Arginine Solution"—begin with one gram per day and after several weeks gradually increase to six grams daily if needed; and split each day's dose into three equal parts. Side effects are rare. They conclude that given such a modest price for arginine, and considering all the benefits that it can provide, one "would be hard pressed to find a better health care bargain available anywhere today."

Bach Flower Remedies

Devi, Lila. *The Essential Flower Essence Handbook: Remedies for Inner Well-Being.* Carlsbad, CA: Hay House, 1998. 346pp. $13.95 (paper).

Flower essences are herbal tinctures that strengthen and balance the emotional and psychological levels of our being and are prepared by extracting the life force from blossoms by means of sunlight and pure spring water. Flower essences work by introducing into our energy fields the elevating vibrational examples of different enabling qualities of the plant kingdom. Devi explains the basis for vibrational flower therapy and the psycho-emotional nutrients of the different fruits and vegetables from whose blossoms essences are extracted. Separate chapters deal with the unique articulation of lettuce ("the unruffler"), coconut ("the uplifter"), cherry ("the good cheer messenger"), corn ("the energizer"), and so on. An intriguing book that is based on the belief that flowers are conscious, intelligent forces that have been given to us for happiness and healing.

Shaw, Nan. *Bach Flower Remedies: A Step-By-Step Guide.* In a Nutshell Series. Boston: Element Books, 1998. 58pp. $7.95.

Bach flower remedies are defined as "simple mixtures of water, flowers and brandy, which work to heal emotional problems, thereby restoring mental harmony and preventing physical illness from taking hold." There are 38 Bach flower remedies that address emotional states in a holistic way, allowing the body to react creatively, instead of passively and destructively, when debilitated by the stresses of life. Based on the work of Dr. Edward Bach, a British medical doctor in the early part of the twentieth century, the remedies are sometimes termed "vibrationary," working on energy rather than material chemistry. The remedies are believed to contain the energy or imprint of the plants from which they were made—no physical part of the plant remains in the remedy. This is a compact, beautifully illustrated guide that employs splendid color photographs and illustrations in describing the remedies—Rock Rose, Water Violet, Beech, etc.—and the principal use and key concept involved. The well-known "Rescue Remedy" to rebalance emotional and physical upsets is made from equal amounts of five remedies. Instructions are given for making your own flower remedies. A final chapter lists common ailments, such as exhaustion, fatigue, fear, hormonal imbalances, and the suggested remedies. A simple and aesthetically pleasing guide.

Carotenoids

Challem, Jack. *All About Carotenoids, Beta-Carotene, Lutein and Lycopene: Frequently Asked Questions.* Garden City Park, NY: Avery, 1999. 96pp. $2.99 (paper).

Carotenoids, readily available in fruits and vegetables, have vitamin-like properties and function as antioxidants. Carotenoids are what make carrots orange, corn yellow, and tomatoes red. In addition to making foods colorful and appealing, they have important health benefits. Beta-carotene is a powerful stimulant of the immune cells; leutein may reduce the risk of macular degeneration; and lycopene may help prevent prostate cancer. A final chapter describes how to buy and use carotenoids available as individual supplements or as mixed supplements. An extensive list of references is provided.

Chitosan

Simontacchi, Carol. *All About Chitosan: Frequently Asked Questions.* Garden City Park, NY: Avery, 1999. 96pp. $2.99 (paper).

Greasy french fries and rich ice cream are no longer a dietary problem! Chitosan, a derivative of chitin, absorbs harmful fats before they are deposited in the bloodstream. Each molecule of chitosan magnetically binds to fatty molecules and passes readily out of the body in the process of elimination. Simontacchi explains chitosan's effect on fats, side benefits such as lowering cholesterol levels, how to incorporate chitosan in a weight loss diet, and suggested dosages—3 to 4 g. of chitosan each day in divided doses. Chitosan should not be taken by pregnant or lactating women, or by children. A short list of references is appended. A possible alternative for those who have already tried calorie- or fat-reducing diets.

Chromium Picolinate

Evans, Gary. *All About Chromium Picolinate: Frequently Asked Questions.* Garden City Park, NY: Avery, 1999. 91pp. $2.99 (paper).

> Chromium works in large part by improving the efficiency of insulin so that diabetics who take this dietary mineral have a much easier time controlling many diabetic complications. Taking chromium picolinate supplements also decreases, it is claimed, total cholesterol and LDL-cholesterol levels. Yet other benefits may include a dramatic increase in muscle mass, a pronounced loss of body fat, and possibly retarded aging. Evans maintains that chromium picolinate is a safe supplement for humans. Contains a glossary, references, and suggested readings. A simple and inexpensive summary in question-and-answer format.

Coenzyme Q10

Sahelian, Ray. *All About Coenzyme Q10: Frequently Asked Questions.* Garden City Park, NY: Avery, 1998. 90pp. $2.99 (paper).

> CoQ10, known as ubiquinol, is a naturally occurring nutrient normally present in every cell of the body and is also available through foods. CoQ10 helps in the production of energy within each cell and serves as an antioxidant to fight free radicals. Sahelian summarizes the (limited) evidence that CoQ10 helps in the treatment of congestive heart failure, coronary artery disease, high cholesterol levels, high blood pressure, periodontitis, and fatigue. A final chapter details a dosage plan for taking CoQ10. Contains a glossary and list of references.

Cordyceps

Halpern, Georges M. *Cordyceps: China's Healing Mushroom.* Garden City Park, NY: Avery, 1999. 116pp. $9.95 (paper).

> Cordyceps is a rare capless mushroom grown at high altitudes in the Himalayas, that feeds off a rare type of cold-temperature caterpillar that hibernates just below the surface of the frozen ground until it becomes a solid mummified form, completely composed of the mushroom. It can now be grown commercially without the caterpillars—known as cultured mycelia. Halpern summarizes what is known about Cordyceps and claims that it can increase vitality and well-being and help protect various organs of the body such as the liver, heart, kidneys, and lungs. Guidelines are provided for the dosages to treat specific disorders. A final chapter tells how to buy Cordyceps, what to

look for, and how much you should take. There are five pages of references.

Creatine

Burke, Edmund R. *Creatine: What You Need to Know.* Garden City Park, NY: Avery, 1999. 44pp. $3.95 (paper).

> Creatine supplements, Burke points out, are being touted as one of the most significant developments in sports-related nutrition since the discovery of carbohydrate-loading three decades ago. Now approved for sale by the FDA, creatine is the ergogenic supplement of choice for athletes looking for an edge in competition. Burke concisely discusses what creatine is, the benefits of creatine supplementation, how to use it, and safety concerns. Specific information is provided on dosing, who should take creatine, forms of creatine, and its use in children. Burke concludes that "based on current data, creatine supplementation appears to be a safe and effective nutritional strategy to enhance exercise performance."

Sahelian, Ray, and Dave Tuttle. *All About Creatine: Frequently Asked Questions.* Garden City Park, NY: Avery, 1999. 87pp. $2.99 (paper).

> Creatine is a popular muscle-building nutrient that enhances performance. Recent research indicates that creatine has other therapeutic benefits in improving cholesterol levels and in treating gyrate atrophy (an eye disease). Sahelian and Tuttle present the basic facts—how creatine works, how much to take and when, side effects, and contraindications.

Williams, Melvin H., Richard B. Kreider, and Jay David Branch. *Creatine: The Power Supplement.* Champaign, IL: Human Kinetics, 1999. 250pp. $21.95 (paper).

> Creatine is a natural dietary constituent of animal foods and is not considered to be an essential human nutrient. Recent research indicates the use of creatine supplementation is an ergogenic aid (substance theoretically designed to improve sports performance). Increasing creatine intake 20- to 30-fold exerts an ergogenic effect on various types of physical performance. The authors review experimental research, laboratory studies, ergogenic effects of creatine on aerobic endurance, and effects on body mass and composition. One chapter discusses health and safety aspects. A highly technical, textbook level treatise on creatine.

DHEA

Cherniske, Stephen. *The DHEA Breakthrough.* 3rd edition. New York: Ballantine, 1998. 356pp. $6.99 (paper).

This is an update of a book with the same title published in 1996 and is a compendium of information on DHEA (dehydroepiandrosterone), a potent hormone readily available in health food stores. Cherniske, an enthusiastic proponent of DHEA, argues that it is not just another treatment fad. "But if it is treated like a fad, hyped to the sky, sold like snake oil, and promoted by greed, we will end up losing something of great value and promise." Replete with multiple references and other documentation, Cherniske has assembled a large array of data showing DHEA's remarkable effects on immunity, aging, brain biochemistry, mind, mood, and behavior. Separate chapters show how DHEA can be integrated into a treatment plan involving exercise, weight management, stress reduction, and nutrition. In this new edition, Cherniske summarizes the latest research information and provides extensive bibliographic notes. An honest and sincere attempt to present a balanced summary of what is known about DHEA.

Sahelian, Ray. *All About DHEA: Frequently Asked Questions.* Garden City Park, NY: Avery, 1998. 90pp. $2.99 (paper).

Sahelian believes that DHEA (dehydroepiandrosterone), available without a prescription since 1995, offers tremendous potential for maintaining health and reversing disease, at the same time as carrying some risks. After production in the adrenal glands, DHEA travels in the bloodstream and enters tissues and cells where it is converted into androgens (such as testosterone) and estrogens. Sahelian, a physician, reviews the evidence that DHEA can slow down aging, improve mood, memory, and sex drive and have beneficial effects on heart disease, cancer, and the immune system. Two brief chapters discuss how to find the right dosage and list cautions and side effects. Evaluation and supervision by a health care provider is recommended. Concise and simple with multiple caveats.

D-Ribose

Burke, Edmund R. *D-Ribose: What You Need to Know.* Garden City Park, NY: Avery, 1999. 43pp. $3.95 (paper).

The energy-rich chemical compound that provides virtually all the energy used by the body is known as adenosine triphosphate, or simple ATP. A simple sugar, D-ribose, also called ribose, stimulates the body's production of ATP. This slender volume concisely explains the benefits of ribose, how it works, and how to achieve ribose supplementation. Those who will benefit most are athletes and people with conditions that decrease blood flow and oxygen availability to their hearts or skeletal muscles. One chapter summarizes the scientific research relating to D-ribose. Contains a glossary and list of references. A somewhat technical explanation.

Echinacea

Conkling, Winifred. *Secrets of Echinacea.* New York: St. Martin's Paperbacks, 1999. 193pp. $5.95 (paper).

At one time, echinacea was the most popular herbal medicine in the United States. Echinacea is an all-American herb and does not grow wild anywhere else in the world. Since 1930, more than 300 articles about echinacea have appeared in scientific journals worldwide. Echinacea is used to fight colds and flu, to assist in wound healing, to reduce the inflammation of rheumatoid arthritis, and to strengthen the immune system. The book is divided into three parts: Part One explains the history of echinacea, how it works and active ingredients; Part Two describes healing powers of echinacea in treating a wide variety of ailments; while Part Three details how to buy and use echinacea effectively and safely. Appendices supply a list of organizations, relevant Web sites, and a short bibliography. The most interesting aspect of the book lies in its description of the history, folklore, and legends of echinacea.

Davies, Jill Rosemary. *Echinacea (Echinacea Angustifolia, Echinacea Purpurea).* Boston: Element Books, 1999. 57pp. $7.95.

A compact guide to the healing properties of echinacea that is now popular for easing cold symptoms and reducing stress. Davies, a British herbalist, provides a concise and panoramic view of the growing, harvesting, and processing of echinacea, how it works, preparations for internal use (tinctures, decoctions, infusions) and for external use (ointment, gargles, and compresses). Formulas and dosages are listed for a variety of ailments such as tonsillitis, urethritis, and skin conditions. A highly attractive book with excellent color photographs and illustrations. A short list of readings and useful addresses (mainly British) is supplied.

Schar, Douglas. *Echinacea: The Plant That Boosts Your Immune System.* Berkeley, CA: North Atlantic Books, 1999. 144pp. $9.95 (paper).

Schar is a member of the Herbalists on Columbia Road (HCR), an herbal medicine think tank in London. His enthusiastic espousal of echinacea stems from his belief that it "offers a logical option and a powerful healing tool to health care practitioners confronting lethal bacteria that will not yield to orthodox treatment." In this somewhat unfocused book, Schar mingles botany, chemistry, medicine, and history to produce a mélange of facts concerning echinacea. The major thrust of Schar's book lies in his description of the history of the use of echinacea by the Eclectic Medical Movement in the United States started by Wooster Beach in 1845 and its usage in the modern age from 1930 to date.

Vukovic, Laurel. *All About Echinacea & Goldenseal: Frequently Asked Questions.* Garden City Park, New York: Avery, 1999. 96pp. $2.99 (paper).

Vukovic, an herbalist, states that "if I had to choose only one herb to keep in my medicine cabinet, it would be echinacea." Her reason is that echinacea is a safe and gentle herb that is remarkably effective for helping the immune system overcome infectious microorganisms. Goldenseal is also a potent antimicrobial. Together, maintains Vukovic, echinacea and goldenseal make a powerful immune-boosting and infection-fighting team that is safer and less expensive than prescription antibiotics. Separate chapters deal with how to use echinacea and goldenseal, and how to choose from the many products on the market.

5-HTP

Sahelian, Ray. *5-HTP: Nature's Serotonin Solution.* Garden City Park, NY: Avery, 1998. 210pp. $10.95 (paper).

Sahelian, a physician, points out that depression, weight gain, insomnia, and anxiety are all linked to vital brain chemicals called neurotransmitters. One of the most important neurotransmitters is serotonin, which is created from a nutrient called 5-HTP (5-hydroxytryptophan). Serotonin can be created from 5-HTP and can readily make its way from the bloodstream to the brain. Separate chapters deal with the use of 5-HTP in treating depression, anxiety, insomnia, fibromyalgia, and other disorders. On a cautionary note, Sahelian concedes that the true promise of 5-HTP will most likely come from its intelligent use in combination with a number of other medicines, nutrients, amino acids, herbs, and hormones. An excellent, informative digest of the essential facts concerning 5-HTP.

Garlic

Fulder, Stephen. *All About Garlic: Frequently Asked Questions.* Garden City Park, NY: Avery, 1998. 96pp. $2.99 (paper).

Reviews, in question-and-answer format, the basic facts about garlic that Fulder (a biochemist) considers to be one of the best preventive remedies of all time. A simple explanation is provided of the use of garlic in reducing blood pressure, lowering cholesterol, improving circulation, treating nagging infections, and cancer prevention. A final chapter shows how to shop for garlic tablets, capsules, and deodorized garlic together with recommended dosages. Finally, the book explains how to take garlic without the bothersome smell that "could fell an ox at 20 paces." Contains a glossary, references and suggested readings.

Ginkgo Biloba

Halpern, Georges. *Ginkgo Biloba: A Practical Guide.* Garden City Park, NY: Avery, 1998. 172pp. $9.95 (paper).

Ginkgo biloba extract is one of the most studied plant-based medicines in Europe and the United States. Ginkgo improves circulation in the body and is effective in treating and preventing a wide range of disorders such as cardiovascular disease, vision problems, brain injury, asthma, impotence, and allergies. There is also evidence that it improves overall brain function and memory, possibly even reversing some of the ravages of Alzheimer's disease. In separate chapters, Halpern details where and how ginkgo is cultivated, its history, and its relationship to the brain, heart, sexuality, and aging. Halpern considers that ginkgo biloba extract "offers the greatest hope for the regeneration of our bodies since Western science discovered the benefits of ginseng and vitamin E," and that it should be as much a part of a person's health regime as vitamin supplements.

Pressman, Alan H. with Helen Tracy. *Ginkgo: Nature's Brain Booster.* New York: Avon, 1999. 206pp. $5.99 (paper).

Pressman refers to a study published in *JAMA* in October 1997 that showed a measurable improvement in memory in Alzheimer's patients taking ginkgo. Utilizing a question-and-answer format, Pressman summarizes the basic facts and discusses ginkgo in relation to Alzheimer's disease, memory, aging, hearing problems, and PMS. His book is a largely favorable judgment on the usefulness of ginkgo that "could become the next aspirin, sitting in medicine cabinets around the country and recommended by establishment doctors as readily as by naturopaths." Contains a glossary and bibliography.

Smith, Tracy. *All About Ginkgo Biloba: Frequently Asked Questions.* Garden City Park, NY: Avery, 1999. 96pp. $2.95 (paper).

Interest in ginkgo biloba stems from its reputation in improving memory and concentration, reducing the symptoms of premenstrual syndrome, and relieving leg cramps. Ginkgo is one of the best-selling herbals in the United States. Flavonoids, such as those found in ginkgo are known to protect blood vessels and strengthen capillary walls and are responsible for the antioxidant activity of ginkgo. Short, concise chapters, arranged in a question-and-answer format, deal with ginkgo and the brain, circulatory system, and sexuality. A final chapter details how to buy and use ginkgo. The recommended dose of standardized extract tablets used in most clinical studies is 40 mg. three times per day with meals over at least 6–8 weeks.

Zuess, Jonathan. *Ginkgo: The Smart Herb.* New York: Three Rivers Press, 1998. 173pp. $10 (paper).

For centuries the Taoist monks of Japan and China have revered ginkgo tea as an elixir of longevity and as an aid to clearing their minds and deepening their meditation. Ginkgo is the number-one selling herb in Europe and is one of the most prescribed medications. Zuess, an Australian physician, describes the history of ginkgo, its use as a brain booster and longevity tonic and its benefits in healing asthma, allergies and PMS. Four chapters provide details on using ginkgo safely, how and where to buy ginkgo, how to use it, and how to avoid side effects. An appendix lists suppliers of ginkgo. Concise and readable.

Ginseng

Davies, Jill Rosemary. *Ginseng (Eleutheroccus Senticosus).* In a Nutshell Series Guide. Boston: Element Books, 1999. 57pp. $7.95.

This compact volume focuses on Siberian ginseng, which is classified as an adaptogen that helps the body to adapt to stress. Ginseng has been used in Chinese and ancient traditional herbal medicine for over 2,000 years. This simple, beautifully illustrated text explains ginseng's history, its anatomy and chemical constituents, how it works in reducing stress levels and restoring energy, how to grow and harvest ginseng, and preparations for use in the form of tinctures, decoctions, capsules, and root wine. A four-page conditions chart lists conditions that Siberian ginseng can help treat and the suggested usage form—tinctures, tea, capsules, etc. Contains excellent color photographs and diagrams. A highly informative yet simple summary of the essential facts. Davies is a British herbalist.

Fulder, Stephen. *All About Ginseng: Frequently Asked Questions.* Garden City Park, NY: Avery, 1998. 94pp. $2.99 (paper).

Ginseng has both short-term and long-term uses. On a short-term basis, it can be used as a rapid and safe stimulant; on a long-term basis, it can successfully be used in recovering from periods of stress and burnout, and in convalescence. Separate chapters deal, in question-and-answer format, with ginseng to boost performance, ginseng and stress, and ginseng and aging. Tips are given to assist readers in shopping for ginseng roots. Contains a glossary, references, and suggested readings. A concise discussion.

MoraMarco, Jacques. *The Complete Ginseng Handbook: A Practical Guide for Energy, Health, and Longevity.* Lincolnwood, IL: Contemporary Books, 1998. 231pp. $12.95 (paper).

MoraMarco, a licensed acupuncturist, states that his book "is based on the knowledge and wisdom of thousands of years of ginseng usage, as well as on many well-documented modern scientific and medical studies." The content of his book focuses on the benefits of ginseng, how ginseng enhances both mental and physical performance, the role of ginseng in sexual health, and how ginseng can bring health benefits in the treatment of anemia, CFS, heart disease, cancer, and other ailments. Two chapters show how to select the right ginseng (Asian, Siberian, or American) and where to purchase it. A useful summary of the basic facts.

Glucosamine and Chondroitin

Sahelian, Ray. *All About Glucosamine & Chondroitin: Frequently Asked Questions.* Garden City Park, NY: Avery, 1998. 96pp. $2.99 (paper).

There are other ways of treating osteoarthritis apart from anti-inflammatory drugs! Sahelian considers that two natural substances, glucosamine and chondroitin, are among the best of them. Glucosamine sulfate successfully alleviates pain, joint tenderness, and swelling. Chondroitin makes cartilage resistant to the pressures that it experiences from bearing weight. Both substances help cartilage to regrow. Sahelian, using a question-and-answer format, describes osteoarthritis and connective tissue problems and offers guidelines for usage of glucosamine and chondroitin. Simple, informative, and inexpensive.

Grape Seed Extract

Clouatre, Dallas. *All About Grape Seed Extract: Frequently Asked Questions.* Garden City Park, NY: Avery, 1998. 91pp. $2.99 (paper).

People who live in countries where wine is a regular accompaniment to meals have a lower incidence of heart attacks than people who drink no alcoholic beverages at all. Grape seed extract produced by modern extraction techniques concentrates many of the benefits of red wine. The extract contains flavonoids that possess antioxidant, anti-inflammatory, anticarcinogenic, and antiviral properties. The benefits offered by grape seed extract are discussed in relation to a number of conditions such as allergies, arthritis, PMS, and cardiovascular diseases. One chapter indicates dosages and availability of grape seed extract. But a glass of wine is more tasteful and satisfying than 300 mg. of grape seed extract!

Huperzine-A

Haneline, Patricia G., and Alan P. Kozikowski. *Huperzine A: What You Need to Know*. Avery's Nutrition Discovery Series. Garden City Park: Avery, 1999. 44pp. $3.95 (paper).

Huperzine A is the active constituent with memory-enhancing properties that is extracted from the club moss Huperzia serrata. Chinese scientists have reported that it can improve memory and alleviate some of the symptoms of Alzheimer's disease. Huperzine A can be used alone or in combination with known memory enhancers, including ginkgo and vitamin E. In this slender volume, the authors explain the brain chemicals that are necessary for memory, the physiological changes in the brains of people affected by Alzheimer's disease, how Huperzine A works to improve memory and cognition, what current research shows, and how to buy and use Huperzine A. It should not be combined with Tacrine or Donezepil. A concise and clear explanation of a promising memory enhancer.

Kava

Cass, Hyla, and Terrence McNally. *Kava: Nature's Answer to Stress, Anxiety, and Insomnia*. Rocklin, CA: Prima, 1998. 274pp. $12.95 (paper).

Kava, the authors point out, has the remarkable ability to promote relaxation without affecting mental sharpness, making it the perfect natural supplement for today's frantic, stress-filled lifestyle. Moreover, according to Cass and McNally, it is safe, free of side effects, and nonaddictive. For anxiety, kava is preferred to antidepressants. In higher doses, kava produces restful and restorative sleep. The authors succeed admirably in assembling essential information relating to its chemistry and action, clinical uses, how best to take kava, safety and contraindications, herbal combinations, use of dietary supplements, and "Listening to Kava"—drinking kava "for inducing and sharing an experience of heightened awareness and empathy, of enhanced

well-being, and freedom from doing." An excellent, well-organized, and informative book on kava as a unique herbal remedy for stress, anxiety, and insomnia. Contains lists of recommended readings and resources. Cass is a psychiatrist; McNally is an organizational consultant.

Connor, Kathryn M., and Donald S. Vaughan. *Kava: Nature's Stress Relief*. New York: Avon, 1999. 234pp. $5.99 (paper).

This is a fairly simple and readable explanation of the basic facts about kava in a question-and-answer format that addresses what kava is and its beneficial effects in treating stress, anxiety, and insomnia. Separate chapters deal with side effects and shopping for kava. A useful appendix, "What's on the Shelves," lists manufacturers, brand names, kava content, other ingredients, and prices. A concise, inexpensive summary.

Greenwood-Robinson, Maggie. *Kava: The Ultimate Guide to Nature's Anti-Stress Herb*. New York: Dell, 1999. 239pp. $5.99 (paper).

In the author's opinion, kava is "an incredible stress-reliever—perfect for trying times when you just can't relax or get rid of health-damaging physical tension." Think of kava as a "Stress Band-Aid." Greenwood-Robinson, a nutritional consultant, discusses in a highly informal and readable manner kava as the "wonder drug of the South Pacific," the growing popularity of kava (kava lounges and kava bars), kava experiences (what kava is really like), the "kick that kava gives," and its use in managing stress, easing anxiety, beating depression, and overcoming insomnia. One chapter compares kava with prescription mood drugs, while another chapter details how much, what kind, and where to buy kava. Appendix material answers questions and provides recipes for kava cooking, references, and Web sites (kava in Cyberspace). More detailed and informative than Earl Mindell's *All About Kava: Frequently Asked Questions* (Avery, 1999).

Mindell, Earl. *All About Kava: Frequently Asked Questions*. Garden City Park, NY: Avery, 1998. 96pp. $2.99 (paper).

Nearly $2 billion worth of Prozac is sold every year to the millions that suffer from depression and anxiety. Yet antidepressant drugs can cause multiple unwanted side effects. Kava, used for centuries by South Sea islanders, was observed to create a sense of blissful well-being in those who ate it or consumed it in a ceremonial drink. For those who are debilitated by chronic anxiety or depression, the use of kava supplements can be highly beneficial. Mindell points out that kava should not be taken in combination with prescription antidepressants and anxiolytics. The dosage recommended is from 70 to 210 mg. per day, divided into three equal dosages. Seven pages of references are provided.

Marijuana

Ford, David R. *Marijuana: Not Guilty as Charged.* Sonoma, CA: Good Press, 1997. 253pp. $24.95.

Ford conducts the reader on a tour through the "Malice in Blunderland" of American marijuana policy. Marijuana can reduce nausea, prevent vomiting, and increase appetite in people with cancer, anorexia and AIDS, and can lower eye pressure in glaucoma patients, as well as controlling muscle spasms in people with cerebral palsy and multiple sclerosis. Yet the U.S. government will not permit sufferers to obtain relief legally. Ford expresses outrage at the harmful effects of current laws and policies involving drug testing, loyalty oaths, drug-sniffing dogs, helicopter flyovers, and property foreclosures. The plea is made to legalize marijuana. The book's major intent is to portray the folly of governmental policy rather than to prove the validity of marijuana as treatment. Only one chapter is devoted to marijuana as medicine.

Randall, Robert C., and Alice M. O'Leary. *Marijuana Rx: The Patient's Fight for Medicinal Pot.* New York: Thunder's Mouth Press, 1998. 498pp. $14.95 (paper).

Presented in the form of a personal narrative by Robert Randall and Alice O'Leary, the co-founders of ACT (the Alliance of Cannabis Therapeutics), which is dedicated to reforming the laws prohibiting medical marijuana use. Randall was the first person granted access to the legal use of medical marijuana grown by the U.S. government. The case for the medicinal value of marijuana and the illogicality and inhumanity of denying its use by patients is submerged in a morass of legal and regulatory detail. Less cogent than David R. Ford's *Marijuana: Not Guilty as Charged* (Good Press, 1997).

MSM

Cooney, Craig, with Bill Lawren. *Methyl Magic: Maximum Health through Methylation.* Kansas City, MO: Andrews McMeel, 1998. 253pp. $22.95.

Homocysteine is an indicator of deficient methylation and efforts to prevent atherosclerosis are centered upon counteracting the harmful effects of homocysteine on the arteries. Chronic deficiencies of folic acid and vitamin B6 control the production of homocysteine from methionine. Cooney and Lawren describe the dietary and supplemental strategies needed to keep blood homocysteine levels within the desirable range, involving fresh fruit and vegetables; and whole grain cereals, fresh fish, and meat that supply folic acid and vitamin B6. Three chapters are devoted to the "Methyl Magic Program"—"Food," "Supplements," and "Exercise," while other chapters deal with the effect of methyl deficiency on other diseases such as fibromylagia, heart disease and stroke, cancer, and arthritis. Appendixes detail a "Methyl Power Shopping Trip at the Supermarket" and "Methyl Magic Recipes." This is a very clear explanation of methylation and the role of homocysteine. Cooney is a biochemist; Lawren is a science writer.

Dennison, Margaret. *All About MSM: Frequently Asked Questions.* Garden City Park, NY: Avery, 1999. 95pp. $2.99 (paper).

The organic version of sulfur is known as methyl-sulfonyl-methane (MSM) that is found in the tissues of fluids of all plants, animals, and humans. Research has revealed that MSM is the main healing element in DMSO (dimethylsulfoxide). Sulfur deficiencies are associated with gastrointestinal problems, a poorly functioning immune system, arthritis, acne, and memory loss. Dennison reviews the health benefits of MSM in relation to healthy skin, allergies, disorders of the digestive tract, and other ailments. A final chapter deals with dosage and usage. In a burst of enthusiasm, Dennison states that "if you suffer from any of the problems mentioned in this book, or if MSM sounds if could enhance your health, then you may want to try MSM to alleviate some of your ailments or simply to experience its health-enhancing abilities."

Jacob, Stanley W., Ronald M. Lawrence, and Martin Zucker. *The Miracle of MSM: The Natural Solution for Pain.* New York: Putnam, 1999. 250pp. $19.95.

MSM has become a hot item at health food stores and drug stores. MSM (methyl-sulfonyl-methane) is a nutritional supplement that supplies biologically active sulfur and offers a natural way to reduce pain and inflammation without serious side effects. Drawing upon their own clinical experience and much anecdotal evidence, the authors describe how MSM can relieve common pain problems such as headaches, back pain, fibromyalgia, tendonitis, and carpal tunnel syndrome. Moreover, MSM is useful in treating allergies, asthma, and arthritis. Specific instructions detail how much, when, with what foods, and in what form to take MSM. In an attempt to provide a balanced presentation, the authors stress the need for further research and offer an appendix, "Truth or Fiction—Sifting through MSM Claims." More detailed and objective than Margaret

Dennison's *All About MSM: Frequently Asked Questions* (Avery, 1999).

Omega-3 Oils

Felix, Clara. *All About Omega-3 Oils: Frequently Asked Questions*. Garden City Park, NY: Avery, 1998. 96pp. $2.99 (paper).

Omega-3 oils ("fish oils") belong to a very special group of fats called the essential fatty acids that are necessary to life. These polyunsaturated acids offer impressive benefits in reducing the risk of heart disease, keeping triglycerides at safe levels, lowering blood pressure, serving as natural anti-inflammatory agents, improving circulation in the tiny blood vessels of the eyes, and reducing the overall risk of cancer. Omega-3 fatty acids are found in fish, flaxseed, soy proteins, and nuts such as walnuts. Specific suggestions are offered to increase the availability of Omega-3 in the diet (eating salmon, sardines, herring, lamb, walnuts) and by taking fish oil supplements. The basic message conveyed is that not all fats are bad and that Omega-3 fatty acids can restore an imbalance of dietary fats. A simple summary in question-and-answer format.

Pycnogenol

Passwater, Richard A. *All About Pycnogenol: Frequently Asked Questions*. Garden City Park, NY: Avery, 1998. 96pp. $2.99 (paper).

Pycnogenol, a pine bark extract, is a potent antioxidant, an immune booster, an anti-inflammatory, a cardiovascular protectant, and an anticarcinogen. Pycnogenol is a dietary supplement that is available in tablets or capsules. Many of the nutrients it contains are bioflavonoids, which are found in fruits, vegetables, nuts, grains and in beverages such as tea and wine. Passwater explains how the substance works as an immune booster, and its protective effects against heart disease. Evidence exists that pycnogenol is also useful in controlling hay fever and other allergies. One chapter discusses dosages and how to take pycnogenol. A useful summary.

SAM-e

Brown, Richard, Teodoro Bottiglieri, and Carol Colman. *Stop Depression Now: SAM-e, the Breakthrough Supplement That Works as Well as Prescription Drugs in Half the Time with No Side Effects*. New York: Putnam's, 1999. 267pp. $19.95.

SAM-e ("sammy") is scientific shorthand for S-adenosyl-L-methionine, which is now available in the United States after being widely available in Europe for several decades. SAM-e is approved for use as a prescription drug in Spain, Italy, Russia, and Germany. In Italy, SAM-e outsells Prozac. Unlike other antidepressants, SAM-e is not a drug. Nor is it an herb like St. John's wort. Instead, it is a substance normally produced by the human organism. The authors (a psychopharmacologist and a medical writer respectively) present the evidence supporting their claim that SAM-e works as well or better than other antidepressants, that it works faster, and with fewer side effects. They state that there is "compelling evidence that . . . SAM-e . . . may just become the treatment of choice not only for depression but also for osteoporosis and fibromyalgia." The "Stop Depression Now" program outlined describes how to take SAM-e in conjunction with modifications in diet and lifestyle. Two chapters show how SAM-e can help in controlling postpartum and menopausal depression and fibromyalgia. A 23-page bibliography is appended. Highly informative.

Clouatre, Dallas. *All About SAM-e: Frequently Asked Questions*. Garden City Park, NY: Avery, 1999. 96pp. $2.99 (paper).

This short summary of the basic facts about SAM-e (S-adenosyl-L-methionine) claims that supplementing with this versatile substance can have important effects on health including mood elevation, blood detoxification, and cartilage formation. Evidence exists reporting its beneficial effects in treating osteoarthritis, depression, fibromyalgia, several liver disorders, migraine headaches, and learning and memory deficits associated with advancing age. SAM-e acts a methyl donor that contributes to methylation. Improving the methylation process by increasing the availability of methyl donors reduces the production of homocysteine (a toxic amino acid) and thereby lowers the risk of damage to important blood vessels. Methyl groups attach to DNA to provide protection against the activation of genes responsible for many diseases. This compact book is of more use in providing an understandable explanation of the process of methylation than in offering a practical prescription for boosting overall health.

Clouatre, Dallas. *SAM-e (S-adenosyl-L-methionine): What You Need to Know*. Avery's Nutrition Discovery Series: Garden City Park, NY, 1999. 44pp. $3.95 (paper).

This is a summary of the essential facts concerning SAM-e, including its origin, mode of action, and typical uses for liver health, fibromyalgia, arthritis, and depression. Clouatre claims that SAM-e in supplemental form has been shown to improve brain and nerve health, and can lead to significant improvement in cases of depression. Moreover, SAM-e may also be beneficial in cases of migraine headache, postpartum depression, and drug rehabilitation. For most purposes supplementation with 200 to 400 mg. of SAM-e twice a day will prove adequate. Four pages of selected references from the professional literature are intended to substantiate the claims made.

Grazi, Sol, and Marie Costa. *SAMe (S-adenosylmethionine): The European Arthritis and Depression Breakthrough.* Rocklin, CA: Prima, 1998. 248pp. $14 (paper).

Research shows that SAM-e is somewhat effective in treating osteoarthritis, either alone or in conjunction with other drugs or supplements such as glucosamine. The evidence is somewhat less strong for its value in treating depression. Grazi adopts a cautious note in documenting the value of SAMe in relation to a number of diseases including osteoarthritis, depression, fibromyalgia, Parkinson's disease, and Alzheimer's disease. A serious attempt to present an objective assessment.

Saw Palmetto

Janson, Michael. *All About Saw Palmetto and Prostate Health: Frequently Asked Questions.* Garden City Park, NY: Avery, 1999. 95pp. $2.99 (paper).

Janson, a physician, summarizes the evidence that saw palmetto (berries obtained from serenoa repens, a small palm tree) relieves the symptoms of benign prostatic hyperplasia (BPH). Saw palmetto appears to be a safe, natural alternative to terazosin (Hytrin), finasteride (Proscar), and surgical treatments such as TURP. The typical dosage according to Janson, is 160 mg. of standardized extract twice a day. There are almost no side effects and no known negative interactions with drugs or other dietary supplements. Janson includes a short list of references and suggested readings. Similar but less detailed than Ray Sahelian's *Saw Palmetto: Nature's Prostate Healer* (Kensington, 1998).

Winston, David. *Saw Palmetto for Men and Women: A Medicinal Herb Guide.* Pownal, VT: Storey Books, 1999. 119pp. $12.95 (paper).

Saw palmetto is best known for its beneficial effects in treating benign prostatic hyperplasia (BPH), a common nonmalignant but uncomfortable enlargement of the prostate that causes bladder frequency and discomfort. Winston, an herbalist, advocates the use of saw palmetto in combination with supportive herbs such as nettle root and white sage, together with dietary changes for the treatment of BPH. Saw palmetto is also useful for other health

conditions including male pattern baldness, polycystic ovary disease, deep cystic acne, and pelvic congestion syndrome. Major emphasis is placed on presenting practical information—tincture formulas, dosages, and converting to metric measurement. The book contains a glossary, selected bibliography, sources of saw palmetto, where to find a competent herbalist, herbal organizations and journals, herbal Web sites, and so on. Factual and useful.

Selenium

Passwater, Richard A. *All About Selenium: Frequently Asked Questions.* Garden City Park, NY: Avery, 1999. 96pp. $2.99 (paper).

The book describes how selenium-containing antioxidant enzymes work in the body. Selenium, a trace mineral discovered in 1817, has antioxidant properties that can protect the body from more than 80 diseases, including cancer, heart disease, premature aging, and arthritis. Passwater, using a question-and-answer format, provides basic information on how antioxidants work, their role in controlling the destructive effects of free radicals, and the health benefits of selenium in preventing cancer, heart disease, arthritis, and a variety of other disorders. Passwater shows how best to use selenium supplements, dosages according to age, safety, and symptoms of toxicity. Contains a glossary, list of references, and suggested readings. A strong endorsement of the health benefits of selenium.

Soy Products

Dolby, Victoria. *All About Soy Isoflavones and Women's Health: Frequently Asked Questions.* Garden City Park, NY: Avery, 1999. 96pp. $2.99 (paper).

Soybeans contain a specific family of phytoestrogens called isoflavones. These natural plantlike estrogens appear to function primarily as antioxidants. When consumed, isoflavones function both as antioxidants and as phytoestrogens in the body. A diet high in soy products (a rich source of isoflavones) can result in a surprisingly low incidence of breast cancer, heart disease, and menopause-related problems such as hot flashes. The benefits of soy are discussed in relation to cancer prevention, menstruation and menopause, osteoporosis, diabetes, and kidney disease. A final chapter shows how to incorporate soy into your life. Contains a short glossary, list of references, and suggested readings. A simple explanation.

Holt, Stephen. *The Soy Revolution: The Food for the Next Millenium.* New York: Evans, 1998. 214pp. $19.95.

"I have taken the work of thousands of researchers in the soybean field," states Holt, "and reported and/or interpreted their findings." The benefits of soybeans and soy supplements are outlined in relation to atherosclerosis, osteoporosis, kidney function, diabetes, prostate disease and hypertension. A detailed and readable statement of the benefits of soy and soy products by a physician who emphasizes that the soybean has been a staple food in Asia for thousands of years and that its medicinal and nutritional values are deeply rooted in traditional Chinese medicine.

St. John's Wort

Bratman, Steven. *Beat Depression with St. John's Wort.* Rocklin, CA: Prima Publishing, 1997. 212pp. $12 (paper).

Bratman (a physician practicing complementary medicine) believes that St. John's wort is a "splendid option for mild to moderate depression." Eschewing the terminology of miracle cures, Bratman considers that a treatment does not have to be miraculous to be thoroughly useful when used in the context of a complementary approach to health care. The basics are well covered—what St. John's wort (*hypericum perforatum*) is; symptoms and causes of depression; and the rising popularity of St. John's wort in Germany and in the United States. Of particular value are two chapters that detail the drawbacks of conventional treatment for depression (Prozac, Zoloft, Paxil, Wellbutrin, Serzone, Effexor), contrasted with the use of St. John's wort as a safe and effective alternative. The limitations of antidepressant drugs are clearly stated and documented. Separate chapters are devoted to how to take St. John's wort, how it compares with drug treatment, how to decide if St. John's wort is right for you, and working with medical doctors and alternative medicine practitioners. An appendix summarizes the research record for St. John's wort. This is a lucid, balanced presentation that points out the limitations of mainstream antidepressants, at the same as presenting the promise of St. John's wort as a safe alternative.

Cass, Hyla. *All About St. John's Wort: Frequently Asked Questions.* Garden City Park, NY: Avery, 1998. 96pp. $2.99 (paper).

Cass, who combines expertise in nutrition and psychiatry, considers St. John's wort "not only as good as prescription medications, but in many cases it is actually more effective and certainly safer" than patented prescription medications. Drawing upon her many years of clinical experience in integrative psychiatry, Cass concisely explains depression, the characteristics of St. John's wort, its use in depression, precautions and side effects, other uses (in viral infections, chronic fatigue syndrome, sciatica), and relevant sci-

entific evidence. Cass concludes that "we find in this herb an unusual combination of safety, effectiveness and a broad range of positive effects, a lack of side effects and low cost." A simple, practical, and inexpensive summary of the basic facts.

Chevallier, Andrew. *St. John's Wort: The Natural Antidepressant and More.* Berkeley, CA: North Atlantic Books, 1999. 143pp. $9.95 (paper).

In this British book, Chevallier (a medical herbalist) points to the wide-ranging effects of St. John's wort (hypericum) on the nervous system, its antimicrobial and immune-stimulant activity, and its ability to control inflammation and heal wounds. The major use of St. John's wort, however, lies in the treatment of depression. The attempt to present a comprehensive picture of St. John's wort falls flat in that the text has no integral theme, and digresses into a discussion of chemistry, botany, history, and summaries of research studies. A very pedestrian presentation.

*Thase, Michael E., and Elizabeth E. Loredo. *St. John's Wort: Nature's Mood Booster.* New York: Avon, 1998. 346pp. $5.99 (paper).

"St. John's wort doth charm all the witches away. If gathered at midnight on the Saint's holy day." Thase, a psychiatrist at the University of Pittsburgh, is concerned that many people are taking St. John's wort on unquestioning faith unaware of the potential dangers of using the herb as depression therapy. To better inform consumers, Thase explains the history, ingredients, safety, effectiveness, and usefulness of hypericum (St. John's wort) as an antidepressant. Two chapters cover how and where to buy St. John's wort, and instructions on how to grow and prepare your own supply. An excellent 25-page section provides an extensive listing and description of information resources such as organizations and Web sites, together with guidance on formulating online searches and evaluating the quality of the information retrieved. Also listed are chatrooms and AOL newsgroups. An excellent compendium that truly assembles almost everything you need to know about St. John's wort. Good.

Tea Tree Oil

Olsen, Cynthia. *Australian Tea Tree Oil: First Aid Handbook.* 2nd edition. Pagosa Springs, CA: Kali Press, 1999. 84pp. $6.95 (paper).

Olsen offers a concise summary of the use and efficacy of tea tree oil (*melaleuca alternifolia*) as a first-aid remedy for a number of skin ailments, and problems relating to the throat and chest, legs and feet, baby and child care, and outdoors and camping. An appendix describes how to make

carbonica, pulsatilla, sepia, arsenicum album, and nux vomica can be used to treat hot flashes, insomnia, and digestive disorders. While offering many homeopathic remedies for common medical problems, there is scant detail as to the sources and dosages of the products identified.

Jonas, Wayne B., and Jennifer Jacobs. *Healing with Homeopathy: The Doctor's Guide.* New York: Warner, 1998. 349pp. $14.99 (paper).

Homeopathy has captured the attention of the American public and continues to gain in popularity. Many pharmacies now stock homeopathic products. The authors define homeopathy as "a system of medicine that uses specially prepared, highly dilute substances to induce the body's self-healing mechanism in a comprehensive manner." The goal of their book is twofold: to give the reader an overview of homeopathy and its history and development; second, to provide the reader with specific information on applying homeopathy to common minor health problems. Separate chapters deal with homeopathy in relation to children's illnesses, women's health problems, common respiratory tract infections, digestive problems, headaches and toothaches, and acute emotional problems and insomnia. This is a paperback version of a book originally published in 1996 under the title *Healing with Homeopathy: The Complete Guide* (Warner, 1996). Jonas is a former director of the NIH Office of Alternative Medicine; Jacobs is a family physician specializing in homeopathic medicine. Lucid and highly readable.

McCabe, Vinton. *Practical Homeopathy: A Comprehensive Guide to Homeopathic Remedies and Their Acute Uses.* New York: St. Martin's Griffin, 2000. 592pp. $19.95 (paper).

McCabe, an advocate of homeopathy, sets himself an ambitious task: "I have tried to write a book that I always hoped someone else would write—a single volume that would give an overview of homeopathic philosophy and a plan to follow for homeopathic practice; it would give solid diagnostic tools for homeopathic practice and a key for the remedies that are most commonly used in acute practice, as well as their doses and potencies." Details are provided on diagnostic symptoms, acute remedies and their use for injuries, emergencies, general aches and pains, and common ailments, and a materia medica. But despite its lofty objective, McCabe offers a cookbook with multiple ingredients but inadequate instructions, which makes the book of little practical use.

Papon, R. Donald. *Homeopathy Made Simple: A Quick Reference Guide.* Charlottesville, VA: Hampton Roads Publishing, 1999. 262pp. $11.95 (paper).

This is a largely successful attempt to make homeopathy more understandable and less esoteric. Responding to his daughter's request at preparatory school for a quick guide to show "which remedy to take for what," Papon prepared a "Repertory" of the various symptoms arranged in order of the various parts of the body affected. The resulting "Five-Minute Prescriber" lists, in 20 separate chapters, 20 parts of the body such as mind, heart, stomach, and back. If you have a headache, then go to the "Head" chapter that lists dozens of symptoms. If the cause is overwork, the indicated remedy is *pulsatilla* (wind flower); if the problem is sinus, then the remedy is *Bryonia alba* (wild hops). One part of the book outlines the major characteristics of the various remedies indicated while another part contains "Secrets of a Practicing Homeopath," and remedies for problems such as candida, menopause, and impotency. Focusing on the top 29 most useful homeopathic remedies, Papon shows how homeopathy can be used. However, diagnosing and self-prescribing with reference to a set of tables is somewhat oversimplified and even hazardous.

Stone, Ursula. *Homeopathy for Back and Neck Pain.* New York: Kensington Books, 1999. 159pp. $4.99 (paper).

The four main homeopathic principles are "like cures like," minimal doses, single medicines prepared according to homeopathic practice, and prescribing based on an assessment of the totality of symptoms. Stone concisely explains terms such as minimal dosing, law of similars, planes of illness and other concepts of homeopathy, and shows how homeopathy can be employed to treat back problems such as pinched nerves, degenerated discs, sciatica, and spinal stenosis. Remedies include the use of some 24 specific homeopathic preparations. One part of the book consists of a materia medica (a catalog of remedies) that shows the use of homeopathic remedies. Stone succeeds more in describing the essentials of homeopathy than in showing how homeopathy can be useful in treating back and neck pain.

Stone, Ursula. *Homeopathy for Headaches.* New York: Kensington Books, 1999. 183pp. $4.99 (paper).

The first part of the book—a description of the principles of homeopathy spanning 37 pages—duplicates word-for-word the first part of Stone's *Homeopathy for Back and Neck Pain* (Kensington, 1999). Part Two discusses how homeopathy can be used in treating headache, while Part Three presents the materia medica (a catalog of remedies). The two volumes could be combined to eliminate what is, in part, a duplicate purchase.

Ullman, Dana. *The Consumer's Guide to Homeopathy: The Definitive Resource for Understanding Homeopathic Medicine and Making It Work for You.* New York: Putnam, 1995. 409pp. $13.95 (paper).

Ullman is a leading spokesman for homeopathic medicine who believes that homeopathic medicines should be considered as the first method of treatment for healing ailments because they are often both effective and considerably safer than conventional drugs. Apart from introducing the reader to the principles and methods of homeopathic medicine, the main value of this book resides in the comprehensive compilation of homeopathic resources including books, tapes, software, homeopathic organizations, sources of homeopathic medicines, training programs, homeopathic journals and newsletters, study groups, and a listing of homeopathic medicines and their common names. An excellent sourcebook on all aspects of homeopathy, despite its publication date.

Wauters, Ambika. *Homeopathic Medicine Chest.* Freedom, CA: The Crossing Press, 2000. 124pp. $12.95 (paper).

"In homeopathy we treat you, the individual, and not the disease." The materia medica used is based on the "provings" of over 250 years of experience as recorded in annals. Classical homeopathy uses one remedy at a time. The choice of remedies by the homeopath is based on observation and on the mental and physical conditions of each case. Two introductory chapters define homeopathy and describe how it works. Separate chapters deal with homeopathic first-aid remedies, first-aid conditions (abdominal pain, arthritis, asthma), with the homeopathic remedy, Bach remedy, and a first-aid materia medica. In addition to summarizing the appropriate use of the materia medica of homeopathy, Wauters (a British homeopath) provides a lucid and concise description of homeopathic therapy.

Massage

Evans, Mark. *The New Life Library: Instant Massage for Stress Relief.* New York: Lorenz Books, 1997. 64pp. $9.95.

Evans, principal of the Bath School of Massage (UK), asks whether "when you come home at the end of the day, do your neck and shoulders feel as if they are set in concrete? Does stress leave your back stiff and aching?" Systematic, caring touch through massage movements encourage the release of endorphins that can be highly beneficial. Professional massage can be an effective treatment for a wide variety of physical problems. Through the use of excellent color photographs, Evans illustrates how to employ self-massage to revitalize and reduce stress, and how to use massage with a partner. A most aesthetically pleasing book that lucidly describes the therapeutic benefits of touch.

Maxwell-Hudson, Clare. *Aromatherapy Massage.* New York: DK Publishing, 1999. 112pp. $13.95 (paper).

A sumptuously illustrated guide to the pleasures and benefits of massage using aromatic oils that help soothe, relax, and refresh the mind and body. Splendid color photographs illustrate full body massage techniques for the face, back, abdomen, and feet; aromatic beauty care (ingredients, equipment, and technique for aromatic facials and scented bathing); and therapeutic remedies—the healing properties of fragrance and essential oils such as eucalyptus oil and lavender oil for relieving insomnia, mental fatigue, stress, and jetlag. A catalog with full-color photographs features some 20 essential oils classified by their uses, therapeutic properties, and sources—jasmine, melissa, geranium, and sandalwood, and so on. A top-notch guide to massaging with essential oils.

Meditation

Bodian, Stephan. *Meditation for Dummies.* Foster City, CA: IDG Books Worldwide, 1999. 348pp. $19.99 (paper).

Bodian, former editor-in-chief of *Yoga Journal*, explains that meditation is the practice and process of paying attention and focusing your awareness. Meditation works and results in less stress, more peace of mind, and a deeper appreciation of the beauty and richness of life. A simple "cheat sheet" that accompanies the book best illustrates the content—meditation lingo, 10 popular meditation techniques, a meditation checklist, 10 tips for getting the most from your meditation, and 10 benefits of regular meditation practice. Serving as a crash course on meditation, the book offers highly specific and practical techniques of relaxing the body and calming the mind, preparing for meditation (posture, stretching, and sitting still), where to sit and what to wear, opening your heart to love and compassion, and navigating roadblocks such as sleepiness, procrastination, and boredom. Separate chapters are devoted to cultivating spirituality, using meditation for healing and performance enhancement, and answers to commonly asked questions. As in other "dummy" books, icons are used to highlight the text pinpointing "Tips," "Traditional Wisdom," "Spiritual Stuff," and so on. Lucid, highly informative and eminently practical. Super!

Mind-Body Medicine

Arem, Ridha. *The Thyroid Solution: A Mind-Body Program for Beating Depression and Regaining Your Emotional and Physical Health.* New York: Ballantine, 1999. 389pp. $24.

While introducing readers to the many ways that the thyroid can affect brain chemistry, Arem (an endocrinologist and thyroid specialist) draws attention to a "hidden epidemic" in that one in 10 Americans—more than 20 million people—suffer from thyroid dysfunction. Arem offers a mind-body approach to identifying and curing thyroid imbalances. Rather than merely describing the various thyroid disorders, the author seeks "to explain the hidden suffering that many patients have difficulty in expressing." Part One of the book describes the thyroid-mind connection and how thyroid imbalance affects mood, emotions, and behavior; Part Two shows how thyroid imbalances may affect weight, sex life, and relationships; Part Three is devoted to women's thyroid problems; while Part Four discusses the diagnosis and treatment of common thyroid disorders. Arem concludes that "the key to correcting thyroid imbalances has changed from simply diagnosing and chronicling physical symptoms to concentrating on the emotional aspects of the disease."

Brownstein, Art. *Healing Back Pain Naturally: The Mind-Body Program Proven to Work.* Gig Harbor, WA: Harbor Press, 1999. 288pp. $19.95.

Brownstein, a physician, has "had the surgery, tried the drugs, felt the despair and the depression." As a former back pain sufferer, he believes that "you can be healed . . . where there is pain, there is life." The mind-body program advocated involves gentle, soothing stretches to make the body flexible, safe and simple exercises, stress management techniques (deep relaxation, breathing, guided imagery, visualization, and meditation), diet and nutrition, and the use of the healing quality of play and recreation. A special section describes what to do for emergency back care when pain becomes incapacitating. This is a holistic approach that fuses together physical strategies with the emotional and spiritual aspects of healing.

Gaynor, Mitchell L. *Sounds of Healing: A Physician Reveals the Therapeutic Power of Sound, Voice, and Music.* New York: Broadway Books, 1999. 260pp. $25.

Gaynor offers a fascinating examination of the use of sound as a complementary therapy in the form of chanting, music, and Tibetan singing bowls. Sound, voice, and music, Gaynor maintains, are potent tools for restoring the inner balance of the body and awakening the spirit. Sound is as powerful a tool for relaxation and mind-body healing as guided imagery. Gaynor shows how to use a variety of techniques—playing the bowls or other musical instruments, and toning or singing—to open and deepen the breath and restore the body to a state of harmony. The techniques used by Gaynor involve the sound of bowls combined with meditation, guided imagery, and vocalization. Other techniques employed include life songs (a unique mantra-like string of one-syllable rhythmic sounds), "Essence" sound meditation that uses the voice and singing bowl or other sound source, and "Energetic Re-Creation" that expands on "Essence" sound meditation. A captivating, extraordinary book by the director of medical oncology and integrative medicine at the Strang-Cornell Cancer Prevention Center in New York City.

Gerrish, Michael. *When Working Out Isn't Working Out: A Mind/Body Guide to Conquering Unidentified Fitness Obstacles.* New York: St. Martin's Griffin, 1999. 242pp. $14.95 (paper).

Gerrish sets out to expose personal fitness blocks that can prevent the achievement of fitness, which he labels UFO's—"Unidentified Fitness Obstacles." Part One of his book reveals what it means to get fit from the inside out; Part Two shows how to address your personal mind/body UFO's (discovering your mental and physical blocks); Part Three exposes the obstacles that can block the achievement of muscular fitness. Separate chapters deal with nutritional UFO's, cardiovascular UFO's, and weight-training UFO's. An approach that combines exercise physiology with psychotherapy.

Harris, Gail. *Body & Soul.* New York: Kensington Books, 1999. 298pp. $29.95.

This is the companion book to the PBS series, *Mind, Body, and Spirit,* which aired in January 1999. Harris states that her book "like the series, is intended as a 'way in' for those who have heard a little about complementary therapies and want to know more, as well as an affirmation and expansion for those who have been interested in health and well-being for years." Harris presents expanded versions of interviews together with personal stories of people who have changed their lives by incorporating "Body & Soul" principles. Those interviewed include Herbert Benson, Andrew Weil, David Eisenberg, Geneen Roth, and Stephen Sinatra. Topics covered include aging well, creating wellness, cancer and the search for healing, mindful eating, East/West medicine, and peak performance. An extensive resource supplement offers advice on how to choose alternative practitioners, a guide to holistic treatments, paying for your care, a whole-self bookshelf, list of professional associations, wellness on the Web, and a glossary. An attractive and literate guide to the basic concepts of the body-mind relationship as viewed by many of the leading experts.

Motz, Julie. *Hands of Life: An Energy Healer Reveals the Secret of Using Your Body's Own Energy Medicine for Healing, Recovery and Transformation*. New York: Bantam, 1998. 309pp. $24.95.

Motz, an energy healer who has worked in the department of cardiothoracic surgery at Columbia Presbyterian Medical Center, describes her healing treatment within the context of the highly mechanized and computerized realm of academic medicine. Her healing method draws on Ayurvedic and Chinese medicine and treats the body and spirit as an interconnected whole. The most interesting aspect of her book lies in her successful attempt to secure the cooperation of a number of senior surgeons who were won over by Motz's persuasiveness and success.

Nacson, Leon. *A Deepak Chopra Companion: Illuminations on Health and Consciousness*. New York: Three Rivers Press, 1999. 110pp. $10 (paper).

Nacson, a longtime friend and colleague of Chopra, offers a "Pocket Chopra" that deals with Ayurvedic medicine, meditation, Karma, purpose, stress, and insight into Chopra's views on healing and expanding human consciousness. The basic notion advocated is that physical health is the balanced integration of the body, mind, and spirit. Nacson provides answers to questions readers themselves would ask Doctor Chopra if they had the opportunity. This is a useful summary of Chopra's teachings, together with short digests of 15 of Chopra's books.

****Ornish, Dean. *Love & Survival: The Scientific Basis for the Healing Power of Intimacy*. New York: HarperCollins, 1998. 284pp. $25.

In this highly acclaimed book, Ornish argues that survival is based on one simple and powerful idea—that our survival depends on the healing power of love, intimacy, and relationships. Research shows that simple changes in diet and lifestyle may cause significant improvements in health and well-being. Yet the most powerful intervention is the healing power of love and intimacy and the emotional and spiritual transformation that often result from these. Ornish suggests pathways to love and intimacy. His book is full of spiritual, emotional, and medical insight. "The heart is a pump that needs to be addressed on a physical level, but our hearts are more than pumps. A true physician is more than just a plumber, technician, or mechanic." The overarching theme is simple and cogent: "anything that promotes feelings of love and intimacy is healing; anything that promotes isolation, separation, loneliness, loss, hostility, anger, cynicism, depression, alienation, and related feelings often

leads to suffering, disease, and premature death from all causes." A landmark book—elegant, lyrical, and based on scientific evidence. Outstanding.

Retherford, Ralph E. *When Chicken Soup Is Not Enough: Revolutionary Healing through the Mind-Body Connection*. Hollywood, FL: Frederick Fell Publishers, 1999. 194pp. $14.95 (paper).

Retherford, the head of a center for mind-body healing in Sonora, California, urges that we shift our attention from physical causes of illnesses to emotional ones in that many of today's common ailments have their roots in mind-body interaction. Retherford provides multiple insightful examples of how emotions convert into physical symptoms; how resentment, unhappiness, frustration, and humiliation can induce pain and illness; and "how we work ourselves sick." The solution lies in abandoning the mechanical model of health and acknowledging that "unconscious material" may be causing illness. A safe and caring environment and a trusting relationship combined with psychotherapy and hypnosis can unlock the door to permanent wellness. Insightful.

Sarno, John E. *The Mind-Body Prescription: Healing the Body, Healing the Pain*. New York: Warner, 1998. 240pp. $22.

Pain disorders have reached epidemic proportions in the United States. Sarno shows that the mind and the body are one and the agony of most pain has a basis in the mind. Part One of his book discusses the psychology that induces physical ailments in that the unconscious avoidance of unwanted emotions can actually stimulate the brain to produce physical symptoms. Part Two reviews various emotionally induced physical maladies such as back and neck pain, tendonitis, and gastrointestinal disorders. Part Three details therapeutic treatment, which focuses on repudiating the physical and acknowledging, and accepting, the psychological. Sarno claims that "for some people simply shifting attention from the physical to the psychological will do the trick." This is a persuasive and well-written analysis of the mind-body connection. However, only one final chapter discusses the author's therapeutic prescription.

Native American Medicine

Alvord, Lori Arviso, and Elizabeth Cohen VanPelt. *The Scalpel and the Silver Bear*. New York: Bantam, 1999. 204pp. $23.95.

This book is the story of a girl from a small, dusty town on a Navaho reservation who left to attend medical school at Stanford and to receive specialized training in surgery. The bear is a sacred animal to Navahos and is represented in many folk tales and myths. Alvord describes her journey and struggle to combine modern medicine with Navaho practices. "I went back to the healers of my tribe to learn what a surgical residency could not teach me." In the Navaho culture, medicine is performed by a *hataalii* who views body, mind, and spirit as connected to other people, to families, to communities, and even to the planet and universe. Healing is not only a one-to-one relationship, but it is also multidimensional. Another basic concept is "Walking in Beauty," which is a way of living a balanced and harmonious life. Alvord—the first Navaho woman surgeon combining Western medicine and traditional healing—offers a fascinating look into Navaho medicine and how it can be integrated with modern surgical practice.

Kavasch, E. Barrie, and Karen Baar. *American Indian Healing Arts: Herbs, Rituals, and Remedies for Every Season of Life*. New York: Bantam, 1999. 309pp. $17.95 (paper).

This is a fascinating reference source that weaves a tapestry of stories, legends, myths, and herbal traditions that illustrate the Native American healing arts. Healing is shown to be linked to the prayers, rites, and ceremonies of the Indian tribes. Here is a valuable source of information on Iroquois childbirth practices, sweat lodge purification rites, squaw balms and papoose roots, earth remedies, and herbal preparations. Appendix material contains a lexicon of herbs, fungi, minerals, and a directory of resources and suppliers together with a selected bibliography. A scholarly compilation.

Mehl-Madrona, Louis. *Coyote Medicine*. New York: Scribner, 1997. 299pp. $24.

This is a very personal narrative by a physician, with a Cherokee grandmother, who combines traditional medical practice with Native American healing rituals and religious ceremonies. "The brightly lit, sterile rooms of Western medicine couldn't have been farther removed from the darkly mysterious sweat lodges where, I have been reading, my Native American ancestors held their healing ceremonies." A fascinating journey from the high-tech, impersonal world of American medicine back to the spiritual healing paradigm of Native American healing.

Squier, Thomas Broken Bear, with Lauren David Peden. *Herbal Folk Medicine: An A-Z Guide*. New York: Owl, 1998. 228pp. $14.95 (paper).

The author is an ex-Green Beret who is the grandson of a Cherokee "root doctor." Squier draws upon the cumulative wisdom of country doctors to bring together the thera-

peutic properties of some 300 herbs and shows how to grow and collect them, with instructions on preparing infusions, decoctions, salves, syrups, elixirs, tinctures, and ointments. An interesting introduction to native American herbal folk medicine.

Reflexology

Dougans, Inge. *The Complete Illustrated Guide to Reflexology: Therapeutic Foot Massage for Health and Well-Being*. Boston, MA: Element Books, 1999. 192pp. $24.95 (paper).

This is another splendid book in the Element Books "Complete Illustrated Guide" series. Utilizing excellent color photographs, illustrations, and diagrams, the text describes reflexology and its place in the healing process. Part One of the book provides background. Part Two shows how reflexology works, with an analysis of the 12 main meridians and the likely symptoms of congestion along their paths. Part Three contains a step-by-step guide to "Practical Reflexology." The grips and pressure techniques that form the basis of the reflexology treatment are explained through clear color photographs. Part Four is a reference section with a glossary and bibliography. This is a lucid and highly understandable explanation of the basic theory and techniques of reflexology.

Hall, Nicola. *Reflexology: A Step-by-Step Guide*. Boston: Element Books, 1999. 58pp. $7.95.

A splendidly illustrated book featuring excellent photographs and diagrams that explain reflexology—a complementary therapy involving the treatment of various disorders by applying pressure to the feet or hands. Precise areas of the feet and hands relate to the particular parts of the body, and the whole body can treated via points on the feet and hands. Separate chapters illustrate how reflexology works, how the treatment is given, how to hold the foot and a step-by-step treatment guide working all the areas of the left and right feet. In each case, the foot is mapped to show the corresponding part of the body that is affected—the reflex area for the head and neck area, for example, are found in the areas of the toes in both feet. A simple and attractive presentation of the basic facts. Concise.

*Oxenford, Rosalind. *Reflexology*. The New Life Library. New York: Lorenz Books, 1997. 64pp. $9.95.

Pressure on points of the body affect other parts lying along the same line and zone within the body. Reflexology acts on parts of the body by stimulating the corresponding reflexes with compression techniques applied by the fingers. If places in the feet where there are congestion deposits can be worked with massage and compression, the corresponding body part will be stimulated and enabled to heal itself. Oxenford, a British teacher of reflexology, explains the zones of the feet and body, the benefits and effects of reflexology, warm-up massage, and reflexology techniques. Relaxation sequences are described for aiding restful sleep, relaxing the neck and shoulders, relieving backache and repetitive strain and reducing pain and stress. Oxenford provides foot and hand charts. A clear explanation of the basic principles and techniques of reflexology, enhanced by the use of splendid, full-color photographs. Good.

Reiki

Vennels, David F. *Reiki for Beginners: Mastering Natural Healing Techniques.* St. Paul, MN: Llewellyn Publications, 1999. 224pp. $12.95 (paper).

Vennels, a sufferer from CFS, describes his miraculous recovery following Reiki treatment from a Reiki master. Reiki, as Vennels explains, is a simple yet profound system of natural healing for body and mind developed by Mikao Usui in Japan in the nineteenth century. One does not have to be a Buddhist to practice Reiki, although Buddhism provides an explanation of what is experienced. Drawing upon much anecdotal evidence, Vennels (a British Reiki practitioner and teacher) offers a simple explanation of how Reiki works, its appropriate use, self-treatment and how to treat others, the Five Principles, Reiki meditation, and stories and accounts of a number of Reiki practitioners. A clear explanation of Reiki, but of very limited practical use.

T'ai Chi

Douglas, Bill. *The Complete Idiot's Guide to T'ai Chi and QiGong.* New York: Alpha Books, 1999. 354pp. $18.95 (paper).

T'ai Chi and QiGong are exercises that form integral parts of traditional Chinese medicine. Both are prescribed for the treatment of stress problems, illnesses, and injuries and can be used to used to heal the physical, mental, emotional, and spiritual body. The goal of T'ai Chi is to move through a series of choreographed movements like a slow martial arts routine proceeding very slowly and in a state of absolute relaxation. Douglas explains how classes are taught, T'ai Chi etiquette, how it works, warm-up exercises, and the art forms currently available. The main point made is that T'ai Chi is much more than a physical exercise in that it can heal every aspect of one's life relationships, and our world.

Touch Therapy

Ford, Clyde. *Compassionate Touch: The Body's Role in Emotional Healing and Recovery.* Berkeley, CA: North Atlantic Books, 1999. 260pp. $14.95 (paper).

Ford maintains that "the body is a road map for the journey of healing and recovery. It can tell us where we have been, where we are, where we need to go, and how best to get there." Moving beyond verbal therapy for psychological trauma and sexual abuse, Ford bypasses talk and "speaks directly to the body in a language it understands." Body therapists, such as chiropractors, massage therapists, and physical therapists do not have to become psychotherapists to help people with emotions expressed through the body. Mind-body healing techniques focus on the mind's relationship to the body and this necessarily involves the body's role in healing and recovery. Therapy done with body and emotions is called by Ford "somatosynthesis." The essential point made is that our body is a crucible for molding and shaping our psyche and that is possible to work with the physical truth of the body to resolve any related emotional truths.

Levine, Andrew S., and Valerie J. Levine. *The Bodywork and Massage Sourcebook.* Los Angeles: Lowell House, 1999. 327pp. $16.95 (paper).

This book opens with the statement that "human touch has the power to heal," and that bodywork and massage have all the power of touch to enhance physical and mental health. The Levines clearly describe massage (Swedish and other types), techniques for releasing points of stress (Shiatsu, reflexology), gentle touch (Trager approach), craniosacral therapy (Rosen method), integrative techniques (Rolfing, Hellerwork), Alexander technique (Feldenkrais), and healing with energy (Reiki, polarity therapy, and therapeutic touch). A highly useful appendix provides a chart listing the key features of the 19 modalities discussed in the book with respect to the degree of touch, clothing worn while receiving the modality, use of massage oils, and duration in minutes. An excellent compilation that brings together in one book basic information on a wide variety of techniques. Andrew Levine is a massage therapist; Valerie Levine is a psychologist.

Toxins and Detoxification

Bennett, Peter, Stephen Barrie, and Sarah Faye. *7-Day Detox Miracle: Restore Your Mind and Body's Natural Vitality with This Safe and Effective Life-Enhancing Program.*

Rocklin, CA: Prima Publishing, 1998. 302pp. $15.95 (paper).

Many chronic health problems are due to low-grade "poisoning" of the metabolism. Stress, toxins, antibiotics, food allergies, excessive use of alcohol, lack of fiber, and too much sugar can poison the body. Detoxification is a therapeutic biochemical, physiological, and nutritional way to reduce the harmful impact of foreign chemicals on the body's cells. The seven-day detoxification program outlined (the "Ecotox" program) employs a variety of techniques to pull toxins out of the body, filter the blood, rehabilitate the intestinal tract, and improve digestion. A typical seven-day home program involves a diet of rice, fruit, and vegetables; nutritional supplements, minerals, amino acids, and antioxidants; daily exercise; and aerobics. A complex prescription loaded with much detail and theoretical assumptions, but not very practical.

Gittleman, Ann Louise. *How to Stay Young and Healthy in Toxic World.* Los Angeles: Keats, 1999. 208pp. $16.95.

Gittleman warns that toxins are "all around us, hiding in the food we eat, the environment and even created by our body's metabolic processes." This results in a weakened immune system and premature aging. Oxidative stress, or free radicals, damage the cells and tissues and can destroy genetic coding. The most toxic underlying cause of free radical proliferation lies in sugar, parasites, heavy metals, and radiation. Gittleman describes each one of the four major toxic invaders and a detoxification program with instructions on how to detoxify the indoor air environment, water, light environment, and food. The detoxification diet program outlined consists of a four-week program specifically designed to flush toxins from the system by supporting liver function (the key detoxifying organ) through special foods and liver-supporting supplementation. The recommended eating plan eliminates all processed foods including white flour, white sugar, artificial sweeteners, margarine, as well as the whole grains from wheat, rye, oats and barley. A drastic solution to achieve a longer life.

Hull, Janet Starr. *Sweet Poison: How the World's Most Popular Artificial Sweetener Is Killing Us: My Story.* Far Hills, NJ: New Horizons Press, 1999. 300pp. $25.95.

The villain is Aspartame. Hull, a nutritionist and environmental scientist, exposes what she considers to be the lethal truth about Aspartame poisoning and the greed of individuals and corporations that put personal profit before public safety. Hull narrates her personal story of blinding headaches, weight gain, shedding hair, and the elevated heartbeat that led her to the hospital and a diagnosis of Graves' disease (thyrotoxicosis) with a recommended destruction of her thyroid with radioactive iodine. Rejecting the recommended treatment option and after searching through medical texts and journals, Hull concluded that her illness was due to an environmental overload of chemicals deposited in the thyroid. After eliminating Aspartame, Hull recovered from Graves' disease. Her book is a detailed summary of the efforts of the Aspartame Consumer Safety Network (founded in 1987) and a digest of the evidence for the toxicological effects of Aspartame. The basic message is "be vigilant to protect your health and do not be seduced by those processing 'sweet poison.'" Appendixes reprint testimony given at Congressional hearings in 1987. A highly readable book that makes an extravagant extrapolation from the author's personal experience to prove the toxicity of Asparatame.

Reuben, Carolyn. *Cleansing the Body, Mind and Spirit.* New York: Berkley Books, 1998. 291pp. $6.99 (paper).

Reuben provides a highly detailed handbook on what toxins such as formaldehyde, vinyl, toluene, dioxine, coal-tar compounds, fluorides, lead acitate, pesticides and herbicides, polychlorinated biphenyl, and so on, are doing to the human body. Evidence of toxic overload includes itching, skin eruptions, foul-smelling gas and feces, bad breath, joint pain, and fatigue. Two-thirds of the book is devoted to detox techniques in the form of cleansing fasts, purging, bowel cleansing, use of herbs as detoxifiers, colonic irrigation, and supplements that detox heavy metals (use of foods, chelation therapy, charcoal, and parasite removal). A separate chapter describes specific methods of detox such as the Hubbard Method, Max Gerson Protocol, and the Ann Wigmore Protocol. Reuben presents much descriptive information but does not state her experience or qualifications.

Vukovic, Laurel. *The 14-Day Herbal Cleansing.* Paramus, NJ: Prentice Hall, 1998. 300pp. $14.95 (paper).

Cleansing, Vukovic believes, is an essential key for health. The liver, kidneys, lungs, skin, lymphatic system, and intestinal tract are continuously working to purify the body. Vuckovic suggests techniques to support the body's natural processes of detoxification. Symptoms of toxicity include fatigue, bad breath, skin rashes, and headaches. A cleansing program to achieve detoxification includes the use of cleansing diets, purifying essential oils, antioxidants, yoga, breathing exercises, aromatherapy, massage, visualization, and meditation. The essential point made is that the natural methods of detoxification advocated are needed to support the body's innate healing abilities.

Traditional Chinese Medicine

Chmelik, Stefan. *Chinese Herbal Secrets: The Key to Total Health.* Garden City Park, NY: Avery, 1999. 192pp. $17.95.

This is a lavishly illustrated book with high-quality photographs and drawings that concisely and clearly explains the basic concepts unique to Chinese medicine—Qi, Yin-Yang, the Five Elements, the Eight Conditions, the Twelve Organs, and so on. Separate sections deal with how herbs can help a number of problems commonly encountered, properties of herbs, useful herbal formulas for particular conditions, and how to ensure good health. Chmelik, a British practitioner of Chinese medicine, succeeds in explaining the use of Chinese herbs for strengthening the Qi, nourishing the blood, aiding digestion, and calming the mind and spirit, but does not provide any practical guidelines for actual use. An intellectually stimulating book of minimal therapeutic value.

Cline, Kyle. *Chinese Massage for Infants and Children: Traditional Techniques for Alleviating Colic, Colds, Earaches, and Other Common Childhood Conditions.* Rochester, VT: Healing Arts Press, 1999. 145pp. $19.95 (paper).

Cline, a specialist in traditional Chinese medicine, describes a sophisticated pediatric massage system that has been used in China for over 1,000 years. His book is intended as an "easily accessible reference source for parents with varying degrees of interest, from those who want only a very simple approach to treating their children to those who want more background and depth." Therapeutic massage is capable of influencing a child's energetic flow in the same way that acupuncture works for adults and is useful for children from birth to approximately 12 years of age. Massage can be used for a large variety of conditions, both acute and chronic. Separate chapters deal with Chinese energetic principles, assessment, techniques, point locations, and massage plans. Appendixes describe massage mediums (water and oil preparations) and external Chinese remedies. A book that stretches the limits of self-help.

L'orange, Darlena. *Herbal Secrets of the Orient.* New York: Prentice Hall, 1998. 380pp. $14.95 (paper).

L'orange, who has degrees in acupuncture, herbology, and anthropology, introduces the reader to simple, basic Oriental health concepts and 108 healing herbs commonly used in traditional Oriental medicine. After describing how to prepare herbal pastes, tablets, extracts, syrups, and pills, L'orange devotes the major portion of her book to showing how more than 100 specific herbs can be successfully employed to heal a variety of ailments. One chapter lists ail-ments alphabetically with suggested remedies. Another chapter contains recipes to incorporate healing herbs and foods into daily life. The recommended treatment for rheumatoid arthritis, for example, is Yi-Jen-Tang or "Coix Combination" that comes down to us from the Tang Dynasty (618–906). Fascinating reading.

Lu, Henry. *Chinese Natural Cures: Traditional Methods for Remedies and Preventions.* New York: Black Dog & Leventhal, 1999. 528pp. $24.98.

Traditional Chinese medicine includes four distinct methods of treatment: herbology, acupuncture, manipulative therapy, and food cures. In addition, it encompasses the remedial exercise Qi-gong and Ta'i Chi. Section One explains the philosophy and methods of traditional Chinese medicine in terms of diagnosis, syndrome classifications, the eight grand methods of treatment, herbology, and traditional food remedies. Section Two lists symptoms and treatments of common complaints such as headache, diarrhea, and obesity. Section Three details food cures with reference to the five energies and five flavors of food. Lu, a specialist in traditional Chinese medicine and acupuncture, presents an excellent description of Chinese medicine but offers minimal guidance in terms of practical application.

Lu, Nan, with Ellen Schaplowsky. *Traditional Chinese Medicine: A Woman's Guide to Healing from Breast Cancer.* New York: Avon, 1999. 358pp. $14 (paper).

Nan Lu, the founding director of the Traditional Chinese Medicine World Foundation, explains the philosophy, history, and principal theories of traditional Chinese medicine (TCM) and how these relate to breast cancer. Lu offers a "Nine-Point Healing Guide" that includes learning the principles of TCM and how the mind, body, and spirit work as a unit, practicing Wu Ming meridian therapy for 20 minutes at least once a day, and continuously sending yourself the message that you are healthy and whole. While clearly describing how several billion people on this planet think about health and healing in a manner vastly different from that of Western society, Lu fails to present a coherent prescription for either prevention or treatment of breast cancer. Reflects alternative rather than complementary medicine.

Williams, Tom. *The Complete Illustrated Guide to Chinese Medicine: A Comprehensive System for Health and Fitness.* Boston, MA: Element Books, 1996. 255pp. $18.95 (paper).

This book is not intended to be a self-help or self-treatment manual but instead aims to demystify and provide comprehensive information about the concepts and principles of the Chinese system of medicine. The first part of the book covers the theories of Chinese medicine as developed from ancient traditions; the second part explains how a condition is diagnosed by a practitioner of Chinese medicine; while the third part of the book concerns treatment. Using high-quality color photographs and diagrams, Williams describes numerous treatment modalities such as acupuncture (what happens and what it feels like), moxibustion, cupping, acupuncture, Chinese herbalism, ginseng, elixirs, and Qigong. Lucid text, further enhanced by superb illustrations and photographs.

Witlocke, Bronwyn. *Chinese Medicine for Women: A Commonsense Approach*. Seattle, WA: Seal Press, 1999. 138pp. $12.95 (paper).

This is a book originally published in Australia in 1997. Witlocke, a Shiatsu therapist, herbalist, and acupuncturist, guides the reader through the main principles of traditional Chinese medicine. In simple terms, Witlocke explains Yin and Yang, Qi, the meridians as channels through which Qi flows, methods to facilitate the harmonious flow of Qi (acupuncture, cupping, moxibustion, Shiatsu, exercise, diet, and herbs), the five phases or elements, and what to expect at a consultation with a practitioner of traditional Chinese medicine. Part Two of the book illustrates how traditional Chinese medicine can be applied to particular conditions such as menstruation, infertility, migraine, common cold, obesity and depression. A clearly written and informative introduction to traditional Chinese medicine with a minimum use of Chinese terminology.

Urine Therapy

Peschek-Böhmer, Flora, and Gisela Schreiber. *Urine Therapy: Nature's Elixir for Good Health*. Translated from the German by Hans-Georg Bakker. Rochester, VT: Healing Arts Press, 1999. 152pp. $9.95 (paper).

Peschek-Böhmer, a German naturopathic healer, rejects the notion that urine is taboo and that "pee is yucky." Addressing the real skeptics, Peschek-Böhmer and Schreiber stress that urine is not full of germs, does not smell, contain viruses and bacteria, or taste bad. Uropoty (drinking of urine) offers enormous health benefits in strengthening the immune sytem and in treating ailments of the throat, chest, arms, back, genital area, legs, skin, and emotional disorders. While listing the benefits of urine in treating sinusitis, candidiasis, gout, and morning sickness, no supporting evidence is provided. There is no bibliography. The major thrust of the book is directed towards dispelling the widespread skepticism and revulsion of most people to the practice. An unusual, unconvincing book.

Yoga

Feuerstein, Georg, and Larry Payne. *Yoga for Dummies*. Foster City, CA: IDG Books Worldwide, 1999. 372pp. $19.99 (paper).

The authors, both yoga masters, intend that their book should "guide you slowly, step-by-step, into the treasure house of yoga." The focus of the book is on Hatha Yoga, which is the branch of yoga that works primarily within the body through postures, breathing exercises, and other similar techniques. Part One of the book tells what you need to know to get off to a good start; Part Two covers getting in shape; Part Three illustrates postures for health maintenance and restoration; Part Four is entitled "Creative Yoga" (designing your own yoga program); Part Five discusses yoga as a lifestyle; and Part Six lists 10 tips for a great yoga practice, 10 great places in the United States to discover yoga, and 10 good reasons to practice yoga. The text is enhanced by black and white photographs illustrating postures, and makes effective use of icons such as "Tip," "Beware," and "Jargon Alert" (a customary feature of the "Dummies" series). Comprehensive and understandable.

Francina, Suza. *The New Yoga for People Over 50: A Comprehensive Guide for Midlife and Older Beginners*. Deerfield Beach, FL: Health Communications, 1997. 286pp. $11.95 (paper).

Francina, a yoga teacher, explores yoga's special benefits for women during the menopausal years, stressing that yoga can strengthen the bones and help prevent osteoporosis and arthritis, and even prevent or reverse heart disease. The modified practices recommended focus on how beginners can adapt the practice of yoga to their special needs, including medical conditions such as cardiovascular disease, arthritis, osteoporosis, and hip surgery. The practice guidelines were tested on students who started practicing yoga after the age of 70, 80, and older. Francina advocates the use of props (ropes, chairs, straps, belts) that help elderly people to stretch, strengthen, relax, or improve body alignment. Gentle yoga especially designed for seniors illustrated by many black and white photographs.

Hirschi, Getrud. *Basic Yoga for Everybody: 84 Cards with Accompanying Handbook*. York Beach, ME: Samuel Weiser, 1998. 71pp. $29.95 (paper).

No more trying to turn pages of a book while standing on one hand! Instead, select the relevant, instructive cards and place them in front of you while you work each yoga position. A concise handbook explains how to mix, arrange, and combine yoga exercises in new ways. The cards are color-coded to show warm-up exercises (red), backbends (green), and so on. Each card shows on its front a silhouette of a posture and an affirmation—e.g., "with all my heart I wish for freedom and ease in my life," while the back of the card provides a smaller silhouette and the name of the posture together with its starting position, static and dynamic variations, and the physical-emotional effects of the work. The manual provides background for the cards and practical advice for using them, with instructions on yoga breathing and imagery exercising. Clever packaging in that the whole set (manual and cards) fits into the hard-bound slipcase provided.

APPENDIX 1

General Information about CAM and the NCCAM*

[June 2000]

This fact sheet provides general information about complementary and alternative medicine (CAM) and the National Center for Complementary and Alternative Medicine (NCCAM). It is designed to give you a quick overview of NCCAM efforts to advance CAM research. When possible, this fact sheet includes the names and telephone numbers of resources that can give you more information.

WHAT IS CAM?

CAM covers a broad range of healing philosophies (schools of thought), approaches, and therapies that mainstream Western (conventional) medicine does not commonly use, accept, study, understand, or make available. A few of the many CAM practices include the use of acupuncture, herbs, homeopathy, therapeutic massage, and traditional oriental medicine to promote wellbeing or treat health conditions.

People use CAM treatments and therapies in a variety of ways. Therapies may be used alone, as an alternative to conventional therapies, or in addition to conventional, mainstream therapies, in what is referred to as a complementary or an integrative approach.

Many CAM therapies are called holistic, which generally means they consider the whole person, including physical, mental, emotional, and spiritual aspects.

CAM'S GROWING POPULARITY IN THE UNITED STATES

A published survey shows that the number of Americans using an alternative therapy rose from about 33 percent in 1990 to more than 42 percent in 1997.[1] People in this study reported using the following therapies most often: herbal medicine, massage, megavitamins, self-help groups, folk remedies, energy healing, and homeopathy. In addition, Americans spent more than $27 billion on these therapies in 1997, exceeding out-of-pocket spending for all U.S. hospitalizations.

A survey published in 1994 reveals that more than 60 percent of doctors from a wide range of specialties recommended alternative therapies to their patients at least once. In addition, 47 percent of the doctors in this study reported using alternative therapies themselves.[2]

Indeed, 75 out of 117 U.S. medical schools offered elective courses in CAM or included CAM topics in required courses, according to an article published in 1998.[3]

*Reprinted from the National Center for Complementary and Alternative Medicine, NCCAM Clearinghouse Web site (http://http://nccam.nih.gov/nccam/an/general); Publication M-42

Another survey found that people used CAM not only because they were dissatisfied with conventional medicine, but because these health care alternatives mirrored their own values, beliefs, and philosophical orientations toward health and life.[4]

Despite the broad use of alternative therapies, health care professionals and the public need more substantial scientific information to demonstrate convincingly whether CAM practices lead to positive clinical outcomes; improve quality of life; and are effective, safe, and/or beneficial. This is where the NCCAM comes into the picture.

WHAT IS THE NCCAM?

In 1998, the Congress established the NCCAM at the National Institutes of Health (NIH) to stimulate, develop, and support research on CAM for the benefit of the public. The NCCAM is an advocate for quality science, rigorous and relevant research, and open and objective inquiry into which CAM practices work, which do not, and why. Its overriding mission is to give the American public reliable information about the safety and effectiveness of CAM practices.

The NCCAM is 1 of more than 20 Institutes and Centers (ICs) composing the NIH. The NIH is one of eight health agencies within the Public Health Service of the U.S. Department of Health and Human Services (DHHS). The NIH is among the world's foremost biomedical research institutions and is the Federal Government's focal point for biomedical research in the United States.

NCCAM'S PURPOSE AND MISSION

The NCCAM conducts and supports basic and applied (clinical) research and research training on CAM. Basic research generally refers to investigations, such as test-tube studies, that take place under controlled conditions in scientific laboratories. Clinical research refers to medical studies of new treatments in people that take place in health care settings, such as hospitals or medical clinics. Scientific inquiry into CAM is a relatively new area of research.

The NCCAM provides information about CAM to health care providers and the public. The Center also develops other programs to further the investigation and application of CAM treatments that show promise.

The NCCAM focuses on the following efforts:
- Evaluating the safety and efficacy of widely used natural products, such as herbal remedies and nutritional and food supplements (e.g., megadoses of vitamins);
- Supporting pharmacological studies to determine the potential interactive effects of CAM products with standard treatment medications; and
- Evaluating CAM practices, such as acupuncture and chiropractic.

The director of the NCCAM is appointed by the Secretary of the DHHS and reports to the director of the NIH. In 1999, Stephen E. Straus, M.D., an internationally recognized expert in clinical research, was named the director of the NCCAM.

Since Fiscal Year (FY) 1993, NCCAM's budget has steadily risen from $2 million to $68.7 million in FY 2000. This funding increase reflects the public's growing need for CAM information that is based on rigorous scientific research.

The Center is located on the NIH campus in Bethesda, Maryland.

NCCAM'S OBJECTIVES

The NCCAM works toward the following goals, grouped under three main headings:

Research
- Collaborate with other NIH ICs and other Federal agencies to advance CAM scientific study.
- Identify and investigate promising, understudied areas.
- Establish a global network for CAM research.

Research Training
- Implement a comprehensive research training plan.
- Provide research training and clinical fellowships.
- Educate CAM scientists about biomedical research methods.
- Educate conventional researchers about the nature and principles of CAM.

Communications

- Establish effective partnerships with CAM researchers, health professionals, and the public.
- Collaborate on CAM information dissemination with other NIH ICs and other Federal agencies.
- Distribute scientifically based information about CAM research, practices, and findings to health care providers and consumers.

NCCAM'S HISTORY AND RELATED LEGISLATION

The NCCAM was initiated through a congressional mandate under the FY 1999 Omnibus appropriations bill signed by President Bill Clinton on October 21, 1998. Before that time, the NCCAM was the Office of Alternative Medicine (OAM). The OAM, established in 1992 within the NIH Office of the Director, facilitated and coordinated the evaluation of alternative medical treatment modalities through research projects and other initiatives with NIH's ICs.

At that time, OAM's primary role was to emphasize the rigorous scientific evaluation of CAM treatments, develop a solid infrastructure to coordinate and conduct research at the NIH, and establish a clearinghouse to provide information to the public.

OAM's expansion into a Center gives the NCCAM greater ability to initiate and fund additional research projects and to provide more information to the public at a time when a growing number of people are interested in CAM therapies and systems of practice.

The 1999 Omnibus legislation also established a White House Commission on Complementary and Alternative Medicine Policy. This Commission will study issues regarding research; training and certification of CAM practitioners; insurance coverage; and other alternative medicine issues. The DHHS will make appointments to and oversee the Commission.

NCCAM'S PROGRAM ADVISORY COUNCIL

The National Institutes of Health Revitalization Act of 1993 provided for the establishment of a Program Advisory Council to advise the OAM director. The Council officially was formed in the summer of 1994, and its first meeting was held in September of that year.

The Council, now called the National Advisory Council on Complementary and Alternative Medicine (NACCAM), meets 3 times a year and currently has 17 members. According to the 1999 Omnibus legislation, at least half of the members are practitioners licensed in one or more of the main subsystems of CAM with which the NCCAM is concerned, and at least three members are consumer representatives. Council members are appointed by the Secretary of the DHHS for overlapping terms up to 4 years.

NCCAM PROGRAMS

Underlying NCCAM's programs is the congressional mandate to study and disseminate information about the safety and effectiveness of CAM therapies and facilitate the integration of safe and effective treatments into an interdisciplinary health care delivery system.

To accomplish such a broad mandate, NCCAM programs support rigorous scientific review, tapping the expertise of scientists from other NIH ICs and other Federal agencies. NCCAM's programs incorporate input from the NACCAM.

Below, we have organized the description of NCCAM's programs into the following five functional areas: extramural research, intramural research training, scientific databases, public information clearinghouse, and liaison with CAM stakeholders.

1. Extramural Research (Grants)

The Extramural Research Program helps design, develop, review, fund, and implement specific CAM research projects and training that occur outside the NIH, in addition to coordinating grants with other NIH ICs.

The goals of this program are to increase the number of NCCAM-supported grants, increase co-funding of the CAM-related activities of other NIH ICs, streamline the management of extramural grants and IC cooperative activities, and maintain information on the status and results of NCCAM-supported research.

The program awards National Research Service Award Institutional Training Grants (T32) to eligible institutions to develop or enhance research training opportunities for individuals, selected by the institution, who are training for careers in specified areas of biomedical and behavioral research. The program supports CAM research-related training of pre-doctoral and post-doctoral students.

A great challenge of the program is to educate potential researchers in CAM to follow methodological procedures that have been long established in the biomedical research communities.

At the same time, conventional researchers interested in CAM need information about the nature, principles, and practices of CAM systems and modalities and their linkage to NCCAM research priorities. In this way, scientific research standards can be applied to CAM research to provide valid and reliable results.

For information about specific products and services of the Extramural Research Program, visit NCCAM's Web site http://nccam.nih.gov/nccam/an/nccamorg/extramural/index.html.

For information about specific extramural research projects, call the NCCAM Clearinghouse at 301-589-5367, or toll-free at 1-888-644-6226.

CAM Research Centers

The NCCAM funds several CAM Research Centers outside the NIH. For up-to-date contact information, specialty areas, and brief descriptions of the Centers, visit NCCAM's Web site http://nccam.nih.gov/nccam/fi/research/centers.html, or call the NCCAM Clearinghouse at 301-589-5367, or toll-free at 1-888-644-6226.

2. Intramural Research Training

The Intramural Research Program supports the work of CAM researchers at scientific laboratories within the NIH. This program provides a foundation for NIH scientists to conduct basic and clinical research in CAM.

The program funds individual post-doctoral fellowships. These fellowships are designed to train a group of investigators who have the skills needed to conduct systematic studies of the safety, efficacy, cost-effectiveness, or mechanisms of action of unconventional methods for treating major diseases and promoting well-being.

3. Scientific Databases

The Scientific Databases Program provides an infrastructure for identifying, organizing, and appraising the scientific literature on CAM practices. The goal is to establish comprehensive, electronic, bibliographic databases of this literature. The literature in these databases is designed to serve as an ongoing source of CAM information for scientists, researchers, practitioners, and the public.

The program also evaluates the scientific literature on CAM practices in conjunction with DHHS's Agency for Healthcare Research and Quality (AHRQ), provides research-based information about CAM practices for dissemination to health professionals and the public, and continues development of a classification system specific for CAM practices. Additionally, the program enhances existing indexing and retrieval capabilities of bibliographic databases for information about CAM practices.

Through the use of rigorous techniques to appraise CAM scientific literature, this program is implementing a process with the AHRQ for developing systematic reviews and meta-analyses of the scientific literature. A systematic review is a report on the science in a particular area of health care. In a meta-analysis, a number of research papers on a specific topic are collected and evaluated scientifically.

To date, this program includes the following two bibliographic databases of CAM information evaluated and selected by the NCCAM for dissemination to the public via the Internet:

- CAM Citation Index http://nccam.nih.gov/nccam/resources/cam-ci
- NCCAM's CAM Citation Index provides bibliographic citations of more than 180,000 journal articles describing CAM research studies and their results. This database includes biomedical research information that also is found in the National Library of Medicine's MEDLINE database. While MEDLINE covers a wide range of biomedical topics, the CAM Citation Index focuses specifically on topics of interest to CAM stakeholders.
- AM Database of CHID http://chid.nih.gov
- Through its Public Information Clearinghouse, the NCCAM maintains the Complementary and Alternative Medicine (AM) Database of the Combined Health Information Database (CHID). The AM Database contains bibliographic summaries of books, journal articles, research reports, audiovisuals, and other materials about CAM. As a single source of information from the Federal Government about a wide range of health topics, CHID is a convenient reference tool for health professionals, patients, and the public.

4. Public Information Clearinghouse

The NCCAM Clearinghouse, established in 1996, is the public's point of contact and access to information about

CAM and NCCAM's programs, conferences, and research activities. Services include a toll-free information line (1-888-644-6226), publications, referrals to other information resources, and the AM Database of CHID. The Clearinghouse is located in Maryland near the NIH campus.

The Clearinghouse collects and disseminates information to the public, media, and health care professionals to promote awareness and education about CAM research and the NCCAM. The Clearinghouse disseminates CAM information that focuses on the scientific research funded, conducted, or collected by the NCCAM, other NIH ICs, and their grantees. The Clearinghouse does not provide medical referrals, medical advice, or recommendations for specific CAM therapies.

Access to the NCCAM Clearinghouse

NCCAM Clearinghouse information specialists respond in English and Spanish to inquiries for information by calling 301-589-5367, or toll-free telephone (1-888-644-6226), TTY/TDY for the hearing impaired (1-888-644-6226), fax (301-495-4957), e-mail (nccam-info@nccam.nih.gov), and postal mail (NCCAM Clearinghouse, P.O. Box 8218, Silver Spring, MD 20907-8218). They answer calls Monday through Friday, from 8:30 a.m. to 5:00 p.m., Eastern time.

After regular business hours, callers either may leave their names and telephone numbers or request fact sheets and other information through the Clearinghouse's Fax-On-Demand system, available through the toll-free number (1-888-644-6226).

Disclaimer Regarding Medical Information and Advice

The NCCAM is not a referral agency for alternative medical treatments or individual practitioners. Therefore, the NCCAM Clearinghouse does not provide medical advice to patients, and it does not provide referrals to alternative health care practitioners.

NCCAM Clearinghouse information specialists are not health care professionals. The information they provide cannot substitute for the medical expertise and advice of a doctor. The NCCAM encourages all patients to talk with their primary health care practitioner about the advantages and risks of CAM treatments.

NCCAM's Customer Service Commitment

The NCCAM Clearinghouse processes requests for general information within 2 business days upon receipt of the requests.

NCCAM Clearinghouse staff members strive to give you quality service. Constructive feedback is welcomed. Please mail comments in writing to the NCCAM Clearinghouse Project Director at the NCCAM Clearinghouse, P.O. Box 8218, Silver Spring, MD 20907-8218.

For more information about the NCCAM Clearinghouse, call the NCCAM Clearinghouse at 301-589-5367, or toll-free at 1-888-644-6226 and ask for a copy of the Clearinghouse's brochure, *Want Information About Alternative Medicine?*

NCCAM Clearinghouse Products

In addition to maintaining the AM Database of CHID, the NCCAM Clearinghouse produces fact sheets, a newsletter, and other publications that provide information about CAM research supported by the NCCAM and other ICs of the NIH. The information is free of charge. For a list of our publications, call the NCCAM Clearinghouse at 301-589-5367, or toll-free at 1-888-644-6226, and ask for a copy of our publications order form.

The Clearinghouse produces NCCAM's newsletter that features CAM updates, NIH research news, and information from the NCCAM. The newsletter is available to the public through the NCCAM Clearinghouse or on NCCAM's Web site http://nccam.nih.gov/nccam/ne/newsletter/index.html.

NCCAM's Media Relations

NCCAM's Media Relations area facilitates accurate coverage of relevant stories with the news media, and provides information about the NCCAM and its current activities to mass media audiences.

5. Liaison with CAM Stakeholders

The International and Professional Liaison Program supports and facilitates cooperative efforts in research and education in CAM approaches worldwide and with professional organizations across the United States. In November 1996, the NCCAM, then the OAM, was designated a World Health Organization Collaborating Center in Traditional Medicine. The 4-year designation includes the NCCAM as part of an international network of 19 established institutions, located in national governments or universities worldwide, that focus on traditional medicine and CAM.

Other NCCAM Activities

A major function of the NCCAM is to facilitate the evaluation of various alternative treatment modalities through ICs within the NIH. This cooperation is based on well-established expertise and encourages collaboration on projects of mutual interest. The NCCAM has identified a network of coordinators at the NIH to assist with issues related to researching alternative medical practices and treatments. In addition, the NCCAM facilitates CAM data review and research with other agencies of the Federal Government.

NCCAM's Web Site

The NCCAM maintains a Web site http://nccam.nih.gov to give you CAM information. Topics on NCCAM's Web site include: the NCCAM; frequently asked questions; Clearinghouse publications; CAM databases; NCCAM research; clinical trial opportunities; research policies, applications, and guidelines; NCCAM's newsletter; press releases; and minutes of NCCAM-sponsored meetings.

Town Meetings

The NCCAM plans to convene a series of regional town meetings for CAM consumers, researchers, practitioners, and the public. The first town meeting, on March 15, 2000, at Harvard University in Boston, Massachusetts, was sponsored in collaboration with the Center for Alternative Medicine Research, Beth Israel Deaconess Medical Center.

The town meetings offer an opportunity for input from professionals, patients, advocacy groups, and local residents who have an interest in CAM, the NCCAM, or other ICs of the NIH.

CAM Conferences and Education

The NCCAM collaborates with other ICs of the NIH to sponsor CAM-related conferences and educational programs. Separate topics covered to date include acupuncture, behavioral treatments, chronic pain, health insurance issues, liver disease, and nursing education.

Cancer Advisory Panel for CAM Research

The Cancer Advisory Panel for Complementary and Alternative Medicine (CAPCAM) is a 15-member panel created in 1998 that includes patient advocates, researchers, and administrators from conventional biomedical and CAM communities. The CAPCAM facilitates the joint review of data from cancer research projects through the NCCAM and National Cancer Institute, another NIH IC.

CAPCAM's mission is to review and assess clinical data submitted by CAM cancer researchers and to advise the NCCAM on the next research steps.

The CAPCAM held its first meeting on July 8-9, 1999, in Bethesda, Maryland. The agenda enabled panel members to explore the scope of their advisory role and to hear presentations of two Best Case Series. The term "Best Case Series" refers to precise clinical information—collected while patients undergo treatment—that indicates some benefit to the patients being studied.

The second CAPCAM meeting was held on December 13, 1999, in Bethesda, Maryland. Speakers from within the NCCAM and NIH discussed the Best Case program for analyzing data from CAM cancer medicine practitioners. Guest speakers discussed the benefits of psychosocial treatment (e.g., group therapy) to patients with certain types of cancer and the current efforts to study the use of CAM as a complement to standard radiation oncology procedures.

Trans-Agency CAM Coordinating Committee

NCCAM's Trans-Agency CAM Coordinating Committee is a group of representatives of several other Federal agencies and departments. The Committee is designed to help the NCCAM coordinate scientific input for CAM research and explore research partnerships.

FOR MORE INFORMATION

Please send requests for information about complementary or alternative medicine to:

NCCAM Clearinghouse
P.O. Box 8218
Silver Spring, MD 20907-8218
301-589-5367 (Telephone)
1-888-644-6226 (Toll-Free, TTY/TDY, and Fax-On-Demand)
1-301-495-4957 (Fax)
nccam-info@nccam.nih.gov (E-Mail)
http://nccam.nih.gov (NCCAM Web Site)

REFERENCES

1. Eisenberg, D.M., Davis, R.B., Ettner, S.L., Appel, S., Wilkey, S., Van Rompay, M., Kessler, R.C. "Trends in Alternative Medicine Use in the United States, 1990-1997: Results of a Follow-Up National Survey." *Journal of the American Medical Association.* November 11, 1998. 280(18):1569-75.

2. Borkan, J., Neher, J.O., Anson, O., Smoker, B. "Referrals for Alternative Therapies." *Journal of Family Practice.* 1994. 39(6):545-50.

3. Wetzel, M.S., Eisenberg, D.M., Kaptchuk, T.J. "Courses Involving Complementary and Alternative Medicine at U.S. Medical Schools." *Journal of the American Medical Association.* September 2, 1998. 280(9):784-7.

4. Astin, J.A. "Why Patients Use Alternative Medicine: Results of a National Study." *Journal of the American Medical Association.* May 20, 1998. 279(19):1548-53.

APPENDIX 2

Major Domains of Complementary and Alternative Medical Practices*
[September 2000]

Complementary and alternative healthcare and medical practices (CAM) are those healthcare and medical practices that are not currently an integral part of conventional medicine[1]. The list of practices that are considered CAM changes continually as CAM practices and therapies that are proven safe and effective become accepted as "mainstream" healthcare practices. Today, CAM practices may be grouped within five major domains:[2] (1) alternative medical systems, (2) mind-body interventions, (3) biologically-based treatments, (4) manipulative and body-based methods, and (5) energy therapies. The individual systems and treatments comprising these categories are too numerous to list in this document. Thus, only limited examples are provided within each.

I. ALTERNATIVE MEDICAL SYSTEMS

Alternative medical systems involve complete systems of theory and practice that have evolved independent of and often prior to the conventional biomedical approach. Many are traditional systems of medicine that are practiced by individual cultures throughout the world, including a number of venerable Asian approaches.

Traditional oriental medicine emphasizes the proper balance or disturbances of qi (pronounced chi), or vital energy, in health and disease, respectively. Traditional oriental medicine consists of a group of techniques and methods, including acupuncture, herbal medicine, oriental massage, and qi gong (a form of energy therapy described more fully below). Acupuncture involves stimulating specific anatomic points in the body for therapeutic purposes, usually by puncturing the skin with a needle.

Ayurveda is India's traditional system of medicine. Ayurvedic medicine (meaning "science of life") is a comprehensive system of medicine that places equal emphasis on body, mind, and spirit, and strives to restore the innate harmony of the individual. Some of the primary Ayurvedic treatments include diet, exercise, meditation, herbs, massage, exposure to sunlight, and controlled breathing.

Other traditional medical systems have been developed by Native American, Aboriginal, African, Middle-Eastern, Tibetan, Central and South American cultures.

Homeopathy and naturopathy are also examples of complete alternative medical systems. Homeopathy is an unconventional Western system that is based on the principle that "like cures like," i.e., that the same sub-

---

*Reprinted from the National Center for Complementary and Alternative Medicine, NCCAM Clearinghouse Web site (http://http://nccam.nih.gov/nccam/fcp/classify/)

stance that in large doses produces the symptoms of an illness, in very minute doses cures it. Homeopathic physicians believe that the more dilute the remedy, the greater its potency. Therefore, homeopaths use small doses of specially prepared plant extracts and minerals to stimulate the body's defense mechanisms and healing processes in order to treat illness.

Naturopathy views disease as a manifestation of alterations in the processes by which the body naturally heals itself and emphasizes health restoration rather than disease treatment. Naturopathic physicians employ an array of healing practices, including diet and clinical nutrition; homeopathy; acupuncture; herbal medicine; hydrotherapy (the use of water in a range of temperatures and methods of applications); spinal and soft-tissue manipulation; physical therapies involving electric currents, ultrasound, and light therapy; therapeutic counseling; and pharmacology.

II. MIND-BODY INTERVENTIONS

Mind-body interventions employ a variety of techniques designed to facilitate the mind's capacity to affect bodily function and symptoms. Only a subset of mind-body interventions are considered CAM. Many that have a well-documented theoretical basis, for example, patient education and cognitive-behavioral approaches are now considered "mainstream." On the other hand, meditation, certain uses of hypnosis, dance, music, and art therapy, and prayer and mental healing are categorized as complementary and alternative.

III. BIOLOGICAL-BASED THERAPIES

This category of CAM includes natural and biologically-based practices, interventions, and products, many of which overlap with conventional medicine's use of dietary supplements. Included are herbal, special dietary, orthomolecular, and individual biological therapies.

Herbal therapies employ individual or mixtures of herbs for therapeutic value. An herb is a plant or plant part that produces and contains chemical substances that act upon the body. Special diet therapies, such as those proposed by Drs. Atkins, Ornish, Pritikin, and Weil, are believed to prevent and or control illness as well as promote health. Orthomolecular therapies aim to treat disease with varying concentrations of chemi-

cals, such as, magnesium, melatonin, and mega-doses of vitamins. Biological therapies include, for example, the use of laetrile and shark cartilage to treat cancer and bee pollen to treat autoimmune and inflammatory diseases.

IV. MANIPULATIVE AND BODY-BASED METHODS

This category includes methods that are based on manipulation and/or movement of the body. For example, chiropractors focus on the relationship between structure (primarily the spine) and function, and how that relationship affects the preservation and restoration of health, using manipulative therapy as an integral treatment tool. Some osteopaths, who place particular emphasis on the musculoskeletal system, believing that all of the body's systems work together and that disturbances in one system may have an impact upon function elsewhere in the body, practice osteopathic manipulation. Massage therapists manipulate the soft tissues of the body to normalize those tissues.

V. ENERGY THERAPIES

Energy therapies focus either on energy fields originating within the body (biofields) or those from other sources (electromagnetic fields).

Biofield therapies are intended to affect the energy fields, whose existence is not yet experimentally proven, that surround and penetrate the human body. Some forms of energy therapy manipulate biofields by applying pressure and/or manipulating the body by placing the hands in, or through, these fields. Examples include Qi gong, Reiki and Therapeutic Touch. Qi gong is a component of traditional oriental medicine that combines movement, meditation, and regulation of breathing to enhance the flow of vital energy (qi) in the body, to improve blood circulation, and to enhance immune function. Reiki, the Japanese word representing Universal Life Energy, is based on the belief that by channeling spiritual energy through the practitioner the spirit is healed, and it in turn heals the physical body. Therapeutic Touch is derived from the ancient technique of "laying-on of hands" and is based on the premise that it is the healing force of the therapist that affects the patient's recovery and that healing is promoted when the body's energies are in balance. By passing their hands over the patient, these healers identify energy imbalances.

Bioelectromagnetic-based therapies involve the unconventional use of electromagnetic fields, such as pulsed fields, magnetic fields, or alternating current or direct current fields, to, for example, treat asthma or cancer, or manage pain and migraine headaches.

NOTES

[1] The term conventional medicine refers to medicine as practiced by holders of M.D. (medical doctor) or D.O. (doctor of osteopathy) degrees, some of whom may also practice complementary and alternative medicine. Other terms for conventional medicine are allopathy, Western, regular, and mainstream medicine, and biomedicine.

[2] These are the categories within which NCCAM has chosen to group the numerous CAM practices; others employ different, broad groupings.

APPENDIX 3

Frequently Asked Questions (about CAM)*
[March 2000]

WHAT IS COMPLEMENTARY AND ALTERNATIVE MEDICINE?

Complementary and alternative medicine (CAM) covers a broad range of healing philosophies, approaches, and therapies. Generally , it is defined as those treatments and healthcare practices not taught widely in medical schools, not generally used in hospitals, and not usually reimbursed by medical insurance companies.

Many therapies are termed "holistic," which generally means that the healthcare practitioner considers the whole person, including physical, mental, emotional, and spiritual aspects. Many therapies are also known as "preventive," which means that the practitioner educates and treats the person to prevent health problems from arising, rather than treating symptoms after problems have occurred.

People use these treatments and therapies in a variety of ways. Therapies are used alone (often referred to as alternative), in combination with other alternative therapies, or in addition to conventional therapies (sometimes referred to as complementary).

Some approaches are consistent with physiological principles of Western medicine, while others constitute healing systems with a different origin. While some therapies are far outside the realm of accepted Western medical theory and practice, others are becoming established in mainstream medicine.

HOW CAN I FIND MORE INFORMATION ABOUT COMPLEMENTARY AND ALTERNATIVE MEDICAL PRACTICES?

Ask your healthcare provider about complementary and alternative medical treatments and practices in general, and about those particular practices used for your specific health problems.

Increasingly, healthcare providers are becoming familiar with alternative treatments or are able to refer you to someone who is. For scientific information about the safety and effectiveness of a particular treatment, ask your healthcare provider to obtain valid information for you.

If your healthcare provider cannot provide information, medical libraries, public libraries, and popular bookstores are good places to find information about particular complementary and alternative medical practices.

Other resources for information are the 25 Institutes and Centers (ICs) at the NIH. For information on a wide range of specific diseases or medical conditions, call (301) 496-4000 and ask the operator to direct you to the appropriate NIH office.

---

*Reprinted from the National Center for Complementary and Alternative Medicine, NCCAM Clearinghouse Web site (http://http://nccam.nih.gov/nccam/fcp/faq/index.html)

Also, you may want to ask practitioners of complementary and alternative healthcare about their practices. Many practitioners belong to a growing number of professional associations, educational organizations, and research institutions that provide information about complementary and alternative medical practices. Many organizations are developing Internet Web sites. Most internet browser programs will have a mechanism for searching the World Wide Web by keyword or concept.

Remember that these organizations may advocate a specific therapy or treatment and may be unable to provide complete and objective health information.

If you have access to a computer with an Internet connection, you may be able to search medical libraries and databases for specific conditions and alternative medical treatments. The NCCAM's online database, the Complementary and Alternative Medicine (CAM) Citation Index (CCI), is comprised of approximately 180,000 bibliographic records describing much of the CAM research that has been published over the last 35 years. The CCI's user-friendly, menu-driven interface allows for searches by various diseases or conditions, alternative medicine techniques or systems, and types of literature.

You may also try accessing and searching MEDLINE, one of the many computer databases available at the National Library of Medicine. Also, you may want to contact the NCCAM Clearinghouse to obtain the fact sheet, "Alternative Medicine Research Using MEDLINE."

HOW CAN I FIND A PRACTITIONER IN MY AREA?

To find a qualified complementary and alternative medical healthcare practitioner, you may want to contact medical regulatory and licensing agencies in your state. These agencies may be able to provide information about a specific practitioner's credentials and background. Many states license practitioners who provide alternative therapies such as acupuncture, chiropractic services, naturopathy, herbal medicine, homeopathy, and massage therapy.

You may also locate practitioners by asking your healthcare provider, or by contacting a professional association or organization. These organizations can provide names of local practitioners, and provide information about how to determine the quality of a specific

practitioner's services. Contact the NCCAM Clearinghouse to obtain the fact sheet, "Considering Complementary and Alternative Therapies," which provides helpful hints and questions to consider when choosing an alternative healthcare practitioner.

Also, you may find complementary and alternative healthcare practitioners by asking people you trust, like friends and family members, who may have experience with practitioners of complementary and alternative medicine.

CAN I RECEIVE AN ALTERNATIVE TREATMENT AT THE NATIONAL CENTER FOR COMPLEMENTARY AND ALTERNATIVE MEDICINE (NCCAM)?

The NCCAM is not a treatment facility and cannot answer specific medical questions. The NCCAM cannot make referrals to individual practitioners or recommend particular therapies for patients.

WILL MY EXPERIENCE HELP IN THE EVALUATION OF COMPLEMENTARY AND ALTERNATIVE MEDICAL THERAPIES?

Many people write to the NCCAM with their own testimony about a successful treatment or a particular healer or healthcare practitioner. To have this information reviewed, people may ask their practitioners whether he/she is collecting information on the success of their treatments. A practitioner can collect and organize the information and present it to the NCCAM once there is sufficient data to make a case for the effectiveness of a particular treatment.

WILL THE NCCAM EVALUATE MY OWN INVENTION OR TREATMENT?

Many people contact the NCCAM with ideas for alternative medical cures. To have a method or cure tested, one must formulate a research protocol. This entails collaborating with individuals who have expertise in research and evaluation, if one does not possess this expertise.

The NCCAM supports rigorous research into a range of alternative medical treatments either by awarding grants or by setting up studies. For further information, please contact the NCCAM Clearinghouse to obtain the "Research Information Package."

CAN COMPLEMENTARY AND ALTERNATIVE MEDICINE BE INVESTIGATED USING THE SAME METHODS USED IN CONVENTIONAL MEDICINE?

People sometimes ask whether the NCCAM uses the same standard of science as conventional medicine. Complementary and alternative medicine needs to be investigated using the same scientific methods used in conventional medicine. The NCCAM encourages valid information about complementary and alternative medicine, applying at least as rigorous, and, in some cases, even more rigorous research methods than the current standard in conventional medicine. This is because the research often involves novel concepts and claims, and uses complex systems of practice that need systematic, explicit, and comprehensive knowledge and skills to investigate.

Appendix 4

Considering CAM?*
[March 2000]

APPROACHING COMPLEMENTARY AND ALTERNATIVE THERAPIES

The decision to use complementary and alternative treatments is an important one. The following are topics to consider before selecting an alternative therapy: the safety and effectiveness of the therapy or treatment, the expertise and qualifications of the healthcare practitioner, and the quality of the service delivery. These topics should be considered when selecting any practitioner or therapy.

ASSESS THE SAFETY AND EFFECTIVENESS OF THE THERAPY

Generally, safety means that the benefits outweigh the risks of a treatment or therapy. A safe product or practice is one that does no harm when used under defined conditions and as intended.

Effectiveness is the likelihood of benefit from a practice, treatment, or technology applied under typical conditions by the average practitioner for the typical patient.

Many people find that specific information about an alternative and complementary therapy's safety and effectiveness may be less readily available than information about conventional medical treatments. Research on these therapies is ongoing, and continues to grow.

You may want to ask a healthcare practitioner, whether a physician or a practitioner of complementary and alternative healthcare, about the safety and effectiveness of the therapy or treatment he or she uses. Tell the practitioner about any alternative or conventional treatments or therapies you may already be receiving, as this information may be used to consider the safety and effectiveness of the entire treatment plan.

The practitioner may have literature with information about the safety and effectiveness of the therapy. Credible information may be found in scientific research literature obtained through public libraries, university libraries, medical libraries, online computer services, the NCCAM Complementary and Alternative Medicine Citation Index (CCI) and the U.S. National Library of Medicine (NLM) at the National Institutes of Health (NIH).

The NCCAM CCI is comprised of approximately 180,000 bibliographic records describing much of the CAM research that has been published over the last 35 years. The CCI's user-friendly, menu-driven interface allows for searches by various diseases or conditions, alternative medicine techniques or systems, and types of literature.

*Reprinted from the National Center for Complementary and Alternative Medicine, NCCAM Clearinghouse Web site (http://http://nccam.nih.gov/nccam/fcp/faq/considercam.html)

For information about researching alternative medical therapies using the NLM, please contact the National Center for Complementary and Alternative Medicine (NCCAM) Clearinghouse and request the fact sheet, "Alternative Medicine Research Using MEDLINE."

For general, nonscientific information, thousands of articles on health issues and complementary and alternative medicine are published in books, journals, and magazines every year. Articles that appear in popular magazines and journals may be located by using the Reader's Guide to Periodical Literature available in most libraries. For articles published in more than 3,000 health science journals, consult the Index Medicus, found in medical and university libraries and some public libraries.

Be an informed health consumer and continue gathering information even after a practitioner has been selected. Ask the practitioner about specific new research that may support or not support the safety and effectiveness of the treatment or therapy. Ask about the advantages and disadvantages, risks, side effects, expected results, and length of treatment that you can expect.

Speak with people who have undergone the treatment, preferably both those who were treated recently and those treated in the past. Optimally, find people with the same health condition that you have and who have received the treatment.

Remember that patient testimonials used alone do not adequately assess the safety and effectiveness of an alternative therapy, and should not be the exclusive criterion for selecting a therapy. Controlled scientific trials usually provide the best information about a therapy's effectiveness and should be sought whenever possible.

EXAMINE THE PRACTITIONER'S EXPERTISE

Health consumers may want to take a close look into the background, qualifications, and competence of any potential healthcare practitioner, whether a physician or a practitioner of alternative and complementary healthcare.

First, contact a state or local regulatory agency with authority over practitioners who practice the therapy or treatment you seek. The practice of complementary and alternative medicine usually is not as regulated as the practice of conventional medicine. Licensing, accreditation, and regulatory laws, however, are increasingly being implemented.

Local and state medical boards, other health regulatory boards or agencies, and consumer affairs departments provide information about a specific practitioner's license, education, and accreditation, and whether there are any complaints lodged against the practitioner. Check to see if the practitioner is licensed to deliver the services the practitioner says he or she delivers.

Appropriate state licensing of education and practice is the only way to ensure that the practitioner is competent and provides quality services. Most types of complementary and alternative practices have national organizations of practitioners that are familiar with legislation, state licensing, certification, or registration laws.

Some organizations will direct medical consumers to the appropriate regulatory agencies in their state. These organizations also may provide referrals and information about specific practitioners. The organizations usually do not function as regulatory authorities, but promote the services of their members.

Second, talk with those who have had experience with this practitioner, both health practitioners and other patients. Find out about the confidence and competence of the practitioner in question, and whether there have ever been any complaints from patients.

Third, talk with the practitioner in person. Ask about the practitioner's education, additional training, licenses, and certifications, both unconventional and conventional. Ask about the practitioner's approach to treatment and patients. Find out how open the practitioner is to communicating with patients about technical aspects of methods, possible side effects, and potential problems.

When selecting a healthcare practitioner, many medical consumers seek someone knowledgeable in a wide variety of disciplines. Look for a practitioner who is easy to talk to. You should feel comfortable asking questions. After you select a practitioner, the education process and dialogue between you and your practitioner should become an ongoing aspect of complementary healthcare.

CONSIDER THE SERVICE DELIVERY

The quality of the service delivery, or how the treatment or therapy is given and under what conditions, is an important issue. However, quality of service is not necessarily related to the effectiveness or safety of a treatment or practice.

Visit the practitioner's office, clinic, or hospital. Ask the practitioner how many patients he or she typically sees in a day or week, and how much time the practitioner spends with the patient. Look at the conditions of the office or clinic.

Many issues surround quality of service delivery, and each one individually does not provide conclusive and complete information. For example, are the costs of the service excessive for what is delivered? Can the service be obtained only in one place, requiring travel to that place? These issues may serve as warning signs of poor service.

The primary issue to consider is whether the service delivery adheres to regulated standards for medical safety and care.

Contact regulatory boards or agencies described in the previous section to obtain objective information. You also may gather information by talking with people who have used the service, and through healthcare consumer organizations.

CONSIDER THE COSTS

Costs are an important factor to consider as many complementary and alternative treatments are not currently reimbursed by health insurance. Many patients pay directly for these services. Ask your practitioner and your health insurer which treatments or therapies are reimbursable.

Find out what several practitioners charge for the same treatment to better assess the appropriateness of costs. Regulatory agencies and professional associations also may provide cost information.

CONSULT YOUR HEALTHCARE PROVIDER

Most importantly, discuss all issues concerning treatments and therapies with your healthcare provider whether a physician or practitioner of complementary and alternative medicine.

Competent health care management requires knowledge of both conventional and alternative therapies for the practitioner to have a complete picture of your treatment plan.

APPENDIX 5

NCCAM CAM Research Centers*
[September 2000]

OVERVIEW OF THE SPECIALTY CENTERS

The National Center for Complementary and Alternative Medicine (NCCAM) provides funding to nine research centers which evaluate alternative treatments for many chronic health conditions including: Addictions, Aging, Arthritis, Cardiovascular Disease, Cardiovascular Disease and Aging in African Americans, Chiropractic, Craniofacial Disorders, Neurological Disorders, and Pediatrics. The Centers are designed to efficiently evaluate promising alternative medical practices by establishing mechanisms for investigators to have their research ideas reviewed, developed and executed in a scientifically rigorous manner.

The first year goals for each Center included the development of an organizational structure and operating plan. The second and third years will focus on the execution and evaluation of programmatic objectives. Each Center will assess and evaluate research opportunities in their specialty area, and develop a prioritized research agenda. These Centers will allow alternative medicine practitioners and research scientists to conduct specific joint research projects. Results of this research will be published in the scientific literature and disseminated to the public.

Research Center	Specialty
Center for Addiction & Alternative Medicine Research	Addictions
Center for CAM Research in Aging	Aging and Women's Health
Center for Alternative Medicine Research on Arthritis	Arthritis
CAM Research Center for Cardiovascular Diseases	Cardiovascular Diseases
Center for Natural Medicine and Prevention	Cardiovascular Disease & Minority Aging
Consortial Center for Chiropractic Research	Chiropractic
Oregon Center for Complementary and Alternative Medicine	Craniofacial Disorders
Oregon Center for Complementary and Alternative Medicine in Neurological Disorders	Neurological Disorders
Pediatric Center for Complimentary and Alternative Medicine	Pediatrics

*Reprinted from the National Center for Complementary and Alternative Medicine, NCCAM Clearinghouse Web site (http://http://nccam.nih.gov/nccam/fi/research/centers.html)

Center for Addiction and Alternative Medicine Research

Specialty: Addictions

Principal Investigator: Thomas J. Kiresuk, Ph.D.

Address:

Center for Addiction and Alternative Medicine Research (CAAMR)
Minneapolis Medical Research Foundation
914 South Eighth Street, Suite D917
Minneapolis, MN 55404
Phone: (612) 347-7670
Fax: (612) 337-7367
Web: http://www.mmrfweb.org/caamrpages/caamrcover.html

Description: This Center supports the rigorous scientific evaluation of complementary and alternative medicine (CAM) treatments for addictions and their health and psychological complications. Several projects are underway, including: pre-clinical trials of an herbal compound formulated to help prevent alcoholic relapse; pre-clinical trials of electroacupuncture to map the neural substrates of opioid dependence; and a clinical trial of an herbal compound for the treatment of hepatitis-C symptoms. A training program for pre-doctoral, post-doctoral and faculty scientists and/or CAM practitioners has been established, and materials are available to researchers and practitioners for guidance in research design and grant applications.

Center for CAM Research in Aging

Specialty: Aging & Women's Health

Principal Investigator: Fredi Kronenberg, Ph.D.

Address:

Center for CAM Research in Aging & Women's Health
Columbia University College of Physicians & Surgeons
630 West 168th Street, Box 75
New York, NY 10032
Fax: (212) 543-2845
Web: http://cpmcnet.columbia.edu/dept/rosenthal/

Description: The Center for CAM in Aging will initially evaluate dietary and herbal treatments in postmenopausal women. The scope of work will be expanded through the Developmental Research Program to include other CAM modalities. The Center contains three highly interactive clinical research projects and one basic science project, supported by administrative, biostatistical, and clinical research cores. It will develop an interdisciplinary research program that targets significant health problems of aging, and will conduct the timely education and training of future CAM researchers.

Center for Alternative Medicine Research on Arthritis

Specialty: Arthritis

Principal Investigator: Brian M. Berman, M.D.

Address:

Center for Alternative Medicine Research on Arthritis
University of Maryland School of Medicine
Division of Complementary Medicine
2200 Kernan Drive
Baltimore, MD 21207-6693
Web: http://www.compmed.ummc.umaryland.edu/

Description:

This Center will support a multi-disciplinary team of researchers and develop institutional and regional collaborations to conduct clinical and basic science research exploring the potential efficacy, safety, and cost-effectiveness of CAM therapies. The Center will investigate the cost effectiveness of and long-term outcomes following acupuncture treatment for osteoarthritis of the knee; the effectiveness of mind/body therapies for fibromyalgia; the mechanism of action and effects of electroacupuncture on persistent pain and inflammation; and the mechanism of action of a herbal combination with immunomodulatory properties.

CAM Research Center for Cardiovascular Diseases

Specialty: Cardiovascular Diseases

Principal Investigator: Steven F. Bolling, M.D.

Address:

Center for Complementary and Alternative Medicine Research in CVD
715 E. Huron Street
Suite 1W
Ann Arbor, MI 48104
Phone: (734) 998-7715
Fax: (734) 998-7720

Description: The University of Michigan Complementary and Alternative Medicine Research Center for Cardiovascular Diseases will focus on the investigation of complementary and alternative medicine (CAM) modalities to treat and prevent cardiovascular disease. Additionally, the center will stress CAM education and promotion of validated CAM treatmetnts for cardiovascular well-being. Initial projects are designed to allow for scientific validation of specific CAM techniques. These include the use of a herbal supplement, Hawthorn extract, in the treatment of congestive heart failure and applying the Reiki biofield energy healing technique in diabetic peripheral vascular disease and autonomic neuropathy. Furthermore, the influence of spirituality upon outcomes in patients having coronary artery bypass surgery will be examined as well as the impact of traditional Chinese medicine techniques of Qi Gong on post-CABG pain, healing, and outcome.

Center for Natural Medicine and Prevention

Specialty: Aging, Minority Health & Cardiovascular
Disease
Principal Investigator: Robert H. Schneider, M.D.
Address:
Center for Natural Medicine and Prevention
College of Maharishi Vedic Medicine
Fairfield, IA 52557
Phone: (515) 472-1129
Fax: (515) 472-1167
Email: CNMP@mum.edu
Web: http://www.mum.edu/CNMP/
Description: The Center will provide a unique and well-established platform for evaluation and translation of CAM modalities, especially Vedic medicine, for the prevention of cardiovascular disease (CVD) in older African Americans and other high risk populations. Proposed research projects, to name a few include: a basic study of mechanisms of meditation on atherosclerotic CVD (arterial vasomotion, cardiac autonomic tone and psychosocial risk factors; a randomized clinical trial of effects of meditation on carotid atherosclerosis, CVD risk factors, physiological mechanisms, psychosocial risk factors and quality of life in older Black women with CVD; a randomized trial on mechanisms and clinical effects of a traditional herbal antioxidant compared to conventional vitamin supplementation on carotid atherosclerosis, endothelial function, oxidative stress, CVD risk factors, and quality of life. The Center includes core facilities for administration, training, pilot/developmental studies, biostatistics, and quality of life.

Consortial Center for Chiropractic Research

Specialty: Chiropractic
Principal Investigator: William C. Meeker, D.C.,
M.P.H.

Address:
Consortial Center for Chiropractic Research
Palmer Center for Chiropractic Research
741 Brady Street
Davenport, IA 52803
E-mail: info@c3r.org
Web: http://www.c3r.org
Description: Faculty and administrators from five chiropractic institutions, the University of Iowa, and Kansas State University have formed the Consortial Center for Chiropractic Research (CCCR) to provide an infrastructure to examine the potential effectiveness and validity of chiropractic health care and to provide the appropriate clinical, scientific, and technical assistance to chiropractic researchers in developing high-quality research projects. Specific aims of the CCCR include developing research workshops, seminars, and educational materials; providing an institutional focus for formal training in research methodology, bioethics, biostatistics, clinical trial design, epidemiological and health services studies, and basic laboratory methods; establishing a network of chiropractic clinicians and investigators in specific topic areas; prioritizing research topics related to chiropractic treatment of musculoskeletal conditions; developing a mechanism for scientific/technical merit review of research proposals; and implementing selected research projects.

Oregon Center for Complementary and Alternative Medicine Research in Craniofacial Disorders

Specialty: Craniofacial Disorders
Principal Investigator: B. Alexander White, DDS,
D.Ph.
Address:
Center for Health Research
Kaiser
3800 N. Interstate Avenue
Portland, OR 97227-1110
Description: The Center will conduct research on potential efficacy, effectiveness, acceptability, effects on health care resource use, and psychosocial and other health outcomes associated with CAM practices for cranofacial disorders (CFDs) as well as the physiological and psychological mechanisms underlying some of these practices. Proposed Phase II clinical trials include: CAM approaches to TMD pain management; alterna-

tive medicine approaches among women with TMD; and complementary naturopathic medicine for periodontitis.

Oregon Center for Complementary and Alternative Medicine in Neurological Disorders
Specialty: Neurological Disorders
   Principal Investigator: Barry S. Oken, M.D.
Address:
   Oregon Center for Complementary and Alternative Medicine
   in Neurological Disorders
   Oregon Health Sciences University
   3181 SW Sam Jackson Park Road - Mail Stop CR-120
   Portland, OR 97201
   Email: orcamind@ohsu.edu
   Web: http://www.ohsu.edu/orccamind/
Description: The Center will initially focus on the use of CAM antioxidants and stress reduction as treatments for neurodegenerative and demyelinating diseases. Many of these diseases have oxidative injury as a causative or contributory factor and several CAM approaches have direct or indirect antioxidant effects. The Center will achieve its goals by facilitating four research projects and maintaining four core facilities that integrate the research strengths of conventional medicine and CAM practitioners and researchers. It will promote the exploration of new areas of CAM research and lead research on CAM therapies for neurological disorders.

Pediatric Center for Complementary and Alternative Medicine
Specialty: Pediatrics
   Principal Investigator: Fayez K. Ghishan, M.D., D.C.H.
Address:
   University of Arizona Health Sciences Center
   Department of Pediatrics
   1501 N. Campbell Avenue
   P.O. Box 245073
   Tucson, AZ 85724-5073
   Phone: (520) 626-5170
   Fax: (520) 626-3636
Description: The goal of the Center is to study integrative approaches in pediatrics. Three projects are planned to start in the first year of the grant. These projects will investigate the role of alternative approaches to three very common pediatric problems, including recurrent abdominal pain, otitis media, and cerebral palsy. The Center has established a pediatric research fellowship in CAM and research methodologies.

APPENDIX 6

Want Information about Alternative Medicine?*
[November 1999]

The National Center for Complementary and Alternative Medicine (NCCAM) is one of the Centers of the National Institutes of Health (NIH). NCCAM's mission is to conduct basic and applied research; provide research training; disseminate health information; and conduct other programs with respect to identifying, investigating, and validating complementary and alternative medicine (CAM) treatments, diagnostic and prevention modalities, disciplines, and systems.

A few of the many CAM practices include the use of acupuncture, homeopathy, herbs, therapeutic massage, traditional Oriental medicine, and vitamins and minerals to promote well-being or treat health conditions.

For more information about the NCCAM, visit their Web site at http://nccam.nih.gov.

NCCAM CLEARINGHOUSE

To give you more information about CAM, the NCCAM established the NCCAM Clearinghouse. We provide the following services:

Toll-Free Information Line
Publications

---

*Reprinted from the National Center for Complementary and Alternative Medicine, NCCAM Clearinghouse Web site (http://nccam.nih.gov/nccam/fcp/factsheets/brochure/brochure.htm) Publication M-24

Referrals to Other Information Resources
Health Information Databases

The NCCAM Clearinghouse does not provide medical referrals, medical advice, or recommendations for specific CAM therapies. We encourage all patients to consult their doctor to discuss both the potential benefits and risks of complementary and alternative health care practices.

Toll-Free Telephone and Fax-On-Demand Service

Our Information Specialists answer the NCCAM Clearinghouse's toll-free telephone line, 1-888-644-6226, in person, Monday through Friday from 8:30 a.m. to 5:00 p.m. Eastern time. This number is TTY/TDY accessible for speech- or hearing-impaired callers, and we can respond to both English- and Spanish-speaking callers. Whenever you call 1-888-644-6226, even if it's after business hours, you can easily access our automated Fax-On-Demand system to have certain Clearinghouse publications sent directly to your fax machine.

Publications About the NCCAM and CAM

The NCCAM Clearinghouse provides free publications, including NCCAM's newsletter. We can give you information about the NCCAM, the different types of CAM practices, and searching scientific databases for CAM information. Some of our publications provide more information about specific CAM practices, such as acupuncture and use of St. John's wort.

We encourage you to visit NCCAM's Web site at http://nccam.nih.gov to read many of our publications online.

Referrals to Additional Information Resources

Our Information Specialists can refer you to other organizations and resources for more information about CAM. These resources have been screened using criteria for relevance, accuracy, and service quality.

AM Database on *CHID Online*

The NCCAM Clearinghouse maintains the Complementary and Alternative Medicine (AM) Database, which is part of the Combined Health Information Database (CHID). The AM Database contains bibliographic citations (summaries) of books, journal articles, research reports, audiovisuals, and other materials about CAM. As a single source for information from the Federal Government about a wide range of health topics, CHID is a reference tool for health professionals, patients, and the public. CHID and the AM Database are available on the Internet at *CHID Online* http://chid.nih.gov.

CAM Citation Index

NCCAM's Complementary and Alternative Medicine (CAM) Citation Index consists of approximately 180,000 bibliographic citations about CAM research from the National Library of Medicine's MEDLINE database. The CAM Citation Index is available on NCCAM's Web site at http://nccam.nih.gov/nccam/resources/cam-ci/.

CUSTOMER SERVICE COMMITMENT

The NCCAM Clearinghouse strives to give you high quality service. We welcome your feedback and suggestions. Please mail your written comments to the following address:

Project Director
NCCAM Clearinghouse
P.O. Box 8218
Silver Spring, MD 20907-8218

CONTACTING US

You can reach the NCCAM Clearinghouse by calling our toll-free telephone number or by sending your request by mail, e-mail, or fax.

NCCAM Clearinghouse
P.O. Box 8218
Silver Spring, MD 20907-8218
1-888-644-6226 (1-888-NIH-NCAM) (Toll-Free, TTY/TDY, and Fax-On-Demand)
1-301-495-4957 (Fax)
nccamc@altmedinfo.org (E-mail)
http://nccam.nih.gov (NCCAM Web site)

Appendix 7

MEDLINE and Related Databases (and Alternative Medicine)*
[June 2000]

UNDERSTANDING SCIENTIFIC INFORMATION ABOUT YOUR ILLNESS

Obtaining valid scientific literature may demand complex and time-consuming searches of libraries and computer databases. Understanding the literature, once it has been retrieved, can be equally challenging. Unlike popular literature, scientific literature contains terminology and concepts which may be unfamiliar to the nonscientist. Another difficulty for people trying to understand scientific literature lies in the wide variety of types of scientific research. It is a good idea to have a healthcare professional, friend, or someone familiar with science help with the comprehension of the literature once it is obtained.

TYPES OF RESEARCH

Many types of scientifically valid research exist. These include studies that use biological substances (sometimes called in vitro research), studies on animals, and studies using humans (called clinical research). There also are reviews of studies, such as meta-analyses, where a number of research papers are collected and analyzed.

One important type of clinical research is the randomized controlled trial. This type of clinical research provides scientific evidence about the efficacy or effectiveness of a therapy. The trial generally uses two groups of people. One group receives the treatment while the other does not. If possible, neither the researchers nor the subjects know who receives the treatment (this is called a double-blind study). Many studies are put through peer review before they are published in a scientific journal.

Peer review is the analysis of research by a group of professionals in a specific scientific or medical field. More information on research methodologies and understanding research may be obtained from public and medical libraries, including the National Library of Medicine (NLM).

NATIONAL LIBRARY OF MEDICINE

The NLM is the premier source of medical science research information in the world. To make research information as accessible as possible, NLM has indexed 20 million printed references into a computer-based bibliographic retrieval system called MEDLARS (Medical Literature Analysis and Retrieval System).

---

*Reprinted from the National Center for Complementary and Alternative Medicine, NCCAM Clearinghouse Web site (http://http://nccam.nih.gov/nccam/what-is-cam/medline.html)

MEDLARS includes more than 40 online electronic databases and databanks. The database of greatest interest to alternative medical researchers is MEDLINE (MEDLARS Online).

MEDLINE contains more than 11 million records dating back to 1963. Although the full text of each article is not in the database, approximately 60 percent of the citations contain author-generated abstracts or summaries of the articles. The complete article may be ordered through a special feature called Loansome Doc.

MEDLINE ACCESS

MEDLINE is readily accessible via the World Wide Web. The NLM Web Site provides two methods of MEDLINE searching: Internet Grateful Med® and PubMed.
For additional information, contact the National Library of Medicine, 8600 Rockville Pike, Bethesda, MD 20894. Telephone: (301) 496-6308.

CONDUCTING SEARCHES ON ALTERNATIVE MEDICINE SUBJECTS

MEDLINE uses a "key word" indexing system called MeSH (Medical Subject Headings) to access information. To search for a subject on MEDLINE, you may enter your own term, or you may select from the MeSH keyword list of approximately 18,000 terms.

Currently, there are 25 main headings in MEDLINE under the term alternative medicine. More specific terms are listed under those main headings. For example, meditation is a more specific term under the heading relaxation techniques.

Many alternative medicine terms are not yet included in MeSH. Although many articles relating to alternative medicine from conventionally focused peer-reviewed journals are in MEDLINE, researchers may have difficulty finding them.

NLM is aware of the increasing interest in alternative medicine and the need for adequate MeSH terms. The National Center for Complementary and Alternative Medicine (NCCAM) is working with NLM to review the current terms, making suggestions for new terms, and improving the indexing for alternative medicine. Currently, almost 40,000 citations can be retrieved by searching under the term "alternative medicine."

These are the MEDLINE main headings under the term Alternative Medicine:

Acupuncture
Anthroposophy
Biofeedback
Chiropractic
Color Therapy
Diet Fads
Eclecticism
Electrical Stimulation
  Therapy
Homeopathy
Imagery
Kinesiology, Applied
Massage
Medicine, Traditional
Mental Healing
Mind-Body Relations
Moxibustion
Music Therapy
Naturopathy
Organotherapy
Radiesthesia
Reflexotherapy
Rejuvenation
Relaxation Techniques
Therapeutic Touch

ALTERNATIVE MEDICINE JOURNALS CURRENTLY IN MEDLINE

The NLM procedure for reviewing and accepting journals of current interest is appropriately rigorous. Not all journals concerning alternative medicine are indexed on MEDLINE. For example, MEDLINE only abstracts 3 of the 16 journals available on chiropractic. Some of the journals relating to alternative medicine indexed in MEDLINE are

Acupuncture and Electro-Therapeutics Research
Alternative Therapies in Health and Medicine
American Journal of Chinese Medicine
Biofeedback and Self Regulation
Chen Tzu Yen Chui (Acupuncture Research)
Chinese Medical Journal
Chung-Hua I Hsueh Tsa Chih (Chinese Medical Journal)
Chung-Kuo Chung Hsi I Chieh Ho Tsa Chih
Chung-Kuo Chung Yao Tsa Chih (China Journal of Chinese Materia Medica)
Journal of Manipulative and Physiological Therapeutics
Journal of Natural Products
Journal of Traditional Chinese Medicine
Planta Medica

OTHER DATABASES AT THE NLM

Other databases are available through the NLM if MEDLINE does not satisfy your requirements. Users can search for many specific topics in biomedical science, including cancer, AIDS, toxicological and chemical data, health services research, and other specialized areas of health and disease. They are available through the Internet Grateful Med®.

NLM PUBLICATIONS

The NLM produces a wide variety of publications to assist health professionals, researchers, librarians, and the general public to use the many available resources. The publications include indexes to biomedical literature, newsletters, reports about library activities, bibliographies, and manuals for using NLM programs.

All publications are available online through the NLM's Internet Home Page, or you can visit the Library at the National Institutes of Health, 8600 Rockville Pike, Bethesda, MD, 20894.

THE CRISP DATABASE

The CRISP (Computer Retrieval of Information on Scientific Projects) System is a major biomedical database containing information about research supported by the U.S. Public Health Service. Most of this research falls into the category of an extramural project. Extramural projects generally are conducted by investigators outside the government, such as scientists at universities, hospitals, and other research institutions. Intramural research programs are conducted by employees of the NIH and the FDA.

Government institutions that fund research projects include: the Agency for Health Care Policy and Research, Centers for Disease Control and Prevention, the FDA, the Health Resources and Services Administration, the NIH, and the Substance Abuse and Mental Health Services Administration.

The CRISP database is accessible through the NIH Internet Home Page under Grants and Contracts. You may search by project title, principal investigator's abstract, or term descriptors. A CRISP thesaurus will become available from the Office of Extramural Research in the fall of 1999.

You may enter your own term, but the search will not be exact. For example, projects listed when searched by the term "alternative medicine" will list government-funded projects that the NCCAM considers as complementary and alternative medical treatments, as well as other treatments that are not considered "alternative" for that medical condition.

For more information contact the Research Documentation Section of the Office of Extramural Research, National Institutes of Health , 6701 Rockledge Drive, MSC 7772, Bethesda, MD 20892-7772. Telephone: (301) 435-0650. Fax: (301) 480-2845. E-mail: DRT@CU.NIH.GOV

CLINICALTRIALS.GOV

The U.S. National Institutes of Health, through its National Library of Medicine, has developed ClinicalTrials.gov to provide patients, family members and members of the public current information about clinical research studies.

IF YOU DO NOT HAVE ACCESS TO A COMPUTER

A variety of options are available if you do not own a computer and want to do online research. Try your local public library (many local libraries have Internet access or a connection to NLM), a medical or academic library at a local college or university, and/or your healthcare practitioner (many practitioners will have a computer, or will have access to one).

AUTHOR INDEX

by Dottie Jahoda

TITLE INDEX

by Dottie Jahoda

Subject Index

by Dottie Jahoda